The Medical Assistant

Marelyn Joyce Fabian
7508 St Clair Ave.
Cleveland 3, Ohio
Ex-1-3503

The Medical Assistant

A GUIDEBOOK FOR THE NURSE, SECRETARY,
AND TECHNICIAN IN THE DOCTOR'S OFFICE

MIRIAM BREDOW *Dean of Women*
Eastern School for Physicians' Aides
New York

Blakiston Division
McGRAW-HILL BOOK COMPANY, INC.
New York   Toronto   London   1958

THE MEDICAL ASSISTANT

Copyright © 1958 by the McGraw-Hill Book Company, Inc. Printed in the United States of America. All rights reserved. This book, or parts thereof, may not be reproduced in any form without permission of the publishers.

Library of Congress Catalog Card Number: 57-12891

To my husband
HEINRICH F. WOLF, M.D.
who has shared so much of his knowledge with me

Preface

About 75 per cent of all doctors today employ one or more aides in their offices. The present book was written to provide a training and reference text for this increasing number of medical assistants. In the past, a young woman who was attracted by the medical profession might study specialized courses and become a medical secretary. As a medical secretary she usually took care only of secretarial duties, and a registered nurse attended to the office nursing. Gradually, however, as the shortage of nurses increased, the medical secretary was called upon to help with the behind-the-scene preparations, and soon she was assisting the doctor with his patients. The career of the medical office assistant evolved.

As a result, books for the medical secretary, including the author's "Handbook for the Medical Secretary," included some information on office nursing. It became evident, however, that a book is now needed which covers the entire range of situations in which the assistant may be called upon to help the doctor in general practice as well as in special fields, in the laboratory as well as in the x-ray department. The present book is written from this inclusive point of view and is intended to serve as a training manual for medical assistants, whether they are being taught in school or in a doctor's office, and an instructional manual for assistants on the job. Although there are countless schools of nursing, only a handful of schools train medical office assistants, and their graduates supply only a fraction of the demand. Thus many doctors are faced with the necessity of training their own assistants. It is hoped this book will lessen the doctor's share of the training.

The book is written for the person with no medical training and attempts to teach (1) what the assistant has to do, (2) how she should do it, and (3) why she should do it. In addition, it includes basic theoretical information that is essential for the assistant to know if she is to carry out her duties competently. Many of the procedures to be followed might be used in several different specialties. Some duplication, therefore, has been unavoidable; but since most topics have been discussed only once, the assistant should consult the index whenever a particular subject is sought.

Many physicians have expressed interest in this book and have been unstinting with their advice. For their specific help in the preparation of different parts, my sincere thanks are due especially to Drs. David Nathan Hale, Werner Hochstetter, Leonard Leroy Hyams, and Earl C. Shaw.

Valuable suggestions and assistance were given most generously by Jules Burns, Lydia Ost, and Marion Roos, R.N., to whom the author wishes to express appreciation. The author is also grateful to Peter A. Moschetta and Frank O. Waters, Jr., for their kind permission to use excerpts from their forthcoming manual, "Medical Laboratory Techniques." She is further indebted to many firms for their cooperation in supplying illustrations and descriptive literature of their products. Too numerous to mention here, their names will be found throughout the book.

Miriam Bredow

Contents

Preface   vii

Introduction   1

CHAPTER 1 **On the Job**   3

    The Assistant's Position · Transmission of Disease · Privileges · Duties · The Doctor and the Medical Office Assistant · Grooming

2 **The Personal Equation**   13

    Personal Psychology · Patient Psychology · Public Relations

3 **Protection through Sterilization**   23

    Bacteriology · The Need for Sterilization · Principles of Sterilization · Methods of Sterilization

4 **Helping with Examinations**   45

    Methods of Examination · Setup for Examination · The Examination · Preparation of the Patient · Draping the Patient · Routine Tests · Special Tests

5 **The Doctor Prescribes Treatment**   67

    Nature of Diseases · Types of Treatment

6 **Principles of Medication**   75

    Types of Drugs · Narcotics and Their Handling · Medications · Emergency Drugs · Anesthetics · Antiseptics · Solutions · Storage · Labeling

7 Techniques of Giving Injections — 94

Reasons for Injections · Types of Injection · Giving Injections · Care of Syringes and Needles

8 Surgery in the Office — 108

Preparation of the Patient · Office Anesthesia · The Operating Room · The Assistant's Role · Dressings · Bandages

9 Application of Physical Therapy — 124

Ultraviolet Light · Heat · Galvanic, Sinusoidal, and Faradic Currents · Diathermy · Ultrasonic Therapy · Massage · Exercises · Hydrotherapy · Electrosurgery

10 Preparations for X-rays — 140

Danger of X-rays · Attitude toward the Patient · Preparation of the Patient · Administrative Routine

11 Treatment and Diet — 149

Constituents of Food · Dietary Requirements · Various Diets · Prescription of Diet · Discussing the Diet

12 Assisting the Specialist I — 160

Diplomates · Allergy · Gynecology and Obstetrics · Neurology and Psychiatry

13 Assisting the Specialist II — 184

Ophthalmology · Orthopedics · Otolaryngology

14 First-aid Rules — 206

Emergencies · Do's and Don'ts · First-aid Supplies

15 Medical Secretarial Duties — 219

Receiving the Patient · Appointment System · Telephone Hours · Out-of-office Visits · Handling the Telephone

CONTENTS

16 Patients' Records   237

The Medical History · Personal Health Record · Filing of Medical Histories · Filing Practices · Patients' Ledger Cards

17 Financial Matters   252

The Doctor's Fee · Bills · Collections · Bookkeeping

18 Insurance in Medical Practice   269

Health Insurance · Workmen's Compensation Insurance · Medicare · Malpractice Insurance

19 Housekeeping Hints   279

Care of Office · Care of Equipment · Supplies · Laundry · Removal of Stains · The Doctor's Bag

20 Laboratory Techniques   291

Urinalysis · Hematology · Bacteriologic Smears

21 Special Tests   325

Basal Metabolism Test · Electrocardiography

APPENDIX **Medical Terminology**   367

Abbreviations · Analysis of Medical Terminology · Vocabulary of Medical Terms

Tables   415

INDEX   421

Introduction

Today the doctor depends more and more on a medical office assistant, who often may not be a nurse, to act as the public relations agent between him and his patients and to help him in many clinical situations and with a great variety of technical detail. This poses a problem for the young woman who is either new in this profession or has been working with a doctor in a different specialty, since every branch of medicine requires special tasks and specialized knowledge on the part of the doctor's assistant.

Like the nurse, the medical assistant should have a knowledge and understanding of the principles or physiological functions on which the procedures in the doctor's practice are based. The gap between the medical knowledge of a physician and that of a nonmedical person—in this instance the medical assistant—is vast.

Without some acquaintance with the medical principles underlying the examinations and treatments in which she assists, the aide is of limited use to the doctor. If efficient teamwork between the doctor and his aide is to develop—teamwork that will result in better service for the patient and less work for the doctor—the assistant must know what the doctor aims to accomplish. Only then will she be the able, competent helper he needs and has a right to expect. Theoretical medical information forms part of the training of a registered nurse, yet she is not expected to practice medicine. The aim is to help the nurse understand what the doctor wants her to do and observe during treatment of the patient. The inclusion of theoretical medical material in this book has this objective for the medical assistant.

The medical assistant will find that her role and responsibilities will vary, depending on the specialty of the doctor by whom she is employed. In addition, she will need to remember that doctors have different opinions in regard to the duties of an assistant, as well as different duties they may wish her to perform. Some doctors will delegate a great many tasks to her, while others attend to almost everything themselves. Each assistant's work, therefore, will depend on the preferences of the individual doctor.

As the career of the medical assistant continues to expand, her status is acquiring professional recognition. A number of state societies of medical assistants have been formed, and there are two national registries. Their aim is to set up standards of training, entrance examinations, and requirements for membership and eventual certification. Information regarding membership may be obtained from the president of the American Association of Medical Assistants, 510 North Dearborn, Chicago 10, Illinois. The American Medical Association has been taking an interest in the formation of new local chapters and has published a booklet with practical information on how to start such an organization. The booklet may be obtained by writing to Director of Special Services, American Medical Association, 535 North Dearborn Street, Chicago 10.

The ambitious and intelligent assistant will want to know more about those topics with which she will be most concerned or which interest her most. A brief bibliography of suitable supplementary reading is appended to most chapters in this book. If she is interested in knowing more about medical historical events, Castiglioni's "A History of Medicine" (Knopf) and Mettler's "History of Medicine" (McGraw-Hill) will be useful.

Each medical specialty is represented by many publications. The advertisements in medical periodicals will be found especially useful for acquainting the novice with the names of instruments, machines, and drugs used in a particular specialty.

The most important terms for each specialty will be found in the Appendix.

1
On the Job

The patient who visits the doctor rarely meets him upon first entering the office. Most doctors are busy with other patients and do not act as their own receptionists. It is the doctor's office assistant whom the patient sees first. It is she who greets him, who makes him feel welcome and at home. He may be ill, in pain, handicapped by an injury, or apprehensive about his health because of disquieting symptoms. The medical office assistant's job begins with her first contact with the patient. Her friendly but professional attitude creates the atmosphere to which the patient responds.

The Assistant's Position

As a rule the assistant spends some time with the patient before the doctor is ready to see him. She obtains certain information from the patient; she may help to prepare him for the doctor's examination or treatment; she may make various tests or administer certain treatments. When the doctor examines or treats the patient, she is at his side, assisting in such a way that the process is completed quickly and smoothly, saving the doctor many motions and the patient unnecessary delay.

According to a recent survey, the results of which were published in *Medical Economics*,[1] medical office assistants as a group perform practically every semimedical service there is; however, practices in individual offices vary widely. The article concludes that every service which is performed by the doctor and which could be done by his assistant costs him ten times as much as it should.

[1] Harold Mickelson and Lois Hoffman, "What Jobs Do Doctors Delegate—and to Whom," *Medical Economics*, April, 1957, pp. 131–139.

Before the patient arrives, the assistant has been busy behind the scene. The consultation, treatment, and examination rooms have been put into perfect order; all necessary instruments have been sterilized and laid out, ready to use; solutions and medications are on hand, fresh linen within reach. Nothing is missing. Everything is as the doctor needs and expects to find it.

Training and experience are necessary to achieve such perfection. Carelessness in the doctor's office may lead to catastrophe. The medical office assistant has far more serious responsibilities than any other secretarial assistant. Without a medical office assistant the doctor is seriously handicapped in attempting to care for the many patients who expect to see him each day. Many doctors are still accustomed to the registered nurse whom they formerly employed and may expect the same services from their assistant. Yet there is a difference between the two professions, and the medical office assistant is well advised to realize this. One of the differences, for instance, is the fact that in a few states, at least, only a licensed person is allowed to give an injection. In these states, a registered nurse, who must have a state license to practice, can give an injection, but a medical office assistant cannot legally do so; a nurse can change dressings and administer medication, but the medical assistant cannot. It follows, therefore, that the latter must make sure of what the medical practice act prescribes and prohibits in the particular state in which she is employed.

Transmission of Disease

Occasionally a young woman is deterred from working in a doctor's office for fear of contracting a disease from patients. Such a fear is entirely unfounded. First of all, few patients with contagious diseases visit a doctor's office; they are in bed. The doctor who visits them at home or in the hospital and the nurses who take care of them do not contract their diseases, because, knowing the circumstances, they can take the proper precautions. There is a far greater danger of catching some illness or infection in one's daily life than in a medical office. Public restaurants, public lavatories, crowded subways or theaters—all are swarming with every kind of germ. To one who is not consciously aware of this, and therefore unable to protect himself, the possibility of infection is always present.

One can better appreciate this situation if he knows something about how diseases are transmitted. We speak of contagious and of infectious diseases. Both kinds, of course, are caused by microorganisms, and the line of distinction is not sharply drawn. The infectious diseases are transmitted only by direct contact with or intake of the pathogenic agent (that is, the microorganism causing the disease). To this group belong typhoid, tuberculosis, and diseases known to be due to streptococci, staphylococci, and diplococci. Contagious diseases, such as poliomyelitis, smallpox, measles, are those transmitted by direct contact with an affected person or with his secretions. Respiratory diseases, for instance, are transmitted by the dissemination of organisms in the breath, cough, or sneeze of the infected person or in discarded handkerchiefs or tissues. In other diseases, infection is spread by contaminated articles passed from one person to another.

Discharges from people with streptococcal infections are only one of several ways in which this infection is spread. Others are floor dust, contaminated food, or milk that has not been properly pasteurized. Some persons carry the germs without being ill themselves. These "carriers" can also spread disease with their discharges. Frequent washing of hands is, therefore, necessary—always before eating and after using the toilet. A good antiseptic agent should be used in the office. But it must be repeated that brief or occasional contact is rarely the cause of an infection.

Persons with infectious diseases that are not contagious are usually not isolated; those with contagious diseases are usually quarantined for the protection of others. With all diseases, however, it is important to remember two points. First, exposure to an infectious agent does not automatically produce the disease. If it did, we would all be constantly sick, for we are continuously in the presence of untold numbers of germs. The average healthy person, however, has an innate resistance or immunity to a great variety of disease-producing microorganisms. Second, a sensible hygienic routine practically eliminates the possibility of contracting a disease from a person known to be infected. The medical office assistant soon develops the habit of washing her hands frequently—certainly before and after touching a patient in any way or handling linen or instruments that have been in contact with a patient. She learns not to put her hands to her face, or even to use her handkerchief, without first washing her hands. Disposable tissues are a great help.

Privileges

The professional field enjoys a special prestige, and anyone employed in it shares this prestige to a certain extent. If the medical profession is esteemed especially highly, it is because the doctor eases human suffering. Furthermore, the intricacies of medicine are so incomprehensible to the nonmedical person that he is bound to have a great respect for anyone who knows the workings of the human body and who knows what such words as *hemoglobinophilic* mean. This esteem extends to anyone working with the doctor.

The person with a desire to get more out of life than material rewards, with a desire to add to the well-being of other individuals, will find work in a doctor's office especially rewarding. There is a great inner satisfaction in helping a sick person get well, lessening pain, or dispelling anxiety. And what interesting work! In a doctor's office no two days are alike, no two patients the same. There is constant change in this stimulating and often exciting occupation.

True, sometimes the hours in a doctor's office are likely to be irregular—long and late. Patients who cannot come during office hours or who have suddenly become ill must be seen and perhaps treated. On the other hand, in an office where a rigid 9 to 5 o'clock schedule is not adhered to, there is the possibility of compensations, such as free time when the work is light or the doctor does not have office hours.

As the assistant works with the doctor for some time, she learns much about each patient—who will get well quickly, who may have a long road to health ahead of him, whose disease is incurable. She becomes the doctor's confidante and shares his interest in each patient. The position of a medical office assistant is truly a worthwhile career for a fine, kind, intelligent young woman.

Duties

What are the duties of a medical office assistant? Naturally they vary. She may be one of a team of assistants, receptionists, secretaries, laboratory technicians, x-ray technicians, or she may be all of these herself. The various duties that she may be called upon to perform are therefore discussed in this book, even though any particular assistant may have an opportunity to work in only one phase of this fascinating career.

Briefly, her duties might comprise such secretarial tasks as making appointments by telephone, receiving patients, setting fees, and collecting payments, keeping the doctor's books, and typing his case histories and letters. Also, since the doctor is likely to have patients who carry health insurance or who are insured under the Workmen's Compensation law, she may have to fill out different forms.

The assistant plays an important part in the medical routine of the doctor's office. She sterilizes his instruments and accessories, prepares setups for examinations and treatments, and assists the doctor during this work. She prepares the patient beforehand by draping him or by taking his pulse, weight, temperature, respiration, and blood pressure. She assists the doctor during the various types of treatment he gives in the office and during minor operations.

She may act as the doctor's laboratory or x-ray technician, performing various diagnostic tests, blood tests, urinalyses, basal metabolism tests, electrocardiography and x-ray examinations.

Finally, she is a housekeeper in charge of the appearance of the office and treatment rooms. She orders supplies and keeps track of them. The medical supplies are in her charge, and she must have an inventory of them at all times.

There is considerable difference of opinion among doctors regarding the amount of work that they feel can be and should be delegated to the medical office assistant. On the one hand, some doctors feel there is much routine work that a well-trained assistant can very well do, thus relieving the doctor of these tasks and leaving him free to see more patients more leisurely. A young doctor just starting out in practice usually does everything himself, including answering the telephone and typing out the bills. But as his practice grows, he turns more and more duties over to an aide. If the assistant proves herself completely dependable, efficient, and able to use good judgment, the average doctor can improve his practice, increase his income, and afford himself more time by delegating a great deal of the work to her.

On the other hand, some doctors are against delegating any work to their assistants. They perform even the tasks which are usually assigned to the assistant, such as receiving patients and making appointments. Many a doctor will tell his patient, "Come in again next Wednesday at the same time," or, "I want to see you punctually at 10 o'clock tomorrow," without checking with his secretary, who may have already scheduled other patients for these hours. In such offices confusion reigns—the doctor is harassed by too much work, and patients have to wait in the office for a long time before they see the doctor.

The work that a medical office assistant is called upon to do, therefore, depends to a great extent on the specialty of the doctor for whom she works and on the individual doctor's preference, as well as on her ability and willingness to shoulder responsibilities. One point, however, is of importance: it must be distinctly understood just what the assistant is expected to do. Her duties should be clearly outlined to her. As she develops on the job, more tasks will be delegated to her. She should make sure that they are precisely stated, rather than have it taken for granted that she will gradually be expected to take on additional jobs.

For a successful career as a medical office assistant, systematize your day. Once you know what is expected of you and what must be done, make a work schedule for yourself and attempt to follow it as closely as possible. Interruptions during the day may prevent you from adhering closely to your plan, but it will help you to check on yourself. Also, until your duties become automatic, such a schedule will serve as a reminder, so that nothing will remain undone. A sample schedule may look like this:

1. Call the doctors' answering service.
2. Check all the rooms for appearance.
3. Fill and connect the sterilizer.
4. Sort and open the mail.
5. Make a list of the doctor's appointments for the day.
6. Pull medical histories out of the file for all patients expected.
7. Prepare trays and setups for the day's appointments.
8. Type yesterday's dictation.
9. Transfer the patients' charges and payments to the patients' ledger cards.
10. Check the supplies and order what is needed.
11. Check the doctor's bag.
12. Do yesterday's filing.

These are some general duties. Each day special reminders may be added, for instance:

Telephone hospital re admittance of patient A. Jackson.
Renew subscription to the *American Journal of Surgery*.

The Doctor and the Medical Office Assistant

For efficient, professional performance, there must be complete harmony between the doctor and his office assistant. And such harmony cannot exist if the doctor feels that the assistant is not putting in a full day's work—that she comes in late, overstays her lunch hour, or leaves ahead of closing hours when the doctor is not there. Nor will there be harmonious cooperation if the assistant feels that the doctor is exploiting her, that he is taking advantage of her willingness to stay overtime. If the assistant is conscientious and dependable about her duties and her obligations to the doctor and she still feels that too much is asked of her, she should discuss this openly with the doctor, rather than harbor a grudge and give poor service. The doctor is probably completely unaware that he is expecting more work and time than the agreement calls for. It should be fully understood just what duties the assistant is to perform and what her working hours are to be. A clear understanding on such matters as duties and working hours saves a great deal of resentment and misunderstanding. Doctors are often vague about such matters, taking for granted that the assistant knows just what she is expected to do.

Here is a piece of advice to all new medical office assistants: Do not be afraid to ask questions of the doctor. He probably does not realize that you are not sure about something, that you need more information about specific points. If necessary, reserve an hour on the appointment calendar for a long chat with the doctor in order to clarify all the points that are still not clear.

The question of hours should be settled at the beginning. A doctor is likely to have some patients who cannot come during the day, and it is well for him and his assistant to agree on days of the week on which to have late office hours. If the assistant stays until 8 or 8:30 P.M. once or twice a week, arrangements can be made for her to leave early on other days. The important thing is to make a schedule that is fairly definite, so that the assistant can plan her personal life also. A full understanding with the doctor on this point is important.

No really good work can be done with equipment that is worn out or in need of repair. The doctor cannot be expected to check on the condition of the assistant's typewriter or notice whether the amount of lighting at her desk is sufficient. It is up to the assistant to speak to the doctor about her working tools and the equipment in her office. She should have a commodious desk which is easily accessible and which she may leave quickly without having to push a typewriter stand out of the way. Her chair should be comfortable and properly adjusted. The telephone should be placed in such a way that the assistant can make notes while talking. As the assistant spends almost one-half of her day in the office, comfortable working conditions will contribute to her contentment in her work.

Grooming

The need for good grooming really goes without saying. Grooming is not a superficial or surface affair; it is part of one's personality. It is hard to imagine a person of impeccable manners who would dress slovenly. Still, it is surprising how often one encounters young and pretty women who detract from their appearance by careless grooming. Grooming applies to the whole person, "from the skin out." A clean, well-fitting uniform is not enough. A daily bath and use of a deodorant, a weekly shampoo, daily care of the hair and nails, clean and polished shoes, straight stocking seams, fresh underwear—all contribute to the total impression. Fingernails should not be too long or too pointed. If any polish is used, it should be of a light shade; and if the polish chips a great deal because of frequent washing of hands, it is better to use a colorless polish. A bottle of hand lotion might be kept in the desk or near the basin and used after washing, to prevent the hands from becoming rough and dry.

Make-up is fine if it is not obtrusive. If a repair job is necessary during the day, it should be done in the rest room or in an empty treatment room, not in front of patients or visitors.

The only jewelry suitable with a white uniform is a string of pearls, or a simple gold chain, and a wrist watch. All other jewelry should be taken off during the day until it is time to put on one's "civilian" clothes. Perfume of any sort may offend a patient or even make him ill. At the most, a light toilet water or Eau de Cologne can be used.

Tobacco stains on the fingers or traces of tobacco smell are repulsive, even to well persons. They are intolerable on a medical office assistant. Smoking in the doctor's office would be in decidedly poor taste for the assistant, a breach of professional etiquette of which she should never be guilty.

Uniforms. A medical office assistant who comes into close contact with patients is expected to wear a white uniform at all times. The uniform is obviously a means of protecting clothing when working with patients or handling medicines. But the uniform has a decided psychological effect, for a patient feels more at ease with a person in a white uniform—less embarrassed to undress or to answer questions and, in general, more willing to cooperate.

Formerly an admonition that a uniform be clean and unwrinkled would have been sufficient. But now that uniforms have entered the fashion field, a brief discussion is in order. There is much to be said for the old-fashioned, starched cotton uniform. It looks professional and is not transparent; however, it does take a lot of care. The cotton uniform wrinkles easily and must be starched and ironed. It is not surprising, therefore, that the many new synthetic fibers, combinations of fibers, and cotton weaves have become popular, with their advantages of fast drying, no starching, and no ironing. Certainly uniforms that are made of a good quality material look well, hang well, and keep their shape. But many of them do need ironing, despite what the advertisements say. The cheaper uniforms often look tired and limp, even after they have just been washed, and if the seams are not pressed, the skirt hangs unevenly.

The less expensive materials are often so sheer that one slip does not give sufficient protection. The assistant should therefore consider her purchase of uniforms carefully. In the long run, good-quality uniforms are the least expensive. Even these may turn yellow if not handled carefully. A special bluing may have to be used. Extreme styles should be avoided, as they are unsuitable for a doctor's office. If uniforms are rented from a linen-supply house, they should be checked before they are accepted. Garments which are the wrong size or which are stained or torn should be rejected.

A white slip should always be worn under the uniform. If you frequently wear a dark dress under which you need a dark slip, you should keep a white slip in the office, together with the uniform. Be sure that the slip is long enough to meet the hem of the uniform, without showing below it, that no buttons are missing, and that there are no ripped seams. A colored handkerchief in the breast pocket detracts from the professional look. The uniform should be kept on a hanger when not in use. White shoes should always be worn with a white uniform, but beige stockings are permissible.

Have some cleaning liquid, a clothesbrush, and a sewing kit for quick repairs in the office. (The cleaning fluid and the sewing kit may come in handy for a patient in distress too!)

2

The Personal Equation

It is often said that the right personality is an absolute necessity for work in the medical field. What *is* the right personality, especially for a medical office assistant? Most important of all, she must like people, must like doing things for others. She must have a cheerful disposition, an even temper. She must be inclined to be methodical and reliable in her entire way of life, and she must have a strong sense of responsibility coupled with a wealth of human kindness.

In addition to possessing these innate character traits, she should, by upbringing and training, be tactful, polite, well mannered, poised, efficient, calm in emergencies, and devoted to her work. Does this sound like a paragon of virtue? It is just what the doctor ordered—for himself.

The reference to "duty, stern daughter of the voice of God" has given us too long the impression that one must be grim about doing one's duty. Nothing could be less true. A person who enjoys his work and gains inner satisfaction from it does his duty cheerfully and gladly. The qualifications that are not inborn, but rather acquired by practice and effort, soon become automatic. There is no strain involved in exercising them.

To the patient, the person who assists the doctor is the "office nurse." If she is cheerful, kind, and efficient, each patient will be devoted to her, and this makes the running of the office a lot simpler. If she is sullen, curt, or disagreeable, the patient will be put into an unpleasant mood himself, and everything will be more difficult. Only a person who has the sympathy and understanding necessary to deal with sick people should undertake to work in a doctor's office. Such a person should be soft-spoken, unselfish, and helpful in her general attitude. At the same time, she must be alert, utterly dependable, and unfailingly accurate. Her manners must be perfect. She must at all times represent the doctor, that is, give the impression of a professional person, with all that this implies. Above all, she must be interested in her work.

Personal Psychology

In the large majority of doctors' offices the medical office assistant is the only employee. At times she may feel lonely and miss the companionship of fellow employees and the chance for personal conversation. At the same time, this situation removes the cause of much of the friction that occurs in so many offices where the rivalries, gossip, and antagonism among employees create tension and irritations. Some doctors, however, do have two or more assistants. They may all be medical office assistants, trained to do the same type of work, and share the work among them; or one may be a laboratory technician, one an x-ray technician, another a receptionist, a secretary, or perhaps a registered nurse. Good, cordial relations among the doctor's office personnel are of the utmost importance in maintaining the professional atmosphere and decorum that each patient expects when visiting the doctor. When people work together, minor irritations are bound to come up. They can be magnified until they become serious incidents that lead to quarrels and resentment. They can also be ignored, glossed over, or quickly straightened out, without leaving any hard feelings. The key word is *cooperation*. If each individual is willing to help the other whenever necessary, no friction need arise. There is no place for the caste system in a doctor's office. If the x-ray technician answers the telephone when the secretary is busy, the secretary in turn helps the x-ray technician when the need arises.

The question of human relationships is a complicated one. Some people are always hard to get along with; almost all of us are hard to get along with occasionally. We are all inclined to take everything personally, because to ourselves we are the most important person in the world. If we meet someone we know, and he greets us briefly and without a smile, we think, "What does he have against *me*? What have *I* done?" The truth is, probably, that the other person was hardly conscious of whom he greeted, being entirely preoccupied with *his* problems. Also, in our own eyes we can do no wrong. We spend hours and hours of our waking time justifying whatever it is we have done that was wrong or merely a mistake. And it would be so simple to admit to ourselves at least, "What a fool I was to do this or that," and let it go at that. We may strive for perfection, but we know we can never reach it. There is no need to have feelings of guilt about making a mistake. The most healing reaction is to admit the mistake and resolve not to make it again.

Interest in psychology has become widespread during the last few years. Many books on this general subject are being published annually and read avidly by the public. There is a great yearning to understand oneself and other human beings. (The study of psychology should work both ways.) In learning to understand one's own reactions, motivations, shortcomings, and abilities, one's adjustment to his environment is greatly helped. We are all impelled by similar longings, fears, doubts, and anxieties, as well as selfish and self-centered thoughts.

It has been said that everyone is, at one time or another, mentally upset or emotionally unbalanced by illness, shock, grief, strain, etc. Learning to recognize such periods for what they are helps greatly in controlling their intensity and duration and hastening the return to normal. At the same time, it helps us to understand that other individuals undergo similar upsets, and with this understanding our reaction will not be one of anger for anger, sullenness for sullenness, but, rather, one of sympathetic consideration.

There are two opposite, contradictory tendencies in every human being. One impels the person to be constructive, helpful, cheerful, to enjoy life and all its vicissitudes. The other causes the individual to be destructive, hostile, revengeful, unhappy, tired of life. These two tendencies are almost constantly in conflict with each other, although there may be periods when one of the two is in complete control. Both are primitive urges and dominate us all our lives.

Religion has, of course, long recognized these opposite impulses and called them simply good and evil. In ordinary life we speak of a person being optimistic or pessimistic, positive or negative, pleasant or disagreeable. Modern psychology has coined the terms "life urge" and "death urge." Sigmund Freud, the originator of psychoanalysis, gave them the names *libido* and *mortido*.

One of the two is predominant throughout the lives of most individuals, although everyone experiences both tendencies at different times. The effort of applied psychology is to minimize the death urge and to develop a healthy life urge. Obviously the person who is dominated by constructive emotions is the person who is going to be successful, who will be liked by others, and who will be happy. On the other hand, the person who is swayed by destructive impulses always finds fault with others, is quick to become angry, and, in extreme cases, may hurt or kill another person or even himself.

What is the practical value of knowing of these impulses? It is this: knowledge is power. If one knows these principles, one can influence the urges that impel one's motivations. The life urge can be fostered by a conscious and assiduous effort to be cooperative and to give praise, sympathy, and understanding to others. The death urge may be suppressed or weakened by constructive effort. The result will be a more integrated, better adjusted personality, with a consequent easing of the inner tensions and conflicts that beset human beings.

Getting along with people—relatives, friends, and business associates—is a knack with which some lucky people are born. Most persons have to study practical rules and apply them consciously. Doctors, teachers, lawyers, and salesmen have all acquired a specific knowledge of people and have developed a definite approach in their dealings with them. We may say that they apply psychology. Psychology, of course, means the study of the *psyche*, which is the Greek word for "mind" or "soul." At present this term refers to all nonphysical manifestations, that is, to mental and emotional processes. In common parlance, however, the word psychology is often used to designate the application of knowledge gained from the study of psychology. We therefore speak, for instance, of patient psychology and mean that which has been learned in the study of the psyche applied to patients.

Patient Psychology

All the principles learned in psychology that are applied to average, well persons must be adapted to meet the needs of patients. A person who is ill, in pain, or worried must be approached with more consideration and understanding. The impairment of a person's health is accompanied by a loss of a sense of security. The doctor's examination and treatments may help to restore some of it, but a strictly professional attitude is not enough. The patient wants emotional security as well. He wants to feel that he is important to the doctor and that the doctor is his friend and is vitally interested in him, not as a case, but as a human being. The patient desires the friendship of everyone connected with the doctor's office, especially the office assistant, with whom the patient often has close contact. The relationship established in the doctor's office is every bit as important to the patient as is the medical care that he is receiving.

What does this mean in practical terms? The assistant should at all times be kind and sympathetic to the patient and show her interest in his particular problem or need. Here is an example: A woman who worked mornings, from 9 to 1, called her doctor frequently for appointments. Every time she called she was offered a morning appointment. Every time she had to explain that she could not come in the morning, and an afternoon appointment was made. Naturally, the patient was irritated by the lack of interest manifested by the doctor's secretary. Imagine her surprise when she called the office of a specialist whom she had visited just once and was told by the assistant, "I know you can't come in the morning, so would 3 o'clock suit you?"

The patient who visits the doctor's office is apprehensive, tense, worried. The strange surroundings bother him. Odors from ether or antiseptics may affect him physically, adding to his discomfort. The sight of medical instruments, bandages, or even cotton may upset him. He has many fears. Most elementary of all is the fear concerning the cost of the treatment the doctor may prescribe. It is a simple but real enough fear. Doctors' bills can play havoc with the family budget and mean financial difficulties for years to come. The prospect of being indebted for a sum which the patient cannot possibly pay within a reasonable time and which may mean financial sacrifice into the distant future is certainly upsetting. The assistant dealing with patients should keep this fear of bills in mind, lest she consider the patient queer or unreasonable.

To this anxiety about cost is added the fear of being hurt by the doctor. Some examinations and treatments are painful, and few people can anticipate pain with equanimity. Is it any wonder the patient is nervous and jittery, perhaps irritable and cross? He will try not to let the doctor see this side of him, but often takes out his irritation on the assistant. Obviously, she must never, under any circumstances, be offended or take any of these outbursts personally. They are aimed at "someone" in the doctor's office, and it would make no difference if her name were Mary, Jane, or Elisabeth, if she were blond or brunet, short or tall.

Finally, there is a fear of death. No one wants to die, not even, strangely enough, those who are incurably ill, in pain, or completely helpless. The thought of extinction is one against which the human organism rebels, no matter how much the mental faculties may at times wish for death. Is it not understandable, then, that patients with serious diseases who come to the heart specialist, the surgeon, etc., require particular consideration and understanding?

The assistant should try to establish a pleasant relationship with every patient who comes to the doctor's office. This may take real effort, but will be a rewarding undertaking. The assistant who obtains friendly cooperation from the patient makes her own work easier and, at the same time, helps the doctor. If she treats patients with impatience or condescension, the relationship will soon deteriorate into open conflict, and the atmosphere in the office will be charged with tension. Even new patients will be affected by such tension.

The patient needs a kind person to help during his ordeal of illness, pain, and perhaps worry. Many surveys made during the last few years have shown that patients are not satisfied with a doctor who just "makes them well." They do not want only a spotlessly clean office and a perfectly working electrocardiograph with an efficient technician; they want friendliness and personal interest from the doctor and from all his office personnel. The doctor may have a big practice, and the patient may come to him because of his reputation. Yet the patient does not stop to figure out that there is little time for personal conversation when the doctor has to see from twenty-five to fifty patients a day. To the patient there is only one patient that counts—himself. A smile, a cheerful remark may be all that is needed. And the assistant must have an unlimited supply of smiles and cheerful remarks. If the patient gets the impression that she is hurried, he immediately suspects that his treatment or examination will be hurried too. If he suspects that he will not receive the proper attention, his resentment is built up at once.

Patients appreciate interest beyond the office visit. A telephone call from the assistant—the doctor hardly has the time—questioning whether the patient feels better, whether the treatment helped, etc., is gratefully received. If the running of the office is properly systematized, such telephone calls can be made between certain tasks. Of course, no such call should be made without the doctor's permission.

One of the chief causes of irritation on the part of patients is having to wait to see the doctor even when an appointment has been made. Most patients are careful to be on time or ahead of time for a doctor's appointment. It is certainly annoying for a patient to have to waste time waiting, especially if he has been given time off from the office. If the assistant takes it for granted that the patient must wait and that he is lucky to be seen by the doctor at all, the doctor will see a very disgruntled person. But if the assistant expresses regret at the delay, perhaps explaining it by telling the patients that there was an emergency call, an unexpected operation at the hospital, or whatever fits the circumstances, she will enlist the patients' sympathy for the doctor. If they have to wait, patients also like to know just how long the wait may be. Nothing is more irritating than to hear the assistant repeat the stereotyped phrase,

"The doctor will see you soon," and then have to wait an hour for one's turn.

Many patients who visit the doctor are very unfortunate persons. The assistant must not display any revulsion or antagonism regarding disfigured, handicapped, or maimed persons or patients with tics or spastic movements. Unless she feels compassion for these unhappy people and a deep, abiding desire to be of assistance to them, if only indirectly through the doctor, her place is not in the doctor's office, nor, in fact, in any area of the medical field.

But the absence of antipathy is not enough. The successful medical assistant must have a positive attitude toward patients. Ideally she should radiate confidence and good cheer, which will automatically reflect in the patient's attitude toward the immediate situation. If the doctor and his assistant are optimistic, the patient will be too; if he is optimistic, his treatment will take better effect, and he will get well sooner or feel better while under treatment. Patients value a kind, friendly attitude more than anything else in a doctor's aide.

Public Relations

Every contact between the assistant and a patient or any person who enters the doctor's office subtly affects the doctor's reputation. An assistant who is unfriendly or who gets on people's nerves by being overtalkative, aggressive, affected, or just plain boorish in her manners might soon drive patients away. In any case, she would be the cause of much unfavorable comment among patients and their friends. Of this comment, the listener may remember only the doctor's name and decide to stay away or not seek out this particular doctor when in need.

On the other hand, an intelligent assistant with a true understanding of her position builds up the doctor's reputation and, incidentally, his practice by creating an atmosphere of friendly good will in his office. This is what is known as good public relations. The medical office assistant is the doctor's public relations agent whose principal aim is to create good will for her doctor-employer. She knows all his patients by name and humors their little foibles and

THE PERSONAL EQUATION

preferences. She helps to build up the doctor's practice. She keeps his office running smoothly and saves him time and trouble, worry and work.

A pleasant, sympathetic, friendly attitude is, of course, an elementary requirement. But there are also some "tricks of the trade" to build up good public relations. All good salesmen keep in mind the fundamental principle that nothing interests people as much as themselves. Evidence of interest in the patient and his special personal problem is one of the strongest pillars of good public relations. Everyone likes to hear his own name (elementary but true). Therefore names should be memorized and used to greet patients on arrival and mentioned frequently in speaking to them.

Next, learn something about the patient's personal life—how many children he has, their names and ages, and any other member of his family who is important in his life. Become acquainted with his business or the type of work he does. Find out about his hobbies. You may not have the opportunity to ask him, but you can be a good listener. Then file away what you have learned for future reference—if not in your memory for quick recall, perhaps in a more conventional filing system, namely, a card index. Have a card for each patient or use a section of the regular ledger card. Jot down some pertinent facts which you can consult before a patient is expected. For example:

Mr. Benson's son is taking part in a high-school debate. Make a note of the date and, when Mr. Benson returns to the office after that date, inquire how the boy made out in the debate.

Mrs. Gray's daughter expects a baby in February. If your card shows this entry, when Mrs. Gray comes in after February, you can inquire whether the baby was a boy or girl.

The patient will give the doctor credit for your interest and the doctor will give credit where credit is due.

Many state medical societies have developed public relations programs, which offer suggestions on how the doctor can build up good will. The doctor needs the help of his office assistant to carry out a public relations program. For instance, some pediatricians make it a rule to send birthday cards to their little patients. This pleases the parents very much. A simple recall system will make sure that the birthday is not forgotten, but the assistant is the one who must take charge of it. Special events such as engagements, weddings, and silver anniversaries call for a card from the doctor if he or his assistant has been informed of them. The assistant is usually delegated to purchase the card, and it is she who must remind the doctor to send it. In the case of a death in the patient's close family, a note of condolence is in order. (Printed cards are in poor taste.)

All this does not mean that there are no problem patients. In fact, every office has them, and they are typical. They are habitually late; they refuse to cooperate; they repeatedly disobey instructions; and at the same time, they reproach the doctor, often via the assistant and in front of other patients, for a lot of imagined wrongs. Such patients must be dealt with tactfully but firmly. The first step is to take them into a private room, as they often subside when they have no audience. The next step is to point out to them that perhaps their recovery is retarded through their own fault. Sometimes a suggestion that they transfer to another physician has salutary results, but the doctor's authorization should be obtained before taking this step.

Just as the assistant fosters good public relations by greeting each patient in a way that indicates she is glad to see him, so, at parting, she should show interest in seeing him again. The patient should leave the office feeling that he was of importance to everyone and that he is expected again. Thus his confidence, good will, and friendship will be gained.

BIBLIOGRAPHY

Laird, Donald A., and Eleanor C. Laird: "The Technique of Handling People," rev. ed., Gregg Publishing Division, McGraw-Hill Book Company, Inc., New York, 1956.

Newton, Roy, and Frederick G. Nichols: "How to Improve Your Personality," 2d ed., Gregg Publishing Division, McGraw-Hill Book Company, Inc., New York, 1954.

3

Protection through Sterilization

Sterilizing the doctor's working tools is one of the main tasks of the medical office assistant, and learning the different techniques of sterilization is an essential part of her training. In order to understand better the importance of and the need for sterilization, she should have some knowledge of the different kinds of infectious agents which might occur in a doctor's office and against which sterilization provides protection. A rudimentary acquaintance with bacteriology would therefore seem one of the requirements of her education. Ignorance or carelessness could be dangerous.

Bacteriology

Anyone familiar with the history of medicine will be impressed by the fact that although a great deal was known about anatomy, certain diseases, and even many therapeutic agents thousands of years ago, the discovery of infectious microorganisms and their role in the production of disease is barely a hundred years old. The study of these microorganisms and the application of the knowledge gained is called bacteriology. While some of the most ancient physicians may have suspected that there were forms of life too small to be seen by human eyes and that some of these might be harmful to man, the majority of doctors, until the middle of the nineteenth century, did not recognize the association between bacteria and the changes and infections we now know they cause.

It was not until 1675, that Antonj van Leeuwenhoek, of Holland, constructed a lens strong enough to detect some of the larger bacteria. Yet this discovery produced no scientific consequences whatsoever. It remained for Pasteur, in the latter half of the nineteenth century, to prove that microorganisms in the air, invisible to the naked eye, entered food and were responsible for spoilage, fermentation, and transmission of disease. Pasteur is now looked upon as the father of bacteriology.

His student, Joseph Lister, who lived from 1827 to 1912, in attempting to keep microorganisms out of wounds or kill them after they had gotten into wounds, developed the modern aseptic technique. In about 1849, Ignaz Semmelweis, a Viennese physician, insisted that doctors and nurses attending women in childbed wash their hands, so as not to carry infections from one patient to another. He was ridiculed and, in despair, died in an insane asylum. In 1843, Oliver Wendell Holmes, of Boston, announced that "childbed fever" was contagious. Robert Koch, a German physician, at the turn of the century isolated a microorganism that is now called the tubercle bacillus and proved that this was the cause of tuberculosis. He formulated the criteria that are still used today for determining whether a certain microorganism is the cause of a particular disease.

Since these early discoveries, all of them startling and controversial at first, bacteriology has grown rapidly and is now one of the most important branches of biological research.

About fifteen hundred species of bacteria are known, of which about a thousand have been classified. Some hundred are known to medicine, and of these only some forty or fifty are infectious to man. Present-day bacteriology is a segment of the science called microbiology (*mikros*, "small"; *bios*, "life"; *logia*, "study of"), which is the study of microscopic life encompassing the following:

1. Bacteria
2. Rickettsiae
3. Viruses
4. Fungi
5. Animal parasites

The term *bacteriology* generally implies the study of the first four types, and this chapter covers only these four. All four types are often included under the general term *bacteria*, although the new fields of virology (viruses) and mycology (fungi) are rapidly developing into distinct, separate sciences. The animal parasites belong in the field called parasitology, which includes the study of the organisms that cause malaria and such human infestations as trichinosis, pinworm, and tapeworm.

Bacteria. These are single-celled microscopic plants rich in nucleoprotein. They have a cell wall which gives them shape, and they reproduce by a process called binary fission (splitting in two). A single cell in suitable environment (optimum temperature, correct nutritional elements, moisture, etc.) reproduces by dividing into two cells called daughter cells (asexual division). These grow to the size of the original parent cell and in turn reproduce to form four cells, then eight, sixteen, and so forth. This complete cycle of birth, growth, and reproduction takes place in 15 to 30 minutes. It is this ability of logarithmic, rapid reproduction that makes bacteria potentially very dangerous.

In most cases the bacterial cell can be stained readily with simple dyes, such as methylene blue, gentian violet, or safranine. This easy-staining characteristic is very important, as it enables a research technician to distinguish bacteria in tissue or smears.

Bacteria are divided into three major morphologic (shape, appearance) groups:

1. Cocci (singular, coccus)—spherical bacteria
2. Bacilli (singular, bacillus)—rod-shaped bacteria
3. Spirilla (singular, spirillum)—spiral organisms

Among the cocci there are three types: staphylococci, diplococci, and streptococci. Staphylococci (grapelike clusters of cocci) are widely distributed in nature and found on the skin, in glands, and in mucous membranes. Some staphylococci are extremely dangerous. The most common pyogenic (pus-producing) organisms known to man, they are usually involved in "pimples," boils, stitch abscesses, and in osteomyelitis. Diplococci (cocci forming pairs of cells) are the organisms that cause such diseases as pneumonia and gonorrhea.

Streptococci (cocci forming chains of cells) also include some very dangerous types, for instance, those that cause epidemic sore throat ("strep throat"), scarlet fever, septicemia (blood-stream infection), and rheumatic heart disease.

To the bacilli belong those organisms that cause diseases such as tuberculosis, brucellosis, typhoid and paratyphoid fever, and bacillary dysentery. The spirilla include the organisms that cause syphilis, relapsing fever, and cholera. Figures 3–1 to 3–3 illustrate some cocci, bacilli, and spirilla.

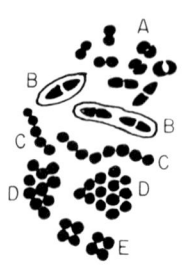

Fig. 3–1. Some forms of cocci. A. Diplococci. B. Encapsulated diplococci. C. Streptococci. D. Staphylococci. E. Tetrads.

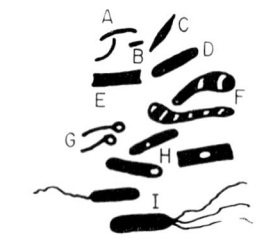

Fig. 3–2. Some forms of bacilli. A. Slender, curved. B. Slender, short. C. Pointed (fusiform). D. Rounded ends. E. Concave ends. F. Irregular (pleomorphic), banded. G. Slender bacillus with large terminal spore. H. Other forms of sporulating bacilli. I. Bacilli with flagella.

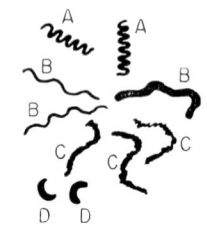

Fig. 3–3. Some forms of spirilla. A. Treponema. B. Borrelia. C. Leptospira. D. Vibrio.

Some bacteria produce spores. By contraction of the cytoplasm, or protoplasm, and elimination of water, the mass of material in the cell consolidates, a hard shell is formed, and a spore results. A spore, then, represents a concentrated form of matter that originally formed a bacterial cell. It results when the environment is unsuitable to sustain bacteria in their original form. When brought into a suitable environment the spores germinate and revert to bacterial form. Because of their hard shell, spores are especially resistant to heat and cannot be destroyed easily, a fact which must be taken into consideration in sterilizing procedures.

Rickettsiae. These are amorphous (not having a definite shape) parasites involved in the various "spotted fevers"—typhus, Rocky Mountain spotted fever, tsutsugamushi fever, and several others. They are generally tick-borne.

Viruses. Like the rickettsiae, the viruses (ultramicroscopic parasites) are not true bacteria. They are the cause of a variety of diseases, such as influenza, poliomyelitis, colds, mumps, measles, and many others. They can pass through the pores of porcelain filters, and their isolation and study are extremely difficult. They are difficult to cultivate since they are complete parasites, which means they will live only in the living cells of other organisms. With the advent of modern techniques and the electron microscope, however, even the viruses are yielding up their secrets to research.

Fungi. This form of life represents a low class of vegetable organism. Fungi appear in the form of mushrooms and molds, as well as in microscopic growth, for instance, infections of the skin.

The Need for Sterilization

It is the bacteria, especially the streptococci and staphylococci, with which one is mostly concerned in a doctor's office, as they are found everywhere—in the air, in dust, on every piece of furniture, and on every object that is handled. It must be realized, however, that not all bacteria are disease-producing. On the contrary, bacteria attack dead matter and destroy it.

As a rule, even disease-producing bacteria do not harm us. First of all, an individual must be susceptible to the organism in question. Most of us have a natural or an acquired immunity for certain pathogenic agents, and thus even close contact or ingestion may not produce any infection. Secondly, microorganisms must appear in concentrated masses before we succumb to their attack. A healthy organism can usually resist a few bacteria. The skin has a bactericidal action, saliva is a strong bactericidal agent, and mucous membranes secrete fluids which are toxic to bacteria. In order to produce a typical lesion, a bacterium must enter the blood stream through a break in the skin or enter the organism through one of its orifices—the mouth, nostrils, ears, etc. Even then the organism may form antibodies, which defend the body by attacking the invading microorganisms. Some individuals have a natural or acquired immunity to certain bacteria.

Microorganisms are passed from person to person. In transmission some disease-producing agents gain in virulence and so are capable of causing infection. Hygienic principles and sanitary practices have therefore been developed to a high degree in Western countries and are being adopted by other civilizations. We all know the importance of washing our hands frequently, especially after touching anything that has been handled by many persons—money, public stair rails, library books—and before eating. Every considerate person covers his face with his handkerchief when coughing or sneezing, so as not to contaminate the air and spread disease with the spray of microorganisms that he emits. Today even children, when they cut themselves, ask that the wound be washed and treated with an antiseptic.

In order to prescribe effective treatment for an infection, it is necessary to identify by laboratory methods the bacteria responsible for the pathological condition. Some routine methods used in a doctor's office are discussed in Chapter 20, entitled Laboratory Techniques. The present chapter is concerned only with the need for protection against harmful bacteria, irrespective of type, by means of sterilization.

Principles of Sterilization

After the discovery of the existence of infectious microorganisms, antiseptic methods were used in surgery; that is, an attempt was made to kill bacteria which might be in the wound, on the skin of the patient, or on anybody or anything that came into contact with the surgical patient. Modern methods substitute aseptic techniques for these crude, early attempts. That is, clean hands and sterile instruments and dressings make antiseptic methods unnecessary, for bacteria, having been destroyed beforehand, are not present after surgery begins.

Some common terms employed in connection with sterilization

have often been used interchangeably, although they are by no means synonymous. The following definitions should be remembered so that the terms will be properly used:

Antiseptic: capable of preventing the growth or action of microorganisms, without necessarily killing them
Aseptic: free from all microorganisms
Bactericidal: capable of destroying bacteria
Contaminated: infected or made impure by contact with unsterile objects
Disinfectant: capable of destroying pathogenic microorganisms but usually not spores
Germicidal: capable of destroying germs
Pathogenic: capable of causing a disease
Sterile: free of all living microorganisms

Aseptic conditions are the rule today in every doctor's office. The maintenance of this aspect of medical practice is a primary duty of the assistant. It is her responsibility to see that utmost cleanliness prevails, and she must do her part to prevent the infection of a patient in the office or the spread of an infection from patient to patient.

Every part of a doctor's office—waiting room, treatment and examination rooms—must be kept spotlessly clean at all times. All objects used must be washed after they are handled and, preferably, rinsed before they are used again. It must not be thought that sterilization is a substitute for cleaning. It definitely is not. To "sterilize," by whatever method, a soiled article that has not first been cleaned would be to defeat the purpose of sterilization.

All instruments, glassware, enamelware, and rubber goods must be washed with soap and water after use. The assistant must constantly remind herself to wash her hands whenever they have touched a patient or a utensil that has come into contact with a patient, lest she transmit an infection from one patient to another. Disinfectant soaps are preferable to ordinary scented toilet soap in a doctor's office. Tincture of green soap is the medium of choice.

A hand lotion may be used after each washing to prevent dry, chapped skin.

The normal, healthy skin forms an excellent protection against infection, and therefore, instruments or appliances that come into contact solely with the skin need only be clean, not sterile. Whenever the skin is broken, however, harmful microorganisms can enter the blood stream and cause a wide variety of infections. Instruments and dressings used on open wounds or in operations, however minor, as well as the rubber gloves worn while attending to them, must be sterile. This is also true of syringes and needles, as injections puncture the skin. The orifices of the body present an additional open door to infectious agents, and any instrument introduced for examination or treatment should be sterile.

The purpose of sterilization is, therefore, threefold:

1. To destroy microorganisms
2. To provide an important safeguard in the control of infection
3. To have sterile supplies available for immediate use at all times

The principle upon which sterilization is based is the fact that no living organism can withstand high temperatures or certain chemical poisons if they are applied a sufficiently long time. Resistance to these agents varies, however, some spores, for instance, being very heat-resistant. The height of the temperature and the length of exposure must therefore be carefully gauged. In addition, there is a difference between dry heat and moist heat. If instruments are covered with an oily substance, the germs that may be underneath enjoy a certain protection, and longer exposure to extremely high temperatures may be necessary to destroy them.

The knowledge of what material is sterile and how it becomes contaminated will help to protect the patient, the physician, and the assistant. The proper care of supplies and equipment provides a definite safeguard in the control of infections and has a direct bearing upon the care of the patient.

Methods of Sterilization

There are at present four methods of sterilization in use:

1. Boiling
2. Cold sterilization (by a chemical germicide)
3. Steam under pressure, or autoclaving
4. Dry heat (hot air)

Boiling. In most doctors' offices, sterilization by boiling is the method of choice. A portable sterilizer that runs on electricity is illustrated in Fig. 3–4. This is used for syringes and all small, *blunt*

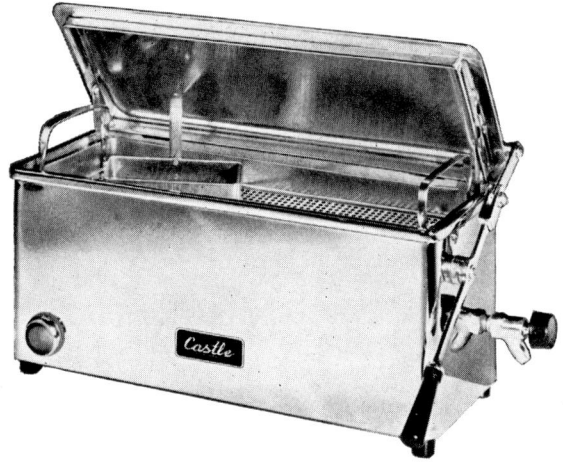

FIG. 3–4. Sterilizer for physician's office. (*Standard Scientific Supply Co.*)

instruments, as well as for glassware, enamelware, stainless-steel objects, and soft-rubber goods.

To sterilize by this method, fill the sterilizer about half full with cold water. It is most practical to use distilled water, as this leaves no sediment; however, in a busy office where the sterilizer may be in use all day, distilled water would probably prove too costly. If tap water is used, sterilizing tablets, of which several kinds are available, or bicarbonate of soda may be added to prevent rusting.

When cleaning the sterilizer, fill it with cold water, a cup of vinegar, or some special sterilizer cleaner and let it boil at least half an hour. Then pour off the water and scrape off any scale that may be left. Wipe the entire interior with alcohol or ether, and the sterilizer is ready to be used again. It should be cleaned at least once a week. The techniques for sterilizing the various instruments and articles which the doctor uses are described below.

Syringes. A syringe consists of three parts: the barrel, the piston or plunger, and the needle (see Fig. 3–5). The needle, in turn, consists of the point, the cannula, and the hub (see Fig. 3–6).

1. Making sure that the syringe is clean, place the barrel and plunger separately in cold water in the tray of the sterilizer. Be sure both parts belong to the same syringe.

2. Close the sterilizer, bring the water to a boil, and let it boil for 7 minutes.

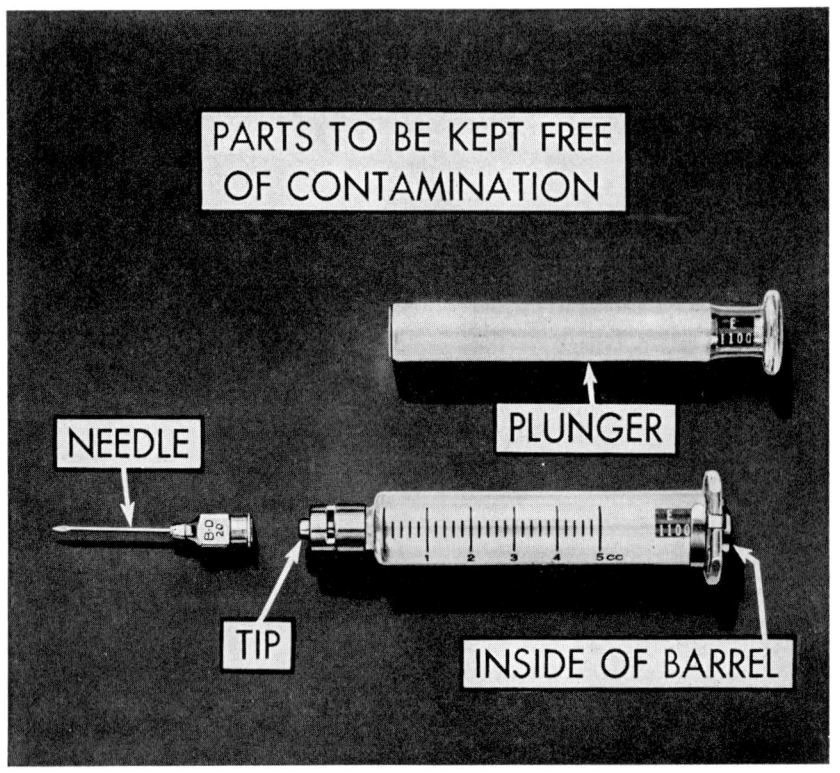

FIG. 3–5. Parts of a syringe. (*Becton, Dickinson & Co.*)

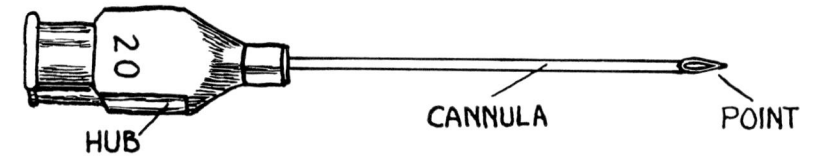

FIG. 3-6. Hypodermic needle.

3. At the end of 7 minutes, place the needles, with the stylet in place, into the sterilizer and boil with the barrel and plunger for 3 minutes. (Some sterilizers have a separate compartment for needles.)

4. Remove from sterilizer with sterile forceps, dry each part of the syringe with a double thickness of sterile towels, and place on a sterile wrapper. Remove the needles with forceps, one at a time; remove the stylet and place it on a sterile cover with the syringe.

5. If the syringe is not to be used immediately, leave the stylet in place and wrap the syringe in a sterile wrapper made of a towel, gauze, or one of the new plastic or fiber materials.

6. Label the package as to contents (size and number of syringes) and date.

Depending on the doctor's needs, the assistant may sterilize syringes just before they are used or she may keep a supply of sterile syringes always on hand.

Blunt Instruments. After cleaning the blunt instruments thoroughly with a stiff brush in soap and warm water, paying special attention to grooves and crevices, place them in the sterilizer. (Clamps should be opened.) Let them boil for 10 to 15 minutes. If they are needed immediately, remove them from the sterilizer with sterile forceps (which are kept in a container of Lysol or another germicide, see Fig. 3-7) and place them on a sterile towel. This method of sterilizing is suggested only if there is no autoclave available.

If the instruments are not needed at once, dry them after sterilization; add a drop of oil to hinges to prevent rusting; and place the instruments in the instrument cabinet until they are needed, when they must be sterilized again. If a complete set of sterile instruments for any particular procedure must be kept on hand, however, the instruments, after being removed by sterile forceps, should be placed on a sterile cover, dried with a sterile towel, wrapped in a sterile pack, and labeled. If any instruments are missing from the complete set, a note to that effect should be made on the label.

Sharp Instruments. As boiling dulls the edges of instruments, sharp instruments should be sterilized in the autoclave or in an antiseptic solution. These methods are discussed later.

Glassware. Glassware that is to be sterilized must first be washed with soap and warm water so that it is mechanically clean before it is placed in the sterilizer. If blood or pus has dried on the glass, soak it for 30 minutes. Place glassware in cold water in the sterilizer, bring it to a boil, and boil for 15 to 20 minutes. Jars, bottles, etc., should be placed on their sides, lest they form air pockets and prevent the boiling water from touching the inside.

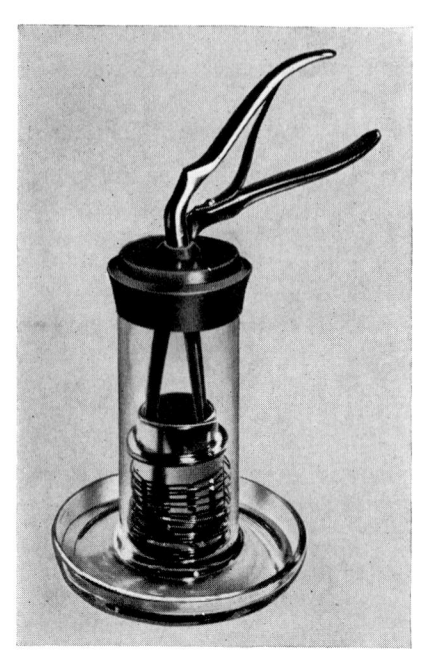

FIG. 3–7. Transfer forceps in glass jar. (*Bard-Parker Co., Inc.*)

Enamel and Stainless-steel Ware. An enamel basin, or any other receptacle, that is worn and chipped should be discarded. Because enamel chips easily, stainless steel is replacing enamel in most medical offices.

1. Scrub the basin thoroughly with soap and abrasive powder and then rinse.

2. Place in the sterilizer and let it boil for 10 to 15 minutes.

3. Lift out with sterile forceps, place on a sterile cover, wrap, and label.

4. If enamelware is to be sterilized before re-use, washing after use is sufficient.

Rubber Goods. First of all, divide all rubber goods into hard and soft articles.

Hard-rubber goods are:

1. Nozzles
2. Pessaries
3. Nose clamps
4. Combs

Hard-rubber goods cannot be boiled but must be sterilized by chemical means.

Soft-rubber goods are:

1. Catheters
2. Dams
3. Rubber tubing
4. Gloves
5. Protective covers

Soft-rubber goods are boilable, but only after they have been mechanically cleaned and rinsed. They should never be boiled together with other materials.

When sterilizing rubber tubing:

1. Clean tubing by forcing warm soapy water through the tube; then rinse. (Tubing used for draining a wound, when no longer needed, is thrown away with the dressing.)
2. When tubing is thoroughly clean, place it in sterilizer and boil 5 minutes.
3. Hang up to drain and dry.
4. *If tubing is to be used immediately,* remove with forceps, hold up to drain, and place on a sterile cover.

When sterilizing rubber gloves:

1. After use, wash thoroughly with green soap and water; rinse.
2. With air or water, test carefully for leaks or tears.

3. Mend holes with rubber cement and rubber patch. (Mending kits for rubber gloves are available.)
4. Tie each pair of gloves together with a narrow gauze bandage.
5. Place in the sterilizer, making sure that water enters all pockets and the gloves remain submerged.
6. Add salt to the water to preserve the softness of gloves.
7. Boil for 20 minutes.

Important: If the gloves are to be used immediately, take them from the sterilizer with forceps, plunge them into a basin with an antiseptic solution, and put them on while the hands are immersed in the solution. If the gloves are to be stored in sterile condition, autoclave them before storing them.

Cold Sterilization. A simpler method of sterilization is that of immersion in a chemical solution of high germicidal potency. Instruments placed into such a solution must be cleaned in the same way as for boiling. They are then placed in a special container with an absolutely airtight cover. (Such a container is shown in Fig. 3–8.) They are left in this container for the amount of time required by the particular solution, usually 15 to 20 minutes.

Manufacturers of germicides claim a high potency for their products, maintaining that they kill bacteria and fungi. If a germicide is used, the directions for each type should be followed with the utmost accuracy. Some germicides must be diluted, but if the dilution is too great, the solution loses its germicidal strength. It is safer to use a germicide that needs no measuring or mixing. Some solutions must be discarded after a certain time, but others can be added to as the volume is reduced.

A few of the older germicides were harmful to instruments and fabrics, but the newer germicides neither stain nor harm fabrics or the operator's hands. For rubber gloves, the solution should usually be diluted. Directions are given with each brand.

The aftercare of materials sterilized in this way is the same as that for boiling. Cold sterilization should be used for sharp instruments and hard-rubber goods if no autoclave is available.

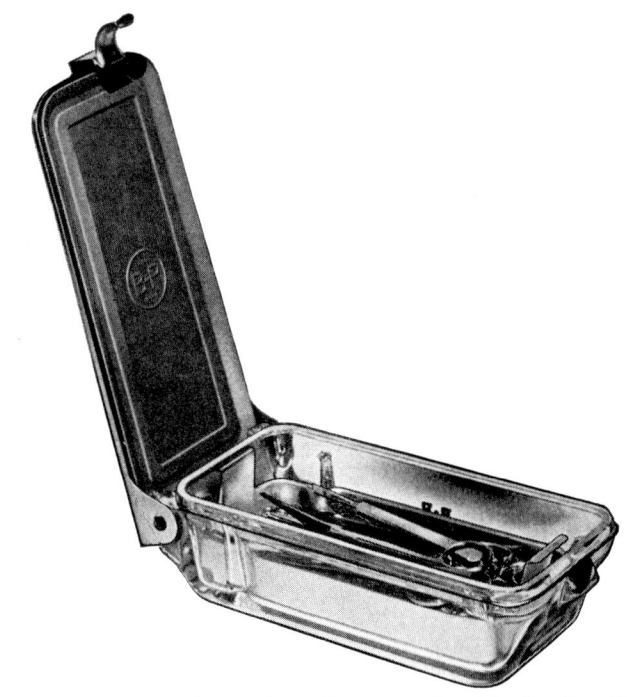

FIG. 3–8. Container for cold sterilization. (*Bard-Parker Co., Inc.*)

If no special germicide is used, sharp instruments can be sterilized as follows:

1. Clean thoroughly with soap and water; rinse well.
2. Place instruments in a 5 per cent phenol solution for 15 minutes.
3. Rinse with a 70 per cent alcohol solution.
4. Remove with sterilizer forceps.
5. Dry with sterile towels.
6. Wrap in sterile cover; label.
7. Protect sharp points with a sterile cotton ball.

Hard-rubber goods and items such as gum plastic, woven silk, and filiform (threadlike) bougies should be sterilized by the cold, or chemical, method. If no special germicide is used, these items should be immersed in a 1:1,000 mercuric cyanide solution for 1 hour. No other method should be used. The items should be rinsed well with sterile water before they are dried.

Autoclaving. The most efficient way of sterilizing surgical supplies is by steam under pressure. This is done in an autoclave. The autoclave works on the same principle as a pressure cooker. That is, the apparatus generates steam under pressure which flows through the sterilizing chamber. Higher temperatures are obtained, and dry materials can be sterilized, as the steam penetrates wrapped packages. Figure 3–9 shows an autoclave, and Fig. 3–10 illustrates the way in which the steam flows through the sterilizing chamber. No living organism can survive a 10-minute exposure to the moist heat of the high temperatures attained by an autoclave. Even the most resistant bacterial spores are destroyed within a matter of minutes. The temperature recommended for autoclaving is 250°F. Hospitals

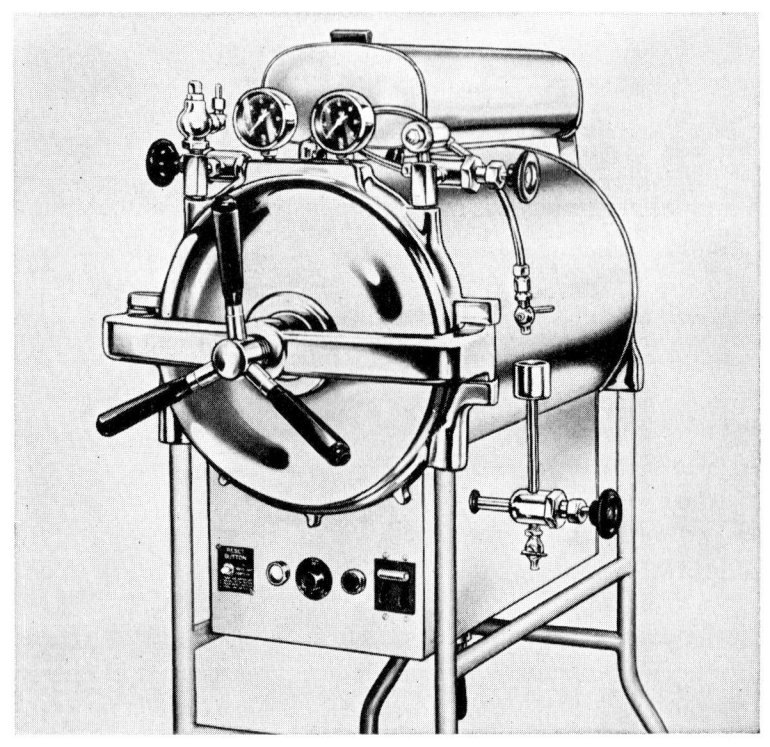

FIG. 3–9. Autoclave. (*Pelton & Crane Co.*)

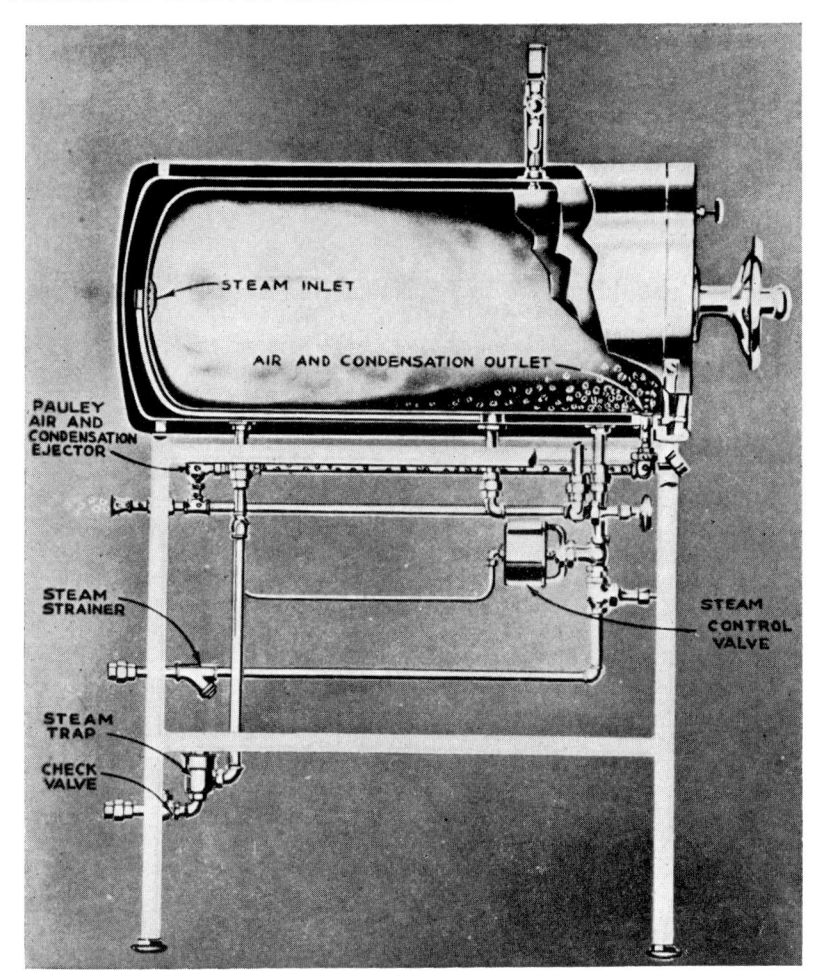

Fig. 3-10. Steam flowing through autoclave. (*Courtesy of LaVerne Ruth Thompson and Clay-Adams Co., Inc.*)

use autoclaving exclusively for sterilizing all surgical and medical supplies.

One of the advantages of an autoclave is the fact that a large amount of utensils, instruments, and packs may be sterilized at one time; however, the autoclave should not be packed too full. Correct techniques for wrapping and loading are essential. There must be space between the objects so that the steam may flow freely through them. Steam should displace the air downward, and the air must circulate around the packages. Modern autoclaves, such as the one illustrated, have a circuit breaker that automatically turns off the current when there is an overload. But this should never occur.

When preparing materials for the autoclave, the following points should be remembered:

1. Packs should not be so large that they do not fit easily into the chamber.
2. All packs must be loosely wrapped.
3. All articles must be completely covered by wrapping and securely fastened.
4. Packages are placed into the autoclave on their edge, not flat, so that the steam can penetrate.
5. Jars and cans are placed on their side, without covers, so that the air can enter.

To sterilize rubber gloves in the autoclave:

1. Wash and test the rubber gloves as for boiling.
2. Powder them with cornstarch on both sides.
3. Use the special envelope container.
4. Turn up the cuff below the thumb.
5. Place the right glove in one pocket, the left glove in the other.
6. Place a small envelope with cornstarch for the hands in the container with the gloves.
7. Close the pockets.
8. Wrap in the outer covering.
9. Mark the size of the gloves (if several sizes are used in the office) and the date of sterilization. Indicate whether they are mended or not.
10. Autoclave for 15 to 20 minutes.
11. Store the gloves for future use.

Figure 3–11 shows several packs prepared for the autoclave. As can be seen, six of the packages are ready to be placed into the chamber, while the other packages have not yet been closed. Note

PROTECTION THROUGH STERILIZATION 41

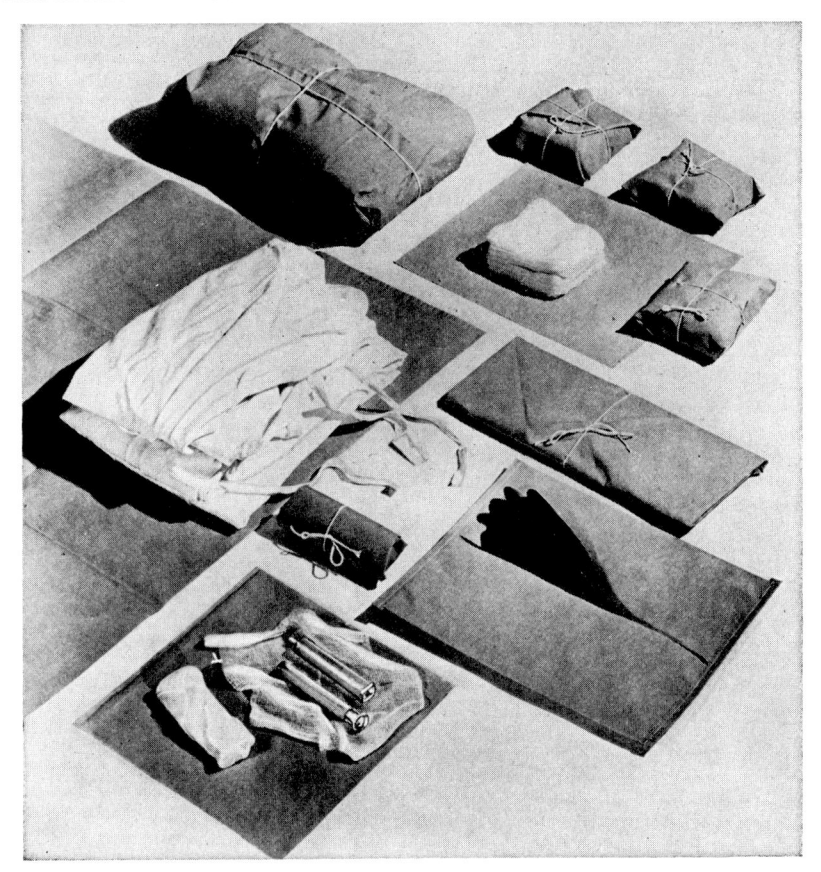

FIG. 3-11. Packs prepared for autoclaving. (*Meinecke & Co.*)

the envelope container in which the rubber gloves are placed, with one pocket for each glove. Figure 3-12 shows an open pack containing a number of syringes and needles. Each pack should be marked with a tag or label that indicates the contents, the date, and the size of the syringes and needles.

Formerly muslin was always used to wrap packages for autoclaving. Now special materials, made of crepe paper or soft fibers, permit more rapid penetration of steam and shorten the period needed for autoclaving. At the same time, they are much less expensive than muslin and can be discarded after use, thereby reducing the cost of laundry and the storage space. They take up less room than

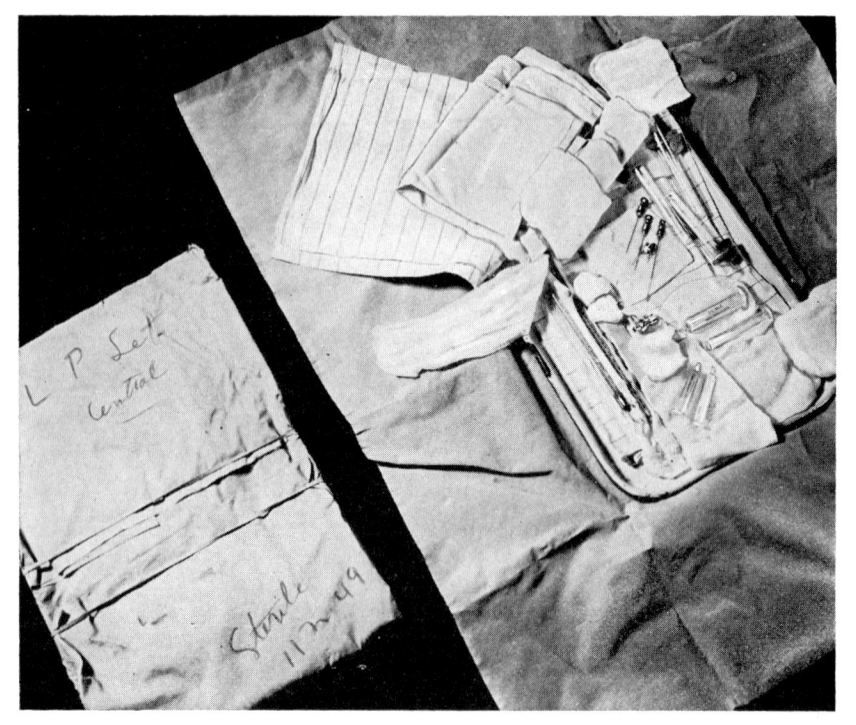

FIG. 3–12. Syringes in pack in preparation for autoclaving. (*Meinecke & Co.*)

textile wrappings, and the manufacturers claim that they remain sterile longer. The packs shown are wrapped in crepe-paper wraps that are sold under the trade name of Sterilwraps.

The load in the autoclave must be timed carefully. The length of sterilization time varies with the materials. Rubber goods should not be sterilized for more than 15 or 20 minutes, as excessive sterilization ruins them. Instruments that are not wrapped and glass- and enamelware are sterilized for 15 minutes. Instruments and dressings that are wrapped should be sterilized for 30 minutes.

The purpose of autoclaving is to sterilize every article completely. In order to have absolute assurance that the contents of any one pack have been properly sterilized, the use of the recently developed sterilization indicators is recommended. These indicators operate on the principle that specifically prepared dyes will change color when exposed to moist heat for a sufficiently long period of

PROTECTION THROUGH STERILIZATION 43

time. An indicator, sold under the trade name of Steam-Clox Indicator, consists of small cardboard tabs with purple markings. One of the tabs is slipped into a metal container and placed in each pack, with the string that is attached to the metal container hanging outside the pack. When the pack is taken out of the autoclave, the metal container is pulled out of the pack by the string, and the indicator is read. If all the purple markings have changed to green, complete sterilization is assured.

Most doctors have found the conventional autoclave too large and complicated for the average office. The recently designed models, however, combine compactness with speed and efficiency. A small autoclave that might be practical for a doctor's office is illustrated in Fig. 3–13. (An even smaller model is available.) It is easy to operate and almost entirely automatic. The boiler is filled with distilled water, the current is turned on, and steam is produced

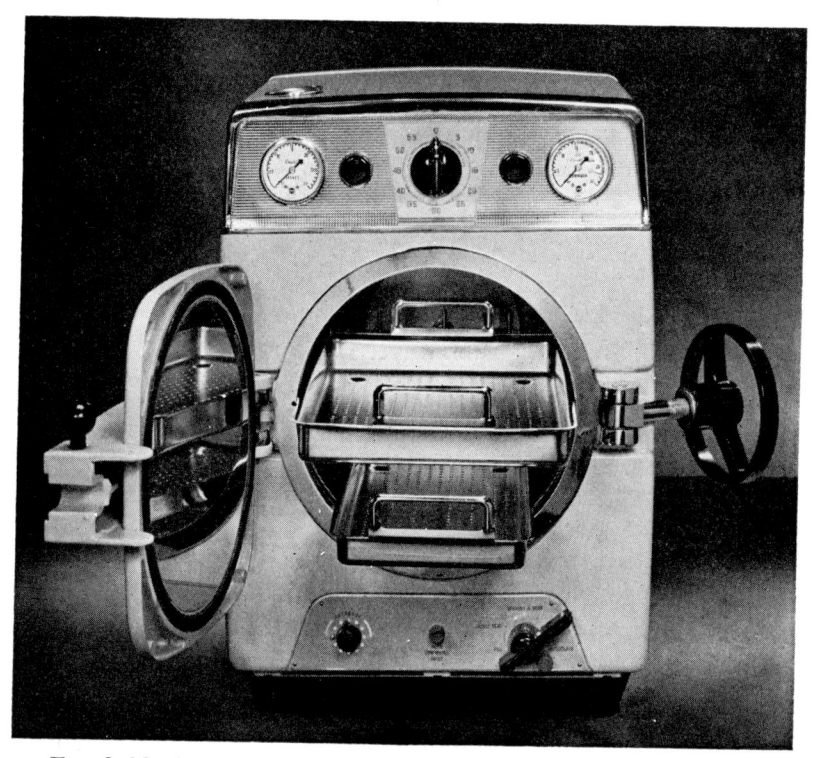

Fig. 3–13. Autoclave for physician's office. (*Wilmot Castle Co.*)

in the sterilizing chamber within a very short time. Control dials permit adjustment of the sterilizing pressure.

Dry Heat. Sterilization by dry heat is a method rarely used in a doctor's office, because it requires much higher temperatures and longer periods of exposure than moist-heat sterilization. Some autoclaves, however, have a special arrangement that permits dry-heat sterilization for instruments that may corrode easily. Oils, powders, petroleum jelly, and such instruments as knife blades are better sterilized by dry heat.

Many surgical supplies today are made of nylon and other synthetic fibers. Most of these materials are specifically guaranteed to be "autoclavable," but this should be checked before any of these supplies are placed into the autoclave.

BIBLIOGRAPHY

Berry, Edna Cornelia, and Mary Louise Kohn: "Introduction to Operating-room Technique," McGraw-Hill Book Company, Inc., Blakiston Division, New York, 1955.

Bryan, Arthur H., and Charles G. Bryan: "Bacteriology Principles and Practice," College Outline Series, no. 3, Barnes & Noble, Inc., New York, 1956.

4

Helping with Examinations

When the patient comes to the physician because he is ill, weak, or in pain, he expects the doctor to determine the cause of his complaints and give him treatment to cure the particular disease from which he is suffering. But it is not always as easy for the doctor to make a diagnosis as the patient imagines. Many diseases have similar symptoms; moreover, the patient's description of his condition is subjective and not always reliable. Just what is the doctor looking for?

To ascertain the patient's disease (to make a diagnosis) may be a simple matter in the case of certain diseases. But a complete examination may be needed to get to the root of the trouble. A complete diagnostic examination includes a physical examination of the patient, x-rays, a basal metabolism test, an electrocardiogram, many laboratory tests, and a variety of other procedures.

The medical office assistant will be especially needed for this part of the doctor's practice. She must prepare the examination room, lay out the instruments needed, get the patient ready for the doctor, perhaps make some of the preliminary examinations herself, assist the doctor during the examination, and attend to the patient during the procedure.

Methods of Examination

There are several methods of examination:

1. *Inspection:* examination by means of sight
2. *Palpation:* examination with hands to outline the size of organs, discover tumors, feel the heartbeat and the vibration of the chest

3. *Percussion:* examination by tapping with fingers, knuckles, or the side of the hand to determine the density of parts or to elicit reflexes

4. *Auscultation:* examination by application of the ears to the body to hear heartbeats and respiration

All these methods are of ancient origin and at one time were performed without the aid of any instruments. Today there are many diagnostic aids. For instance, a percussion hammer is used instead of, or in addition to, tapping with the fingers or the side of the hand. Such a hammer is shown in Fig. 4–1. It consists of a wire handle and a hard-rubber head.

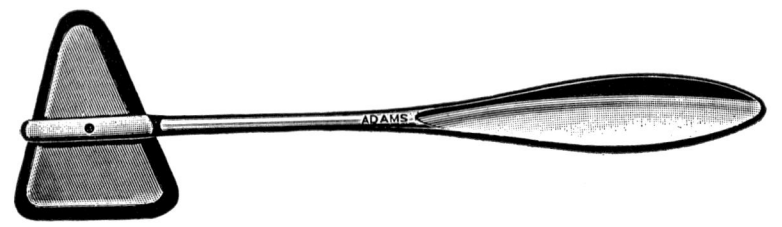

Fig. 4–1. Percussion hammer. (*Clay-Adams Co., Inc.*)

Auscultation is done nowadays with a stethoscope, illustrated in Fig. 4–2. The stethoscope consists of earpieces, rubber tubing, and

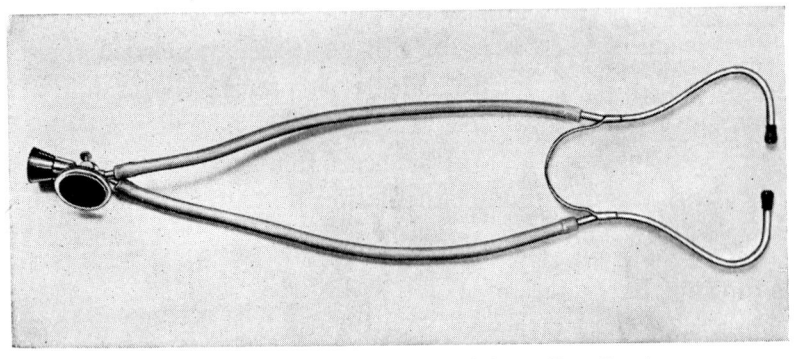

Fig. 4–2. Stethoscope. (*Clay-Adams Co., Inc.*)

a chest piece. Two types of stethoscope are in use, one with a bell-shaped chest piece, called the Ford type, the other with a disk, called the Bowles type. The stethoscope shown is a combination model. A flick of the bar with the thumb changes the chest piece from the disk to the bell, or vice versa.

For visual inspection of internal organs or body cavities, there are a variety of instruments specially designed for the different parts of the body. They can be introduced easily and are electrically lighted, so that the internal part can be observed clearly. In a general examination, two of these instruments are used routinely, namely, the otoscope, for inspection of the ear, and the ophthalmoscope, for inspection of the inner eye. Instruments such as the bronchoscope, for inspection of the bronchi; gastroscope, for inspection of the interior of the stomach; and others are used by specialists for their particular examinations.

Setup for Examination

Every physician has a particular set of instruments that he prefers to use during an examination. The assistant should be thoroughly familiar with these, and all of them should be laid out for the doctor on a stand or table within easy reach. Until the assistant has learned what the doctor needs, she may find it helpful to have a check list to consult each time she prepares the table for an examination. The folllowing is a list of utensils and instruments that may be needed.

1. Head mirror
2. Stethoscope
3. Percussion hammer
4. Tuning fork
5. Flashlight
6. Tongue blades
7. Rubber gloves and lubricant
8. Cotton applicators
9. Kidney basin
10. Tissues or wipers
11. Containers labeled with the patient's name
12. Slides
13. Ophthalmoscope
14. Otoscope

The assistant will soon learn the doctor's particular method. She should hand the items to him in the order in which he uses them. All instruments that have been used should be laid aside for cleaning.

The examination room should be spotlessly clean, well aired, and comfortably warm. The door or curtain must at all times be closed so that no passer-by can look into the room.

If the patient is to be examined on the examination table, the table should have a clean cover, which may be a cotton or muslin sheet, crepe paper, or a rubber sheet on the lower part of the table and a towel at the head.

The Examination

In a routine general examination, any one or all of the following procedures may be carried out:

1. While the patient is sitting, the doctor inspects the neck, chest, and back by percussion, or tapping, and listens for heart sounds with the stethoscope. When examining women, the doctor inspects the breasts also. The chest should be covered with a towel while the doctor examines the back, the back covered while he examines the chest.

2. The patient lies flat on his back, supine position, while the doctor examines the abdomen and the size of the liver and spleen. For this examination the knees are flexed, to relax the muscles of the abdomen. The chest is covered with a towel, the legs and pubic area with a sheet, so as to expose only the abdomen; or a corner of the sheet is put under the chin, with the opposite corner between the legs and the sides wrapped under the patient. The sheet is moved up and down as the doctor inspects different areas.

3. The arms, legs, fingers, and toes are examined, and the movement of the joints is tested.

4. The arteries and veins in the lower extremities are examined. A tuning fork is applied to the toes to test vibratory sensation in the legs. The knee-jerk is tested while the patient sits on the table with his legs hanging down.

5. An internal or pelvic examination is always performed on married women. The doctor inserts two fingers into the vagina and, with the other hand, palpates the abdomen.

6. Blood pressure, height, weight, pulse, respiration, and sometimes the temperature are taken. This part of the examination is often done by the assistant before the patient sees the doctor. The procedures for this part are discussed in detail later.

Preparation of the Patient

It is the assistant's task to receive the patient and prepare him for the doctor's examination. After certain information has been obtained from the patient, such as address, occupation, and whatever the doctor wishes to know (see Chapter 15 for discussion of this phase), the patient is taken to the dressing room and asked to disrobe. He should be given explicit instructions about this, as he may be completely ignorant of what is going to take place and will need to be told exactly what garments to take off.

For an examination of the neck, chest, shoulders, or arms, it is not necessary for the patient to wear an examination gown. A woman need take off only her outer garments, as underwear can usually be slipped off the shoulders. A man would have to take off his coat and shirt.

In the case of a pelvic, vaginal, or rectal examination, a woman usually need only slip off her drawers and girdle and roll down her stockings.

For a general examination, the patient disrobes entirely, and is given an examination gown. As this type of gown fastens in the back, the assistant may have to close it when the patient is ready. In some offices, women are asked to remove all garments except their underslip, shoes, and stockings. The slip takes the place of the examination gown. Most women seem to prefer this.

If a woman patient seems reluctant to have the assistant see her undress, or if the woman attempts to hide her underwear, the assistant should respect this attitude and withdraw as much as possible, and she should not attempt to pick up the patient's belongings.

A woman patient should be instructed to take off all jewelry before the examination, place it in her pocketbook, and take this with her to the examination room.

Some patients, because of injury or pain, may need assistance in undressing. The assistant should offer to help such a patient. She may also show him how to remove his garments in such a way as to cause no pain. In the case of an injured arm, for example, the sleeve is removed from the healthy arm first, so that the coat or dress can be slipped off the injured arm without any pull. When the patient is dressing, the process is reversed. The assistant can point out to a woman with a disability that she may find it more convenient to wear a dress that buttons down the front and need not be pulled over the head.

Usually a specimen of the patient's urine is needed for examination. In some offices it is routine procedure to ask patients, when they make an appointment for an examination, to bring in a specimen. Otherwise it is necessary to give the patient a receptacle and ask him to void into it. If the specimen is taken in the office, it should always be taken before the examination. The specimen is then put into a bottle, and the patient's name, as well as the date, put on the label. If the doctor has a laboratory, the specimen is examined at once; if it is to be sent to an outside laboratory, the bottle must be placed in the refrigerator.

Some women take a long time dressing and undressing, thus tying up the dressing room for other patients. The assistant, in such cases, may offer to help the patient, or she may tactfully suggest that the patient wear fewer or simpler things when she comes to the office the next time.

It may be necessary to talk to the patient to prepare him mentally for the examination. It is impossible to give any general rules about this, as all patients react differently. Some are stoic and show little emotion; others are so nervous and afraid that great understanding is necessary to calm them. A medical office assistant will have many occasions to apply her knowledge of patient psychology when dealing with patients before examinations. If she is able to put them into a peaceful frame of mind by a kind, sympathetic attitude, she will help the doctor greatly and ease his work considerably. Whenever possible, the type of examination to be done and the purpose for which it is being done should be explained to the patient. In this way the patient's cooperation can be enlisted.

Draping the Patient

It is always important to remember that the patient should be made as comfortable as possible, so that he will relax and make the examination easier for both himself and the doctor. Particular care must be taken to see that the patient is warm enough. Even in a warm room, a patient who is nervous because of the impending ordeal, and even more nervous because of anxiety over what the doctor may find, may feel chilly and should be covered with enough towels for warmth or, if necessary, a blanket.

For certain examinations (and treatments) there are standard positions in which a patient is examined. Women are draped with sheets for examinations. This is always the duty of the assistant, and the patient should be draped when the doctor enters the room. Draping the patient has a twofold reason. First, it makes a patient more comfortable to be covered as much as possible. Second, when only the part to be examined is exposed, the patient's modesty is protected—a very important psychological point. Women should be exposed as little as possible, and the assistant should not leave the room while a woman is being examined by a male doctor. Sometimes, holding a patient's hand will reassure and quiet her.

The different draping positions are shown in Fig. 4-3. Some examination tables have stirrups at the lower end to secure the feet. The sheet is draped over the patient in such a way that only the part to be examined is exposed. Obstetric sheet holders may be clamped over each thigh to prevent the sheet from slipping. Some of the standard draping positions are:

1. Sims' position: the patient lies on the left side and chest; the right knee is drawn up; the buttocks are brought up to the long side of the table.

2. Jackknife position: one end of the table is lowered, and the patient lies face down on the table, bracing the legs against the lowered part of the table so that the buttocks are elevated.

3. Trendelenburg's position: the patient lies on the back with head lowered and knees hanging over the end of the table.

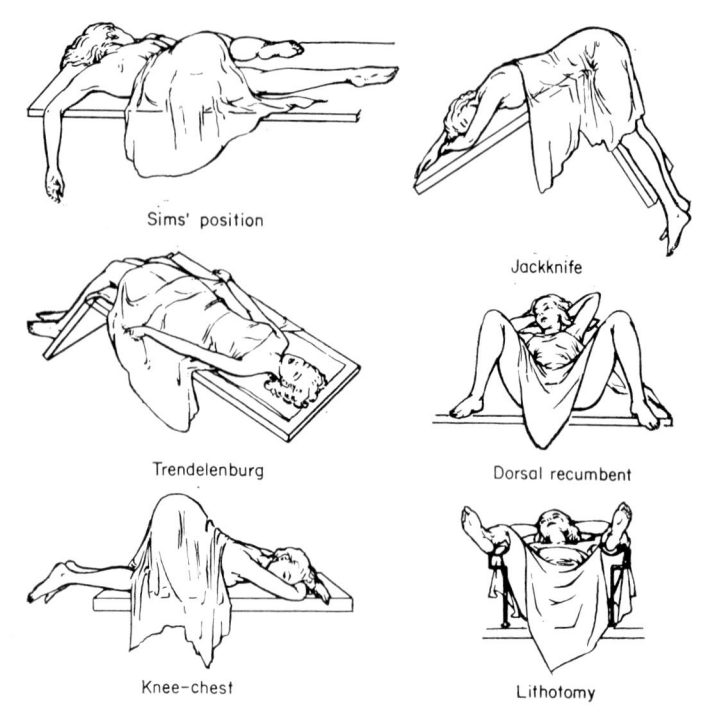

FIG. 4-3. Positions for draping. (*Adapted from Bertha Harmer and Virginia Henderson: "Textbook of the Principles and Practice of Nursing," 5th ed., The Macmillan Company, New York, 1956, Fig. 122, p. 563.*)

4. Dorsal-recumbent position: the patient lies on the back with heels in the stirrups or feet flat on the table. The buttocks are brought to the lower edge of the table.

5. Knee-chest position: the patient lies on the chest and knees, with buttocks in the air.

6. Lithotomy position: the patient lies on the back, as in dorsal-recumbent; arms are crossed under head or over chest; hips and knees are fully flexed and feet are supported in stirrups.

As most of these positions are difficult to maintain for any length of time, the assistant must do all she can to make the patient comfortable. A small pillow may be used for support, a towel to prevent slipping. She may have to hold the patient to keep him in the required position long enough for the doctor to complete his examination or treatment.

Routine Tests

There are a number of tests that in some offices form a routine part of every patient's visit, not only at the initial examination, but each time he comes to the office thereafter. The medical office assistant may give these tests as part of her duties. Even if she only assists the doctor in performing them, she should understand the significance of each procedure.

Blood Pressure. The taking of a person's blood pressure is included in all general examinations and in many special ones. Blood pressure is checked frequently as an indication of a patient's health.

The symbolic importance of the blood is reflected in literature and in everyday expressions in which the term *blood* connotes a nation, a race, an individual. Countless proverbs and sayings refer to blood: blood is thicker than water, blue-blooded, blood brothers, it makes my blood boil—to name only a very few. No doubt the reader can think of many more. The donation of blood by private individuals for blood transfusions has heightened the public's interest in this part of our physiology.

The average healthy person has about 6 quarts of blood in his body. This blood flows through many miles of blood vessels, carrying oxygen, water, and food to all the cells of the body. Blood consists of red cells, white cells, platelets, and plasma. The *red cells* (erythrocytes) carry oxygen and food to all parts of the body. If the circulation fails in any part, the cells in that part die, and necrosis sets in. In the heart muscles circulation failure causes the development of infarcts (the name given to areas in which necrosis has developed); in the legs of old people who, because of arteriosclerosis, develop such narrowing and occlusion of the vessels that no blood, or insufficient blood, can flow in, gangrene sets in.

Each individual cell in the organism takes oxygen from the red cells in the blood and delivers carbon dioxide to it. The blood cells obtain this oxygen from the lungs, where they deposit the carbon dioxide. Another function of the blood is to carry the heat that is produced in the active muscles.

The *white cells* (leukocytes) are the defenders of the body. They protect the organism against infections. If an infection occurs, the white cells swiftly descend on it and envelop it. Other white cells come to their assistance to help carry off dead matter, and for this reason they are often called the scavengers of nature. They do, however, also bring material to the injured spot for reconstruction.

Platelets are an important factor in the coagulation (clotting) of blood. *Plasma* is the medium in which the cells and platelets are suspended. It consists mainly of water, with some proteins, fats, sugar, and mineral salts.

The blood is pumped through the body by the heart at a steady rate, and this represents what is spoken of as blood pressure. The public has become very conscious of blood pressure, and nonmedical persons frequently discuss their blood pressure. Though blood pressure that is regarded as too high or too low may cause them great anxiety, what is regarded as normal blood pressure may give a deceptive sense of complete health.

For the information of the medical office assistant, who should understand the basis of the procedures in which she has a part, the body mechanism which determines a patient's blood pressure is briefly discussed below in simple, nonmedical language.

The blood is driven through the arteries by the heart in almost the same way that a pump drives water through a system of pipes. Each time the heart contracts, the blood in the heart is pushed into the artery. This phase is known as the *systole*. As the stream of blood enters the arteries, they expand; being elastic, they return to their normal size when the heart stops pumping. By doing so they force the blood further on into the blood vessel, because the valve of the aorta (the main artery of the body) is closed. This phase is known as the period of *diastole*.

The maximum amount of pressure exerted by the heart in pushing the blood into the arteries represents a person's blood pressure. In the healthy person this is relatively stable, the average range being between 118 and 130 mm. Hg (mercury) for persons up to forty years old. When a person ages and the arteries become less elastic, more force is needed by the heart to pump the blood through the body, and the blood pressure rises. As hardening of the arteries is a condition common to aging persons, most older persons have a higher blood pressure; since a certain proportion of the older population do have high blood pressure, the *average* range for an older age group will of course be higher than 118 to 130. Older persons who have maintained arterial elasticity and who have escaped hardening of the arteries may still have a blood pressure of about 130. The notion that a person should have a blood pressure of 100 plus his age is sheer superstition and should be discarded.

When the heart rests after pumping the blood into the arteries, the pressure naturally falls. The moment of its greatest relaxation, just before the next contraction, represents the diastolic pressure. A person having a systolic pressure between 118 and 130 would have a diastolic pressure between 70 and 80. In taking the patient's blood pressure, both figures must be taken into account, for again, if the arteries are no longer elastic, they will not return entirely to their normal size, and the pressure will not fall so much.

On the other hand, if the heart is weak, for any reason whatsoever, the force with which it drives the blood into the arteries is weak, and the resulting pressure is low. Though satisfactory reasons for low blood pressure have not yet been established, a blood pressure of 90 to 100 gives no cause for alarm. For some individuals this rate remains stable while they are in perfect health. Low blood pressure occurs both after severe blood losses and with diseases of the adrenal gland.

Blood pressure therefore depends on four factors:

1. Force of the heartbeat
2. Resistance in the arterial system
3. Elasticity of the arteries
4. Volume of the blood

High blood pressure or tension is called *hypertension;* low blood pressure, *hypotension. Systole* represents the period when the blood is streaming into the arteries; *diastole,* when the arteries are closed off from the heart.

The amount of blood pressure is influenced also by emotional states. Excitement, anxiety, worry—all may raise the blood pressure, if only temporarily. Blood pressure depends to some extent on the adrenal glands, and every excitement brings about a spilling over of the adrenal secretion, contraction of the arteries, and consequent rise in blood pressure. Therefore, if a patient seems to have an abnormally high blood pressure, all other tests should be performed and the blood pressure taken again later when the patient may have calmed down. The very fact that the patient is to have an examination, including a blood pressure test, sometimes brings about a rise in blood pressure. Furthermore, the pressure differs according to the person's position, that is, whether he is standing, sitting, or lying down.

Technique. The instrument used to take blood pressure is called a sphygmomanometer. It consists of a small rubber bag enclosed in a long, narrow cloth bandage, called the cuff. This is connected with a rubber bulb at one end and either a mercury manometer or a dial indicator at the other (see Fig. 4–4). A stethoscope is used with each one of these apparatus.

The technique is as follows:

1. Seat the patient comfortably, with the arm (preferably the right) supported on a level surface at elbow height. Apply the cuff on the inside of the bare upper arm, just above the bend, and wrap it closely around the arm.

2. Place the chest piece of the stethoscope on the artery on the inner side of the arm, just below the cuff.

3. Close the valve on the rubber bulb and slowly inflate the cuff by pressing the bulb. Thumping sounds will be heard. Continue inflating the bag until all sounds disappear. As long as any sound is heard the artery is not fully compressed.

4. When there is no more sound, open the valve slowly and release the air from the cuff. As soon as the pressure in the bag is less than that in the artery, blood begins to enter the artery below the cuff, and a snapping sound is heard. Take the reading of the manometer at this moment. This signifies the *systolic* pressure.

5. Continue releasing the pressure in the valve. The snapping sound at first becomes stronger, then changes to a dull thumping,

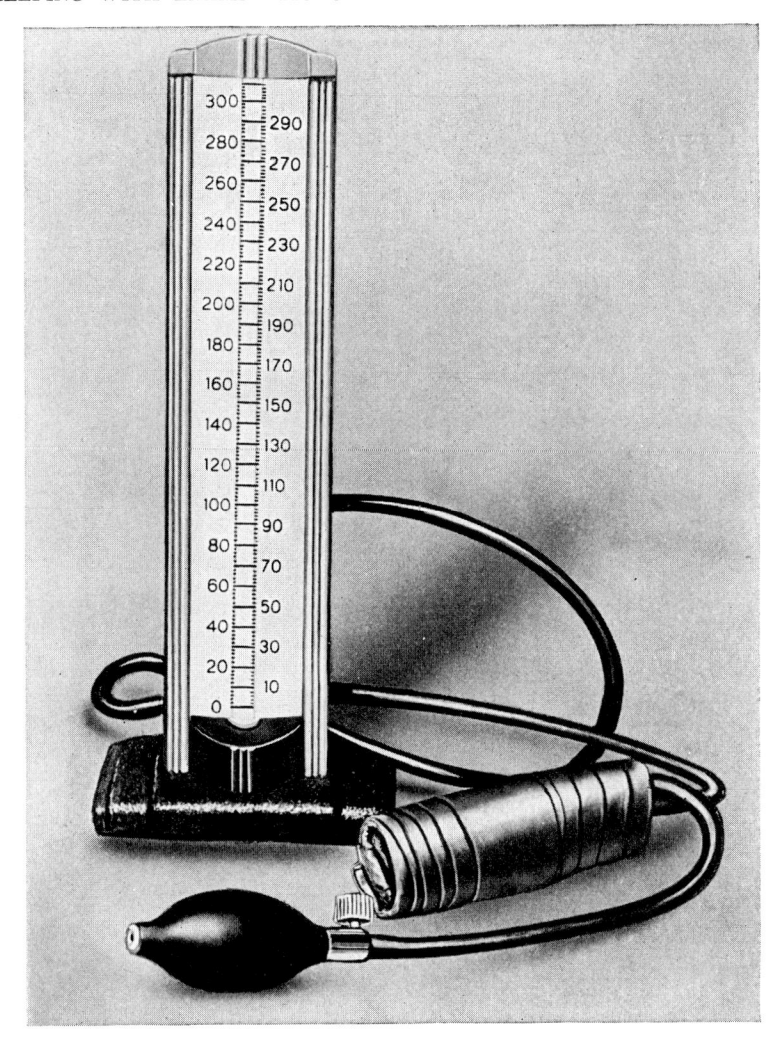

Fig. 4-4. Blood pressure apparatus: mercurial type. (*Becton, Dickinson & Co.*)

and finally disappears. At that point, the artery is fully opened, and the blood flows quietly through it. Take the manometer reading just before the sound disappears. This is the *diastolic* pressure. In recording the blood pressure, both the systolic and the diastolic reading must be given. The customary form is 120/80—expressed verbally as 120 over 80.

Figure 4–5 shows the assistant taking the blood pressure of a patient with a dial indicator. Many doctors consider the mercury manometer more accurate. The apparatus for the blood pressure test must be handled with care. If the rubber tubes are not properly folded when placed back in the case, the glass column may break when the case is closed.

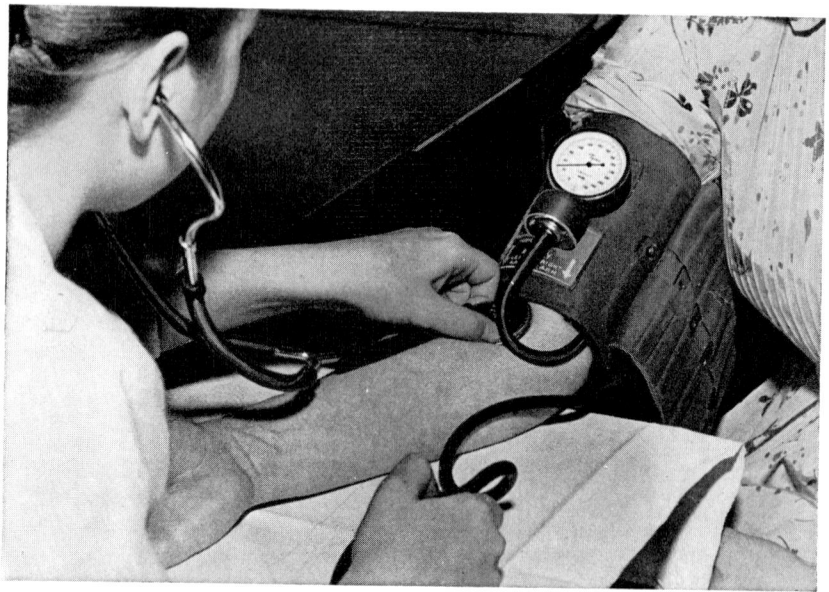

Fig. 4–5. Technique for taking blood pressure. (*Photograph by Roscoe Smith.*)

Weight and Height. Taking a patient's weight during the first examination is a routine procedure. In many cases weight must also be checked at each successive visit, because the loss or gain of weight may be an important indication of the patient's progress. Pregnant women, for example, as well as persons suffering from tuberculosis or obesity, must be weighed at each visit. Children are usually weighed whenever they are brought to the pediatrician's office. (The weight of babies is taken in ounces as well as pounds.)

It is best to weigh a patient in an examination gown. Crepe-paper slippers are provided in some offices. If the patient is weighed each time, it is not necessary for him to disrobe, as the relative weight is of importance, rather than the net weight. Care must be taken, however, to see that the patient is dressed as similarly as possible each time, or the reading will be misleading. The difference in weight between heavy walking shoes and sandals or between a woolen winter suit and a cotton summer dress is considerable and, unless noted on the chart, would result in an inaccurate record.

Weighing should not be done hurriedly. The assistant should ask the patient to stand quietly and wait until the indicator on the scale has come to complete rest.

Most scales have special attachments by which the height can be measured easily and accurately. The patient should take off his shoes. If there is no attachment on the scales, the patient should stand comfortably against a flat wall. A ruler is laid on his head against the wall, and a pencil mark made at that spot. The height from the floor is then measured with a yardstick. Tape measures are not reliable. Pediatricians usually measure the height of their patients on succeeding visits, perhaps twice a year. In such an office a yard measure may be painted on the wall against which the child is asked to stand. Height should be measured in inches and fractions of an inch.

Pulse Rate. The pulse is usually taken at the wrist over the radial artery, which is found on the wristbone, just under the thumb. Place the middle finger lightly on the wrist and locate the pulse. Do not use the thumb, as it has a pulse of its own. When the pulse can be felt distinctly, look at the minute hand on your watch and begin to count each beat. Count for exactly 1 minute. The pulse rate may also be taken at the temporal artery if the patient's arms are wrapped up.

When noting the pulse rate, include a description of the type of pulse beat—weak, strong, fast, slow, regular, irregular, fluttering, faint. *Bradycardia* indicates an abnormally slow pulse; *tachycardia*, an abnormally rapid one.

The rate of 70 to 80 pulse beats a minute is average for healthy persons, but wide fluctuations have been noted. Children frequently have a faster pulse rate. A rate of 60 may be normal for one individual, while in another, 90 might occur regularly.

Respiration. Respiration is so automatic that few people are aware of this important and complicated function. Yet physical as well as emotional states are reflected in the rate and type of breathing. With each inspiration air is taken into the lungs through the trachea, or windpipe. The lungs absorb the oxygen and in the expiration expel the carbon dioxide. The rate of respiration represents the cycle of one inspiration, or inhalation, and one expiration, or exhalation.

Respiration is an important indication of a variety of pathological conditions. The rate of respiration is determined by counting the number of inspirations and expirations during 1 minute. Sometimes these may be counted for a half minute and multiplied by two.

As has been mentioned, respiration is affected very easily, and the fact that the patient knows his respiration is being watched would be sufficient to alter the rate and depth of breathing. It is therefore advisable to observe respiration without the patient's knowledge. This can be done either by placing one's hand on the patient's chest, casually, or by watching respiration carefully while ostensibly still taking the pulse. The minute hand of the watch should be noted.

The normal rate of breathing is about 18 to 20 inhalations and exhalations per minute, though respiration rates vary among different individuals—some breathing more slowly, some more rapidly. The normal relationship between respiration and pulse is 1 to 4. The rate depends upon temperature and the amount of exertion. Respiration becomes more rapid when the body needs more oxygen. At high altitudes we breathe more rapidly, because the air contains less oxygen. The same is true after exertion, because more oxygen has been used up.

When the doctor is checking respiration, the rate alone is not a sufficient index to the patient's condition. The doctor must know whether the breathing is regular, deep, shallow, short, rasping, labored. If the breathing is shallow, it means the patient does not ventilate his lungs sufficiently and does not get enough oxygen into them. Labored breathing is spoken of as *dyspnea* and is accompanied by bluish, or *cyanotic,* coloring. This is generally a sign of heart disease.

A special type of breathing is called Cheyne-Stokes respiration. Characterized by variations in rhythm and depth, it is generally observed in very serious conditions.

Temperature. Among the many wonderful things about living organisms is the fact that in warm-blooded animals a certain temperature is maintained almost constantly and that in human beings this normal temperature moves within a very narrow range and is practically the same for all. External factors may influence this temperature, of course, but the heat-regulating center, located in the basal ganglia of the brain, controls body temperature. This center is similar to the thermostats used in heating houses. In a very hot, humid climate, for instance, the temperature may rise, because perspiration, one of nature's ways to cool us off, does not evaporate, and we therefore feel the heat much more than in a dry climate. If the environment is cold, on the other hand, the blood vessels contract, heat loss is reduced, and we shiver; that is, the muscles contract and produce heat.

During illness, however, this heat-regulating factor is disturbed, and the temperature rises, particularly in the case of infections. For the physician, therefore, a patient's body temperature is an important diagnostic factor.

Meaning of Fever. How often does one hear the expression "He has a temperature and should be in bed!" In that case we all should be in bed, for everybody has a body temperature if he is alive. This expression is not a scientific one, but a colloquialism. What is meant, of course, is that the person has a temperature above normal; in other words, a fever.

"Normal" temperature is usually 98.6° Fahrenheit (37° centigrade), but this means only that the vast majority of people have this particular temperature most of the time. Some persons have a constant, or normal, temperature below or above this figure. The physician can learn a patient's normal temperature only by observing the patient over a period of time. Eating, drinking, smoking, or exercise may raise the body temperature, and cold drinks may depress the mouth temperature. Usually the body temperature is low in the morning and rises during the course of the day, so that there may be a difference of a whole degree between morning and evening temperature.

In spite of these differences, however, a significant change in temperature, especially a rise, that is, fever, is a certain sign of disease. It is for this reason that the temperature is taken when a patient is examined.

Formerly fever was considered a disease in itself. We know now, however, that fever is an effort of the organism to fight off an attack of pathogenic organisms. The intensity of the fever depends not only on the degree and intensity of the attack, but also on the condition of the individual. Although children, for instance, often have a high fever during a slight illness, old people may die of pneumonia without any fever. When the organism fights too violently, that is, when the fever becomes too high, measures must be taken to counteract it. In general, however, it is not the fever that is treated, but the condition that causes it.

Technique. Temperature is measured by means of a thermometer, which in the United States and Great Britain registers in degrees Fahrenheit. In Europe and Latin America temperature is measured in degrees centigrade, 100° representing the boiling point, and 0°, the freezing point. The drawing in Fig. 4–6 shows

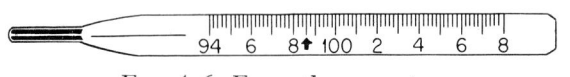

FIG. 4–6. Fever thermometer.

a picture of a clinical thermometer. Degrees are indicated by long lines; fractions, by short lines. The method of action lies in the mercury, located in the bulb at the bottom, which expands when it comes in contact with body heat.

Table 1 (see Appendix) indicates the conversion of centigrade into Fahrenheit and vice versa. Leaders in the medical profession are endeavoring to introduce the use of the metric system into all medical measurements.

There are three methods of taking temperature: oral, axillary, and

HELPING WITH EXAMINATIONS

rectal. Though the oral method is used almost exclusively in doctors' offices in the United States, the axillary method is preferred in Europe. The oral method is impractical for some persons—children, for instance, or persons with colds who must breathe through the mouth. The axillary method is advised for such persons. Not only is the axillary method more accurate than the oral one, but it is also timesaving, as the thermometer, after use, need only be wiped with a cloth moistened with alcohol and shaken down before it is used on the next patient. To a doctor who has a large practice, with many patients waiting, this is obviously a great advantage. Rectal temperatures are the most reliable, though they usually are as much as 1°F. higher than oral temperatures.

A thermometer is a very delicate instrument and must be handled with great care. It is essential to wash one's hands before handling it.

1. Check the reading on the thermometer. It should read 96°F. or lower. If it reads higher, it must be shaken down. This is done by holding the thermometer between the thumb and the index finger and shaking it down with a snap of the wrist. Be careful to stand away from chairs or tables, so that the thermometer will not strike a hard surface. Use hand motion only; hardly move the arm; do not touch the bulb with the hands.

2. Take the patient's temperature.

   a. Oral. Rinse the thermometer in cold water after removing it from an antiseptic solution. Place it under the patient's tongue on the side of the mouth. Tell him to keep his tongue down and lips closed and to breathe through his nose. Keep the thermometer in place at least 3 minutes, preferably 5.

   b. Axillary. Place the thermometer well into the patient's armpit and tell him to cross his arm over his chest and keep it close to his body. Leave the thermometer in place 5 minutes.

   c. Rectal. Cover the end of the thermometer with a lubricant such as petroleum jelly. Insert gently into the rectum until only about half the thermometer is exposed. Leave in place 5 minutes. During this time children and unconscious or irrational patients must be carefully watched. After withdrawing the thermometer, wipe it with facial tissue. It is often advisable to let the patient insert and withdraw the thermometer himself.

3. Read the thermometer. Stand with your back to the light, hold it between the thumb and index finger (never touch the bulb), and rotate it slowly back and forth until the mercury column is clearly seen. The top of the column indicates the scale reading.

4. Note the temperature reading on a chart or the medical history. Always indicate the method by which it was taken.

5. Clean and sterilize the thermometer. Wash it with soap, rinse it in cold water, and place it in an antiseptic solution for about 10 minutes. Never hold a thermometer under hot running water and do not leave it standing indefinitely in an antiseptic solution.

Thermometers come in different shapes. The slender bulb is considered more effective for oral temperatures, and the rounded bulb is held better by the rectal muscles. There is no difference in the quality of their performance.

Good thermometers must pass rigid inspection for proper calibration, so that the reading will be absolutely correct. Cheap thermometers of unknown manufacture may not give reliable readings.

Fever Chart. If a patient's temperature is taken regularly, it is recorded on a fever chart. This is important because the type of temperature curve may help in the diagnosis. We speak of continuous fever if it lasts a number of days and of intermittent fever when it appears in regular or irregular periods. A special type of fever curve occurs in lobar pneumonia, in which the temperature rises with a chill up to 104° or more, continues on that level, and then after several days drops suddenly to below normal.

A sudden temperature drop is called a *crisis*; a gradual one, a *lysis*. In malaria, the temperature rises suddenly, and the fever lasts 3 or 4 hours and ends suddenly. In a hectic fever, the temperature rises suddenly up to 105° or more and may drop within an hour. This type of fever occurs in very severe cases of septicemia and tuberculosis.

It can be seen from these brief remarks that the curve of the fever is of importance, and that the thermometer readings must therefore be entered on a chart. Such a chart is illustrated in Fig.

HELPING WITH EXAMINATIONS

4–7. Pulse and respiration are also entered on this chart. It is not used in a doctor's office very often, as patients with fever are usually in bed and the chart is kept at the bedside. The doctor may, however, keep charts in the office for patients whom he has visited at home.

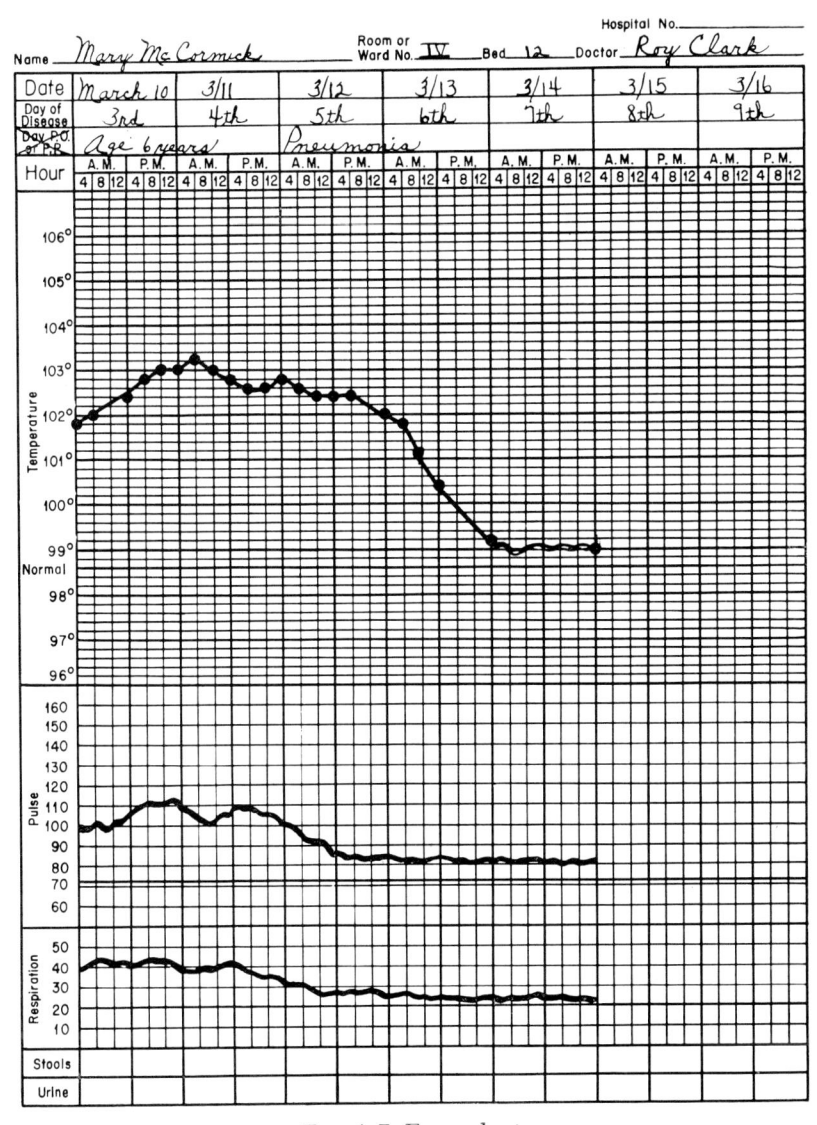

FIG. 4–7. Fever chart.

Special Tests

A complete examination, in addition to the foregoing procedures, includes various diagnostic laboratory tests. As a routine matter the blood and urine are examined for certain substances, the presence of which might be an indication of certain diseases. Smears for bacteriological examination may be taken of any discharge. The basal metabolic rate, that is, the rate of oxygen consumed by a person at complete rest, may be taken. Frequently the heart is examined by means of an electrocardiogram. A doctor may have a laboratory for the routine tests, and he may also own a basal metabolism machine and an electrocardiograph. In this case the medical office assistant is expected to perform the various tests. The techniques are described in Chapters 20 and 21, Laboratory Techniques and Special Tests.

BIBLIOGRAPHY

Harmer, Bertha, and Virginia Henderson: "Textbook of the Principles and Practice of Nursing," 5th ed., The Macmillan Company, New York, 1956.

5

The Doctor Prescribes Treatment

After the doctor has carried out all the necessary examinations, including laboratory tests and possibly x-rays, he makes the diagnosis. And on the basis of his diagnosis he prescribes treatment for the patient. This treatment may take various forms. Except for psychotherapy, which the doctor administers alone and for which no assistant is needed or even wanted, the medical office assistant is expected to perform many tasks in helping the doctor treat his patients.

The efficient and conscientious doctor's aide will want to know just what the doctor is trying to accomplish. Only by understanding the reason for his treatments will she be able to anticipate his needs and thus establish the smooth teamwork that is necessary if she is to be of any real help to him. When a registered nurse assists the doctor, he expects her to have a certain amount of medical knowledge and takes it for granted that she is familiar not only with the meaning of medical terms but also with anatomy, physiology, and pathology. Now that the medical office assistant is replacing the nurse in the doctor's office, she too is often expected to have a background of medical knowledge and an understanding of the basic medical routines carried on in the office. A certain amount of medical knowledge, therefore, is an essential part of her training for this career.

The scope of this book does not include instruction in anatomy and physiology, but there are many good volumes on these subjects written especially for nurses, with clear and simple illustrations to help a person without any previous training gain some understanding of the construction and functions of the human organism. If her training did not include the study of these subjects, the medical office assistant is urged to learn as much about them as possible by perusing at least one of these books. Two titles are mentioned in the bibliography at the end of this chapter. It would of course be impossible for the assistant to study enough books to gain an insight into the entire field of medicine, so a few general remarks on the nature of diseases are included herewith.

Nature of Diseases

Bewildering as the vast labyrinth of pathological conditions may seem to a nonmedical person, there are really less than a dozen disease groups into which all the different complaints and pains and ills may be classified. The medical office assistant should be familiar with these groupings. The apparently limitless variety of sicknesses seems to most observers equaled only by the number of people who suffer from them. Whether the sickness be a cold or cancer, each individual is so differently affected that each would appear to be suffering from an entirely different condition. Yet, the entire field of disease can be narrowed down to a few basic types.[1]

Inflammation. The most common of all pathological conditions is inflammation, which is a defense reaction of the body. When an area is affected, more blood rushes to the defense and the site becomes red and swollen—inflamed. This happens whether the cause is an infection or an injury, whether it is external or internal. Inflammations can develop on the skin, in the internal organs, or in the joints, but the reaction varies according to the location. It also varies according to the age of the patient; that is, younger patients generally have more severe reactions than older persons. A severe inflammation may harm an organism more than the original pathological condition. A fever can go so high that the patient will die of it. Or an inflammation may destroy an organ or its function. To give just one example, if swelling persists in an inflamed joint, connective tissue will grow, because it is better nourished; this will eventually lead to adhesions and finally to a stiff joint.

[1] The material in this section is abstracted from a manuscript by Heinrich F. Wolf, M.D.

THE DOCTOR PRESCRIBES TREATMENT

The doctor's therapeutic aim, therefore, in addition to removing or combating the cause, is to attenuate the inflammation before it does too much harm. The terms *acute* and *chronic* are indications of the relative intensity or duration of a condition. Inflammation, being a defense mechanism, may occur in many conditions and cannot be considered a disease in itself.

Disease Groups. Aside from inflammations, pathological conditions may be classified into the following groups:

1. Infections, local and general
2. Tumors, benign and malignant
3. Blood diseases
4. Deficiency diseases
5. Glandular disturbances
6. Degenerative diseases, involving deterioration or dysfunction of an organ
7. Allergies, the "mystery of medicine"
8. Psychoses, neuroses, and psychosomatic conditions
9. Injuries
10. Congenital conditions

1. Infections, probably the most common of the disease groups, may be caused, as noted previously, by a host of microorganisms, most of which produce a syndrome (complex of symptoms) that is characteristic of the particular pathogenic organism.

2. Tumors are unrestricted growths in the body. In medical terminology they are designated by the ending *oma*, the preceding root generally being the name of the tissue in which the tumor occurs—for instance, lipoma, a growth consisting of fat; lymphoma, a growth of lymph tissue; adenoma, a growth of a gland, etc.

Tumors are divided into two main groups, benign and malignant. The benign ones may grow to a considerable size but do not encroach on other tissues and do not establish branches in other parts of the body. Such tumors, however, may become dangerous because of their excessive size, for instance, a myoma of the uterus. It is also possible that what has appeared to be a benign tumor may suddenly show malignant changes. A lymphoma, for instance, can change into a lymphosarcoma.

Malignant tumors may also develop in different tissues. In growing they destroy vital tissues and so lead to a general breakdown of the organism. Some of the cancerous cells enter the blood or lymph stream and, by a process called metastasis, establish branches in other parts of the organism, where other tumors then develop. Among the malignant tumors are cancers and sarcomas.

3. Blood diseases. Blood consists, as was stated before, of red and white blood cells, plasma, and platelets. The blood picture may be disturbed in two different ways; that is, it may have too many cells or too few. If there are too many red cells (over 6 million per cubic millimeter) we speak of polycythemia; if there are not enough (fewer than 4 million per cubic millimeter in men, 3.5 million per cubic millimeter in women) we have to deal with anemia.

Anemia occurs in two forms, namely, primary and secondary. In primary anemia, either the cell-producing organs are disordered or there is too much destruction of red cells. If the process that destroys the red blood cells is too active, pernicious anemia results, a condition characterized by a progressive decrease in the number of red blood corpuscles, muscular weakness, and disturbances of the gastrointestinal and nervous systems.

Secondary anemia develops when there is a continuous loss of blood (as in bleeding, hemorrhage, tapeworm). In such cases the relative number of white and red cells is not changed. If the bleeding stops and new blood is supplied by blood transfusion, the condition can be reversed.

If the cell-producing organs do not function properly, abnormal white cells are produced, and leukemia results, popularly called cancer of the blood.

Hemophilia, a disease affecting males only, but transmitted by females, is caused by a disturbance in the blood-clotting mechanism and excessive bleeding may result, even from a minor cut.

Platelets have a part in the clotting of blood. If the number of platelets sinks below 50,000 per cubic millimeter, internal bleeding occurs and may lead to death. This condition is caused by a disease of the bone marrow.

If the number of white cells sinks below 1,000 or 2,000 per cubic millimeter, the condition is referred to as agranulocytosis. Such cases are often caused by exposure to radiation (atom bombs or x-rays). Victims of this disease have no resistance to infection, as the white cells which fight infectious organisms are not present in sufficient number.

4. Deficiency diseases are due to a lack of minerals or vitamins in the patient's diet or to an inability of the organism to utilize foods properly. Pellagra, beriberi, and scurvy are deficiency diseases caused by lack of vitamins. Nowadays all such conditions are called avitaminoses.

5. Glandular disturbances affect both the endocrine, or ductless, glands and the lymphatic glands. Among the endocrine glands are the pituitary, the thyroid, the parathyroid, the adrenals, and the pancreas.

The hypophysis (pituitary) is called the master gland, because the functioning of all other glands seems to be controlled by it. It regulates growth and the female reproductive cycle. The thyroid gland, which controls basal metabolism and mental development, also has some role in growth. The parathyroid gland, which lies in front of the thyroid, controls the calcium metabolism.

Adrenals produce epinephrine, which, to some extent, controls blood pressure. The adrenals also balance the activity of the pancreas. The pancreas produces enzymes, which are needed for the process of digestion, and insulin, which controls sugar metabolism.

The various glands influence one another and keep the system in balance. They may be overactive or underactive, and in either case disturbances in the system will occur. These glands produce hormones, which are discharged into the blood and regulate the relationship between the glands. If one of the glands does not function properly, the other glands attempt to counteract this dysfunction. For instance, if the pancreas produces too much insulin, which could kill a person by removing sugar from the blood, the adrenals step in and curb the production of insulin.

6. Degenerative diseases are caused by a deterioration or degeneration of some body parts. Some pathological conditions of this type result from a congenital inferiority of a particular organ, but

most of them are due to the breakdown of an organ because of normal wear and tear, that is, the aging process. Diabetes, nephrosis, muscular dystrophy, heart diseases, and arteriosclerosis—all come under the heading of degenerative diseases. The exact reason why these conditions develop is still largely unknown.

7. Allergy is a condition of hypersensitivity in which an individual reacts with pathological symptoms to a specific substance with which he comes in contact or which he takes internally and which is harmless to the majority of other individuals. This is discussed in more detail in Chapter 12 under Allergy.

8. Neuroses are states of emotional imbalance which affect only a particular aspect of the patient's behavior. He may have difficulty in adjusting to his environment and may suffer from anxiety or depression, but be perfectly rational otherwise. Psychoses are more serious mental disturbances of the total personality in which the patient loses contact with his environment, has delusions about it, or, in severe cases, is oblivious of those around him and disoriented as to time and place. Psychosomatic (from the Greek *psyche*, "soul"; *soma*, "body") conditions are physical symptoms whose origin can be traced to mental causes (nausea at the sight of blood, for example) or, in older usage, behavior aberrations due to physical causes. (See also Chapter 12.)

Types of Treatment

The treatment that the doctor prescribes may take various forms. If he has an assistant, he must be able to rely on her in many ways. It will be her duty to get ready in advance all materials, trays, instruments, and apparatus that the doctor will need and to prepare the patient for the particular treatment—by administering medication to him, seating him, draping him, or performing some other service. The principles of preparation discussed in the preceding chapter apply for treatments as well as for examinations. Furthermore, the office aide must assist the physician during the procedure—handing him instruments, taking discarded materials from him, holding basins, steadying the patient, doing whatever is necessary in a given situation. Successful procedure depends to a great extent upon smooth cooperation between the doctor and his assistant, and only practice will make it perfect. But the assistant should try to learn beforehand just what her role is to be, have her employer explain what he expects her to do, and then try to anticipate his wishes.

The different forms of treatment are:

1. *Medicinal treatments:* administration of medication
2. *Surgery:* the use of the knife
3. *Physical therapy* or *physical medicine:* the use of physical or mechanical agents
4. *Diet therapy:* restricting the patient's diet to certain foods or regulating the amounts taken
5. *Psychotherapy:* verbal discussion of the patient's condition

Medicinal treatments include those in which any type of medication is administered—drug, hormone, vitamin, or chemical compound. Medicinal treatment is given in one of the following ways:

1. *Oral:* by mouth
2. *Parenteral:* by injection (not by the alimentary canal)
3. *External:* by application on the skin (as an ointment) or by inhalation, instillation, or irrigation
4. *Rectal:* as a suppository or enema

Surgery is subdivided into various branches according to the type of operation or the part of the body concerned—abdominal surgery, neural surgery, thoracic surgery, plastic surgery, etc. It is further divided into major surgery and minor surgery. Major surgery usually refers to operative treatment of the vital organs or other extensive operations which require hospitalization. Minor surgery includes operative procedures that do not require general anesthesia or immediate bed rest. The line between the two is not definitely drawn. Some surgeons even maintain that there is no minor surgery—that each incision is a major and potentially dangerous procedure for the patient.

Surgery performed by means of an electric current is usually included under physical therapy. The electric current destroys or cuts superficial tissue and at the same time sears the open surface and thus prevents bleeding. This type of surgery is discussed in Chapter 9, Application of Physical Therapy.

Physical therapy comprises treatment by physical means, such as light, heat, cold, water, electricity, massage, and exercise. Rehabilitation, a branch of physical therapy, is now one of the most important phases of this specialty. Rehabilitation deals mainly with helping handicapped persons learn to lead a useful life. It is carried out in hospitals and institutions only.

Mechanical treatments are also used in orthopedic medicine, namely, fitting of braces and inlays and application of plaster casts. Orthopedics, however, as well as orthopedic surgery, is a special branch of medicine and is not included under physical therapy.

From the foregoing remarks it is evident that a medical office assistant can fill various needs, depending on the specialty of the doctor for whom she works, and that there is a wide field of activity for her services.

BIBLIOGRAPHY

Anthony, C.: "Textbook of Anatomy and Physiology," 4th ed., The C. V. Mosby Company, St. Louis, 1955.

Woerdeman, M. W.: "Atlas of Human Anatomy," McGraw-Hill Book Company, Inc., Blakiston Division, New York, 1950.

6
Principles of Medication

All doctors prescribe medication at one time or another. Many doctors keep some drugs on hand for emergencies and for treatments or minor operations performed in the office. Doctors in outlying communities, where pharmacies may not be accessible, must keep a complete assortment of medications on hand to dispense in the office and on house calls.

Medications are divided into various kinds: those given to supply a deficiency in the organism—vitamins, for instance; hormones, which help regulate malfunctions of the endocrine glands; antihistamines, to counteract allergic reactions; drugs that have a specific action for definite conditions; and—perhaps most important of all—the blessed painkillers, most of which come under the heading of narcotics.

The assistant, who will most certainly be in charge of all the medical supplies, will have various duties in regard to ordering, storing, dispensing, administering, and preparing medications. Quite obviously she should be acquainted with the effects and indications of the different types of drugs used in medical practice. Handling drugs requires a strong sense of responsibility, which can only be developed if the person involved understands, at least to some extent, the action of the various drugs.

Under the Pure Food and Drug Act, all drugs that come into the open market are checked for purity, strength, and composition. Various standard publications provide a list of approved drugs. The medical office assistant, who will at times handle some drugs and perhaps prepare others, should be familiar with at least one such publication, and it is desirable that this be available in the doctor's office for quick reference. The best known publications are listed below.

The official publication is the "United States Pharmacopeia," which is revised periodically and contains detailed information on the most commonly used drugs—their description, standards of purity, strength, composition, appearance, etc. The United States Pharmacopeial Convention has set up standards for drugs, and those that meet these standards may carry the imprint U.S.P.

The American Medical Association issues annually a publication entitled "New and Nonofficial Remedies" (recently retitled "New and Nonofficial Drugs"). This includes new drugs not yet included in the "United States Pharmacopeia," but approved by the Council on Pharmacy and Chemistry of the AMA. "The Physicians' Desk Reference," published by Medical Economics, Inc., is another publication listing drugs and their manufacturers. It is revised periodically.

It must be stressed, though it is a commonplace, that any drug, no matter how benign if given in small quantities, may prove dangerous to health and even fatal if given in excessive amounts or to a person who is hypersensitive to that particular drug. Children have died from an overdose of aspirin; some patients have had severe allergic reactions to penicillin. The assistant, therefore, should never dispense any medication whatsoever without specific instructions from her physician-employer.

Another rule that she must observe unvaryingly and practice so assiduously that it becomes automatic is to check every medicine *three times:*

1. When taking it out of the cabinet
2. When removing contents from the bottle, carton, or vial
3. When discarding the container or replacing it in the cabinet

Too many unnecessary accidents have occurred as a result of medication that has been administered by mistake because the bottles looked alike or had been moved from their customary place or the label simply was not read carefully. Constant vigilance is an absolute *must* for anybody entrusted with the job of handling medicines.

Types of Drugs

Drugs are divided into many different types, the most important groups being the following:

Antibiotics	Heart stimulants
Antidotes	Hemostatics
Antihistamines	Hormones
Antilaxatives	Narcotics
Astringents	Tranquilizers
Cathartics	Vasoconstrictors
Diuretics	Vasodilators
Emetics	Vitamins
Expectorants	

Antibiotic: a medicine made from molds that destroys a great variety of disease-producing bacteria. (The term *antibiotic* is made up from the words *anti*, "opposite or against," and *biotic*, "relating to life.") Some of the best known antibiotics are penicillin, the first one to be discovered; Aureomycin; Terramycin; streptomycin; and the various sulfa drugs. Their discovery has led to the conquest of many infections that formerly were inaccessible to therapy because any chemical agent known to kill the infectious organism was also harmful to the human organism. The antibiotics are, as a rule, harmless, though certain individuals develop severe allergic reactions to them. Many physicians, therefore, make it a rule to apply a patch test before administering an antibiotic, to determine whether the patient can be given the medication safely. In emergencies, of course, the allergic reaction may have to be tolerated in order to save a patient whose life may be threatened by an infection—such as pneumonia, for instance.

Antidote: a substance that neutralizes or precipitates a poison and lessens its toxicity.

Antihistamine: a medicine that reduces the production or counteracts the effect of histamine in the body.

Antilaxative: a medicine that inhibits loose bowels.

Astringent or *Styptic:* a drug that contracts the tissue and, if applied to an open surface (not protected by the skin), stops or retards discharge or bleeding. Silver nitrate and alum are the most commonly used astringents.

Cartharctic: a medicine that promotes or hastens the evacuation of the bowels. Cathartics are often divided into three subgroups: (1) laxatives—mildly purgative, such as cascara, mineral oil; (2) purgatives—calomel, castor oil, any one of the salts; (3) drastic purgatives—croton oil, jalap (hardly ever used any more). Stewed fruits, although not a medicine, may also be used for a mild laxative or regulatory effect.

Diuretic: a medicine that increases the secretion of urine.

Emetic: a substance that produces vomiting.

Expectorant: a medication that promotes the ejection of fluid or phlegm from the lungs, bronchi, and trachea.

Heart Stimulant: a substance that stimulates the heart to beat faster and more strongly, such as digitalis, Coramine, caffeine, camphor (in oil), Adrenalin, strychnine, quinidine.

Hemostatic: an agent that arrests the flow of blood by contributing to its coagulation. Vitamin K is such a substance.

Hormone: a substance produced by the endocrine (ductless) glands that is secreted directly into the blood stream. If a gland is not functioning properly, additional hormones may be supplied to the organism in the form of medication.

Narcotic: a drug which, used in moderate doses, produces sound sleep, relieves pain, and allays sensibility.

Tranquilizer or *Ataraxic:* a drug that calms persons who are agitated and disturbed. It differs from hypnotics and barbiturates in that it does not produce sleep or drowsiness. Patients under the influence of these drugs become quiet and reasonable and accessible to psychotherapy. The most commonly used tranquilizers are chlorpromazine, promazine, reserpine, and meprobamate.

Vasoconstrictor: a substance that causes constriction of blood vessels.

Vasodilator: a drug that dilates the blood vessels and reduces blood pressure. Drugs used are amyl nitrate, nitroglycerine, opium, morphine, and some comparatively new drugs, such as Serpasil.

Serpasil is a derivative of the East Indian plant *Rauwolfia*, which is a source of many other new drugs, including the tranquilizers.

Vitamin: one of the many organic substances that are necessary to the body for many functions and are found in minute quantities in different foods. Vitamins are designated by the letters of the alphabet and subdivided by number (B_1, B_2). Most of them are produced synthetically and can therefore be administered in any desired quantity.

Miscellaneous. New drugs are discovered almost daily, and although many of them are soon discarded, the pharmacological equipment of medicine is constantly being enlarged. These new drugs are found in plants, extracted from animal organisms, or made synthetically in the laboratory. Quite a few of them have been found effective in such a variety of pathological conditions that the name "miracle drug," or "wonder drug," has been given to them—outside of medical circles, of course.

Narcotics and Their Handling

This group of drugs occupies a special place in the pharmacological equipment of the medical profession. The name is derived from the Greek *narcosis*, a "state of deep unconsciousness."

Formerly the term *narcotic* was applied only to cocaine and derivatives of opium, such as morphine, heroin, and codeine. All these drugs are habit-forming, which means that the individual taking or given the drug may become dependent on it, suffers great physical distress if deprived of it, and will go to any length, including crime, in order to obtain it. Marihuana, a Latin-American weed, is also an addiction-forming drug but is not used medically.

In recent years, barbituric acids have been added to the list of hypnotics. These drugs are manufactured synthetically and, though they induce sleep, do not result in drug addiction. They are habit-forming, however, in that a person may have to take an increased amount in order for them to continue to be effective in prolonged use. If taken in sufficient quantity, they may prove fatal. For this reason their sale and administration come under the regulations for narcotics. Veronal, Allonal, Nembutal, and most other medicines ending in *al* are derivatives of barbituric acids. Lately, still other hypnotics have been introduced which are not barbiturates and which are not supposed to be habit-forming.

Because the effect of narcotics is either soothing or exhilarating, anyone who has taken or been given these drugs may become habituated to them and crave them, and thus drug addiction results, with its devastating consequences of ruined health and ruined lives. As medicine could not dispense with narcotic drugs, a method of controlling their use had to be found, and so in 1914, the Harrison Narcotic Act was passed. This Act has been amended a number of times but is still considered to have many loopholes, as attested to by the frequent deaths as a result of an excess of sleeping pills, juvenile delinquency due to drug addiction, and criminal cases with a record of drug addiction. The Harrison law aims at restricting the use of narcotic drugs to legitimate medical practice. It requires all those who handle these drugs—manufacturers, importers, wholesalers, retailers, physicians, dentists, and pharmacies—to register with the Federal government. The agency that is concerned with registration and enforcement of the law is the Bureau of Narcotics of the U.S. Treasury.

Any physician who possesses, administers, or prescribes narcotics is required to register with this bureau. He must be duly licensed in the state in which he practices, and his application for a narcotic license must be sent to the district branch of the U.S. Treasury in which his office is located. Large cities are divided into several districts, but a doctor in a small town may have to send his application to the nearest large city where the U.S. Treasury has a branch office.

The application must contain the doctor's name and address and the number and date of his state license, and it must be signed by the doctor. If any of these data are inaccurate or missing, the application is returned, and valuable time may be lost. The application must be accompanied by a money order or certified check for $1. A large number of applications are returned annually simply because the doctor has forgotten to enclose the money or has neglected to have the check certified.

Once the application has been accepted, a tax stamp bearing his narcotic-license number is issued to the doctor. This should be displayed in his office, and the license number must appear on each prescription blank. The license must be renewed annually, as it expires automatically at the end of the Federal fiscal year, June 30. A doctor who is licensed to dispense narcotics receives a form each year that must be completed and returned with a certified check for $1. It is the assistant's responsibility to see that this form is received, filled out properly, and returned in time.

When the doctor issues a prescription for a narcotic drug, the blank must contain his narcotic-license number, as mentioned before; the patient's name and address; and the date. All prescriptions must be written in ink or indelible pencil or may be typed. The drug prescribed becomes the property of the patient.

Doctors are constantly exposed to the danger of being taken advantage of by a drug addict, as doctors are, of course, a logical source from which a drug addict may try to obtain the drug he craves. Constant vigilance is therefore necessary. For one thing, prescription blanks must be handled carefully. Doctors usually receive large supplies of prescription blanks from the nearest pharmacy free of charge and so become careless with them, use them as scratch paper, and leave them lying around the office and waiting room. An experienced addict may either appropriate the pad or skillfully tear off some blanks when no one is watching. Such persons are adept at forging prescriptions and usually take them to pharmacies in different parts of the city where they think the doctor's handwriting is unknown. If something about a prescription arouses the suspicion of a pharmacist, he may call the doctor's office to verify it. The assistant, who would be the one to take the telephone call, should be able to remember any patient's name and advise the pharmacy whether or not the doctor has written out a prescription for the person presenting it. If the prescription turns out to be a forgery, the assistant, with the doctor's authorization, should notify the nearest branch of the Bureau of Narcotics at once and, if possible, give a description of the guilty person. One way to guard against the possibility of theft is to lock up all prescription pads except one, which the doctor should keep in a drawer of his desk.

Some addicts visit a doctor as patients, describing—usually most convincingly—the symptoms of the condition from which they pretend to be suffering and claiming that they have suffered this condition before and know from experience that morphine, or whatever drug they want, is the only remedy. If it is part of the assistant's duties to take medical histories from new patients, such self-diagnosis and self-prescription should be a warning signal that she should report to the doctor at once, before he sees the patient.

The Bureau of Narcotics suggests that the doctor obtain narcotic drugs for his office practice, not from a pharmacy, but from a regular wholesale or supply house. They should be ordered on official opium order blanks, rather than on prescription forms. Booklets containing ten such blanks, with the doctor's name, address, and license number stenciled on each blank, may be obtained from the Bureau of Narcotics for 10 cents. Each blank is made out in triplicate, two copies of which are sent to the firm from which the drug is ordered and one of which remains in the doctor's office as his record. This record must be kept at least two years so that it will be available for inspection.

Narcotic drugs kept in the doctor's office must be carefully watched. They should always be locked up, and a running inventory kept so that the assistant can know immediately if anything is missing. Whenever the doctor administers or dispenses a drug, *a record must be made*. While the Bureau of Narcotics will accept as a record a notation made on the patient's medical history, to present all files for inspection is a time-consuming matter. It is better to have a special record for drugs dispensed—either a card for each type of drug, on which the amount, date, and name of patient is entered each time, or a book in which the daily record is entered. These records too must be kept two years. Printers of professional stationery carry books specially designed for keeping the narcotics record in permanent form.

On the application for renewal of the narcotic license the amount of drugs on hand must be indicated. If an inspection is made, the agent can quickly determine from the application and the copies of the opium order blanks how much material the doctor had in his possession and, from the dispensing record, how much should be left. As the wholesalers send one of the order forms to the Bureau of Narcotics, it may be quickly noted when a doctor buys an excessive amount of drugs. An inspection will certainly be made in the case of an unusually large purchase of drugs, but routine inspections are made from time to time. The better the records are kept, the less time is consumed by such an inspection.

Addicts also try to obtain drugs by stealing them from a doctor's bag. It is a well-known fact that most doctors carry some morphine, or a similar drug, on their house visits. Doctors are the most frequent victims of thefts in which a car is broken open and the owner's bag stolen. If the doctor returns to the office in a hurry and leaves his bag where visitors have easy access to it, the chances are that it will disappear or at least be opened and rifled. The bag should therefore be placed in a closet at once when the doctor returns, until the assistant has time to empty and check its contents.

Medications

Medication in the doctor's office may be: (1) administered, (2) dispensed, or (3) prescribed. Medication is *administered* when it is actually given to the patient—orally, by injection, by inhalation, etc. It is *dispensed* when it is given or sold to the patient for use later. It is *prescribed* when the patient is given a written order to have filled at a pharmacy.

In many offices the doctor dispenses medication to the patient instead of sending him to a pharmacy to obtain it. Under the law, certain drugs may be dispensed by prescription only, and the assistant should find out which drugs these are.

If she administers any medication to the patient, she should remain with him while he is taking or applying it. She should observe him carefully and call the doctor immediately if the patient shows any signs of an unfavorable reaction.

All medications dispensed, administered, or prescribed should be entered on the patient's medical history, with the date, amount, and type prescribed (the more details, the better). All narcotics should be entered in a special record book—a fact that cannot be repeated too often.

Methods of Administration. The methods of administering medication are varied and depend on many factors. The simplest method is the *oral* one, in which the drug is given in the form of pills, tablets, capsules, or solution.

Certain substances lose their potency when taken orally and passed through the gastric tract. For this reason, or when an immediate result is desired, medication may be administered by *injection*. Preparing the injection tray and perhaps administering some of the injections are among the duties of the medical assistant. The next chapter, therefore, is devoted to a discussion of the technique involved.

Another way of administering medication is by *inhalation*, that is, through the respiratory tract. This is done by means of an apparatus which vaporizes the liquid and thereby disseminates it through the respiratory passages. Such an apparatus works on the same principle as a perfume atomizer. Inhalation medication may also be given in cases of certain heart conditions to produce quick relief. Medication may also be introduced by *instillation*, that is, introduction of a liquid by drops. This may be done into a vein or an eye.

Drugs administered through the *rectum* may be in the form of a suppository; an enema; or proctoclysis, that is, the drip method. The reason for rectal administration may be either that the patient is unconscious or mentally ill or that the effect desired is the slow absorption of the drug through the wall of the colon. It is also done in cases in which the stomach cannot tolerate the medication.

Vaginal application of medication is done by suppository or by douche, in addition to painting with a liquid or applying an ointment, if a local effect on the cervix or the vaginal cavity is desired.

Inunction, or application of an ointment or a lotion to the skin, is another method of administration. This may be done by the assistant. It is recommended that she use rubber gloves when applying ointments frequently. This is particularly important when ointments containing mercury are used.

PRINCIPLES OF MEDICATION

The *sublingual* or *buccal* method is used in giving certain medications that are absorbed through the mucous membranes more directly than in any other way. In the sublingual method, the tablet is placed under the tongue or between the gum and the cheek and left to dissolve. It should not be swallowed or chewed. For throat infections, lozenges or troches are given in the same manner; however, in the latter cases, the medication, instead of being absorbed by the mucous membrane, mixes with the saliva and thus flows through the throat to the affected area.

As can be seen from the above, methods of applying medication are divided into two types: (1) local, or direct application of the drug to the tissue or organ involved; and (2) general, or application of the drug to a site remote from the organ or tissue involved. A drug applied in the second manner must circulate in the blood stream, a process called absorption. (Excretion is the process whereby the drug is eliminated from the body.)

Dosage. Doses of medicine may be made up in a variety of amounts. Both multiples and fractions of grams and grains are used, though the metric system is recommended by organized medicine as the system of choice. Table 2 (see Appendix for tables) shows equivalent values of avoirdupois and metric weights; Tables 3 and 4 give equivalent values of metric and apothecaries' measures for liquids (volume); Tables 5 and 6 give apothecaries' and metric equivalents for solids (weight); Table 7 shows metric and linear equivalents; and Table 8 shows equivalents of common household measures. These tables should always be consulted if it is necessary to find metric equivalents for the measures commonly used in the United States.

In order to administer the correct dosage of medication, the assistant must be familiar with the different systems of measurement used for solids (by weight, in grams, grains, drams, ounces, or fractions of a pound) and liquids (by volume, in minims, drops, drams, ounces, cubic centimeters, teaspoonfuls, tablespoonfuls, or fluidounces). When medication is prescribed in drops, a medicine dropper is used to assure correct dosage; when in solution, a medicine glass, which is marked on the outside to indicate different amounts. Refer to Tables 2 to 7 for systems of measurement. In addition, consult Table 8 which gives ordinary household measuring standards and approximate equivalents. These equivalents may be explained to the patient if he is instructed to take a medicine at home.

If the assistant's duties include the administration of medications, the following rules should be observed:

1. Never pour medicine back into the bottle from which it was taken.
2. *Never* use medicine from an unmarked bottle or box.
3. Never pour medicine from a bottle with a label that is upside down or blurred.
4. Read the label three times.

Prescriptions. Although the assistant never writes out a prescription, for her information a sample is shown to illustrate what items are included. As shown in Fig. 6–1 they are:

Doctor's name and address
Narcotic-license number
Date
Patient's name and address (also age, if patient is a child)
The sign ℞ meaning *recipe*, or "take thou"
The name or names of drugs and the vehicle in which they may
    be mixed: water, alcohol, syrup, or ointment
Directions to pharmacist: whether to make up prescription in
    tablets, pills, capsules, or solution
Directions to patient: how much, how often, and what time to
    administer (Example: 1 tablet half an hour before each meal,
    or t.i.d., meaning three times daily)
Doctor's signature and degree (M.D.)

As indicated above, medications are made up in solution or in pills, tablets, or capsules. Pills are medication that has been molded into small balls. Tablets are medication pressed into a round, flat shape. Capsules are dry powder in a gelatine container. They are swallowed easily because of the container, which is smooth and

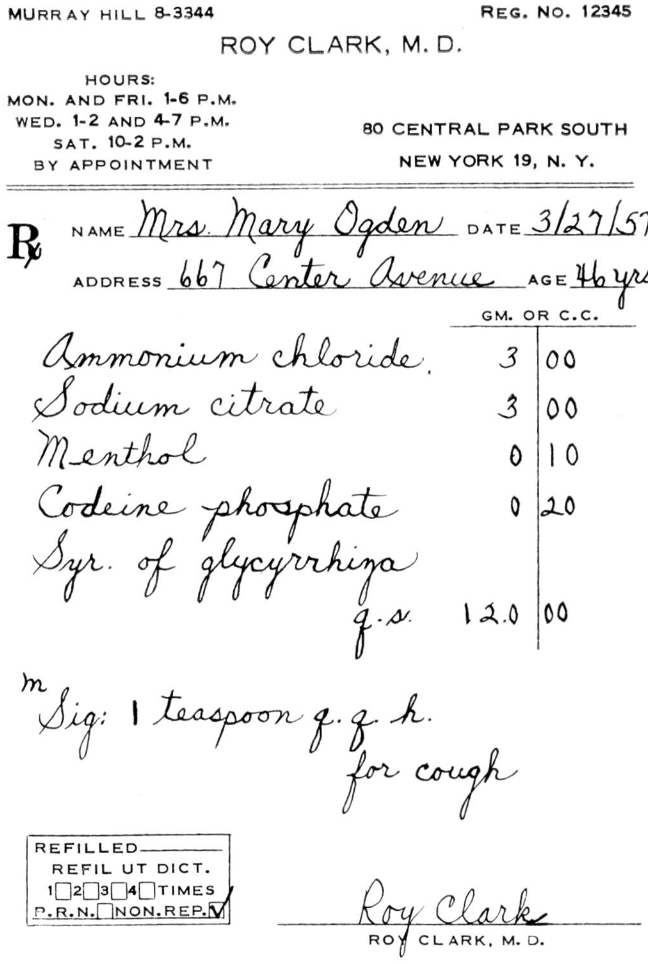

MURRAY HILL 8-3344 REG. NO. 12345

ROY CLARK, M. D.

HOURS:
MON. AND FRI. 1-6 P.M.
WED. 1-2 AND 4-7 P.M.
SAT. 10-2 P.M.
BY APPOINTMENT

80 CENTRAL PARK SOUTH
NEW YORK 19, N. Y.

℞ NAME Mrs. Mary Ogden DATE 3/27/57
ADDRESS 667 Center Avenue AGE 46 yrs.

	GM. OR C.C.	
Ammonium chloride	3	00
Sodium citrate	3	00
Menthol	0	10
Codeine phosphate	0	20
Syr. of glycyrrhiza q.s.	120	00

m Sig: 1 teaspoon q. q. h. for cough

REFILLED ——
REFIL UT DICT.
1☐ 2☐ 3☐ 4☐ TIMES
P.R.N.☐ NON.REP.☑

Roy Clark
ROY CLARK, M. D.

FIG. 6–1. Sample prescription.

dissolves quickly. Capsules are taken more easily than powder mixed with a liquid.

Tablets and capsules are made up in fractions of milligrams. Care must be taken, in filling a prescription, to be sure to allow for the correct number of pills to supply the strength prescribed. Many types of medication today are prepared by the drug manufacturers in the form in which they are sold, so that they need not be made up by the pharmacist. If the prescription reads, for instance, "½ gr.

twice daily," and the tablets are made by the manufacturer in amounts of ¼ gr. each, two tablets will have to be taken each time. On the other hand, if the prescription has been made up in ½-gr. tablets, one tablet twice a day will suffice.

Most prescriptions are written out in longhand by the doctor, but there is no reason why they could not be typed by the assistant and signed by the doctor.

Some prescriptions are marked "not to be repeated," and in that case a new prescription must be obtained from the doctor when the medicine has been used up. Other prescriptions, especially those for nonnarcotic medicines, may be filled repeatedly—prescriptions for vitamins, for instance. If a patient calls up to ask whether it would be possible for the doctor to mail him a copy of his last prescription, the assistant should tell the patient to come to the office, because the doctor would want to check on the patient's present condition before deciding whether the old prescription is still indicated.

To aid the doctor in writing out prescriptions, a file of drug products should be kept, preferably on index cards, with the name of the drug, the manufacturer, and the amounts in which it is packed. For instance, if a certain medication is prepared in vials of twenty-five tablets, it would be much cheaper to prescribe twenty-five tablets than thirty, because if thirty were prescribed, the pharmacist would have to open another vial and would charge accordingly.

Prescription blanks are often supplied by a pharmacy close to the doctor's office, and the patient is usually sent to this pharmacy. A pharmacist eventually learns the doctor's preferences regarding filling prescriptions, and cooperation between the two is in the interest of the patient. Any pharmacy, however, is able to fill any prescription. When the patient is given the prescription, he should be reminded to request a bill from the pharmacy for income-tax purposes.

A doctor who dispenses any medicines himself should order them in bulk directly from the manufacturer, as this results in a considerable saving.

Emergency Drugs

In every office, emergencies may occur for which certain drugs must be on hand. The most important of these and the reasons for their use are the following:

1. Adrenalin—in case of an asthmatic attack.
2. Morphine—in case of a heart attack, to quiet the patient and to alleviate pain.
3. Digitalis—in case of a heart attack, to stimulate the heart muscles.
4. Insulin—in case of a diabetic coma.
5. Emetics—in case of poisoning, to produce vomiting. (Emetics are effective, of course, only if the poisonous substance was swallowed.)
6. Antidotes—to prevent or counteract poisoning when it is too late for an emetic or when the poison was not introduced orally—for example, in cases of snake bite or insect bite (black widow spider).

Antidotes may be given orally, by injection, or as a gastric lavage. There are specific antidotes for a variety of poisons, but few private offices would have all of them; moreover, the poison that was contained in the material ingested is frequently unknown. Some general antidote may therefore be used. The following are the most effective general antidotes:

1. Activated charcoal mixed with water absorbs alkaloids such as strychnine, morphine, atropine, as well as mercuric and arsenic compounds.
2. Tannic acid precipitates alkaloids and metallic poisons.
3. Magnesium oxide neutralizes mineral acids.

A supply of the so-called "universal" antidote, which contains these three ingredients, should always be kept on hand.

Anesthetics

Drugs that produce a loss of feeling are used in a doctor's office whenever local anesthesia is required—for example, in minor surgery. The subject of office anesthesia is discussed in Chapter 8, Surgery in the Office.

Antiseptics

An antiseptic is a substance that prevents the growth of microorganisms. In the doctor's office, depending, of course, on the type of practice, antiseptics are used a great deal. They may be used as a mouthwash (in solution), for sterilizing the skin before an injection, for sterilizing wounds, and for sterilizing instruments. Some of the common antiseptics are alcohol, boric acid, chlorine, creosote, gentian violet, iodine, Lysol, Mercurochrome, permanganate, phenol, and vinegar.

Solutions

Solutions have many uses in a doctor's office, and in some offices the preparation of solutions is one of the assistant's most important tasks. Certain medications are obtained in bulk (powder, tablets, liquid) and are prepared in sterile solutions in the office. Some solutions are used for injections, others are administered orally, and still others are used as lavages, irrigations, inhalations, dressings, or cleansing preparations. Some of the most commonly used solutions are hydrogen peroxide, Burow's solution, bicarbonate solution, boric acid solution, saline solution, and permanganate solution.

Solutions consist of the vehicle in which the substance is dissolved or suspended, called the *solvent*, and the substance itself, the *solute*. Depending on the vehicle, the mixture may be an alcoholic solution, an aqueous solution, a colloidal solution, a suspension, an emulsion, or a "true" solution. When the substance is dissolved completely, the mixture is spoken of as a true solution.

In preparing a solution, the assistant must follow instructions with the utmost accuracy. Sterile water or a sterile saline preparation are the vehicles most frequently used for solutions mixed in the office. Solutions are described in percentages or ratios. For instance, a 10 per cent solution would mean 10 parts of the solute mixed with 90 parts of the solvent. If a 10 per cent solution of a solid material is required, 10 Gm. is dissolved in a certain amount of water and enough water is then added to make 100 parts. Conversion from one system of weights and measures to another may be necessary. Table 9 (see Appendix) presents some percentages for the preparation of solutions.

Storage

For efficient management of the medical supplies, all medications should be kept methodically in a cupboard or closet set aside specially for this purpose. All drugs for *external* use should be kept together; likewise, all drugs for *internal* use. Each bottle or box should have a definite place, so that any particular medicine can be found quickly. When cleaning the supply closet—and it should always be neat and spotless—the assistant should take out the bottles and boxes and arrange them on a table in the same order as in the closet; then, when she has finished cleaning the shelf, she should return them one by one to the same place.

Poisons should be clearly labeled as such and kept in distinctive bottles. Of course, all drugs and every medication—whether in liquid, powder, capsule, or pill form—must be labeled. Ampuls should be kept together with the files used to open them. Oils must be kept in a cool place. Antibiotics usually have to be refrigerated. (If the doctor has a refrigerator, it may also be used for storing food or drinks. The necessity of labeling all medications plainly is therefore obvious.)

Narcotics must be locked up at all times. The narcotics closet should never, even for a moment, be left open. In fact, it is desirable that all medications be kept under lock and key, for not all patients coming to the doctor are honest, and much harm can be caused if medicines are taken and later sold, given to unauthorized persons, or even taken by the patient himself—all these possibilities have actually happened.

Unused drugs tend to deteriorate and must be discarded. A

system of dating drug supplies should be worked out, so that it will be possible at all times to find out how long a certain drug has been in the office. A doctor's office must never run out of medical supplies. As soon as the last half of any material is reached, the drug should be reordered.

Labeling

Color may be used to good advantage in labeling bottles. Labels are available in different shades or with a variety of colored borders, and the assistant can save herself time and confusion by using different colors for different types of medication. For instance, all medicines for internal use may be marked with white labels; all medicines for external use, with red labels. If all bottles with the same color label are kept together, the assistant will turn automatically to the right section when looking for a medicine. Also, if a bottle is put in the wrong place, it may be immediately spotted. In the office of an ophthalmologist, for instance, all dilators have yellow labels; all antiseptics, pink ones. Barbiturates may be indicated by green-bordered labels; antibiotics, by blue-bordered labels; and so forth. A system to suit each office can easily be worked out and adopted.

Labels should be clearly and plainly marked. As ink runs at the slightest drop of moisture, its use is not recommended. If the labels are typed, the typewriter ribbon should be fully inked. Colored marking pencils are useful to an assistant who can print well or who has a clear handwriting. A blurred or spotted label should be replaced at once. If a container is found without a label, the contents should be discarded.

Care must be taken to replace a label immediately when it becomes loose. Most labels are attached with mucilage, which is likely to dry out and allow the labels to drop off. Scotch tape, which is popular, also dries out, becomes yellow, and soon looks unsightly. Painting the freshly typed label with white shellac produces the best-looking and longest-lasting results.

BIBLIOGRAPHY

"United States Pharmacopeia," The United Pharmacopoeial Convention, Inc., Washington, D.C.

"New and Nonofficial Drugs," American Medical Association, Chicago (revised periodically).

"Physicians' Desk Reference to Pharmaceutical Specialties and Biologicals," Medical Economics, Oradell, N.J. (published annually).

7

Techniques of Giving Injections

Although the administration of medicines either orally or externally is as old as the practice of medicine itself, the introduction of a drug or some other substance into the body by means of injection is a modern development. It would have been a dangerous procedure before aseptic techniques were known, and these, as we have seen, are of recent origin.

For a variety of reasons the administration of medication by injection is now the method of choice whenever feasible. One reason is that this method makes it possible to determine the exact amount of medication the patient receives. With other methods the doctor never can be sure that the patient is actually taking the medication as prescribed. The principal reason, however, is that medication enters the blood stream more quickly when injected in undiluted strength and is therefore more effective.

Many patients come to the doctor's office regularly—daily or two or three times a week—over long periods just to receive injections. Giving these injections, or at least preparing the tray for them, is the assistant's duty. In some cases the assistant may have to show a person how to give injections to a patient at home. Diabetics, for example, need daily insulin injections. A thorough knowledge of the procedure of giving injections is therefore one of the most important requirements for a medical office assistant.

Reasons for Injections

Injections are given for several reasons:

1. When an immediate effect is desired
2. When, either because of the condition of the patient or the nature of the drug, the medicine cannot be given by mouth

3. When the effect of the drug would be destroyed by the digestive juices
4. When a local reaction is desired

Although giving injections is now a routine procedure, performed often by relatives of the patient at home, certain dangers do exist and should be recognized:

1. Injury to a vein or a superficial nerve
2. Breaking of the needle in the tissue
3. The possibility of an abscess developing because of:
    a. Improper sterilization of the injection area
    b. A soiled needle or syringe
    c. An operator with unclean hands
4. Injection into a vein instead of a muscle

An injection should not, as a rule, be given to a delirious or irrational person. It is well to explain the procedure to a patient who is about to receive an injection for the first time.

Types of Injection

There are several different methods of injection:

1. Subcutaneous injection—into the tissue between the skin and the muscle
2. Intramuscular injection—directly into the muscle
3. Intradermal injection—into the upper layers of the skin
4. Intravenous injection—into a vein
5. Intra-articular injection—into a joint
6. Injection into a fracture
7. Lumbar puncture

Subcutaneous Injection. This method is the one used most frequently. Insulin injections for diabetes are given in this way. Only aqueous solutions are used for this purpose. To give the injection, the operator lifts a fold of the skin and pushes the needle quickly into the fold; or, with the left hand, she applies pressure next to the site to be injected, to divert the patient's attention to that area, and quickly pushes the needle into the tissue (see Fig. 7-1).

Intramuscular Injection. For this method, the operator requires a thorough knowledge of anatomy, so that he can make the injection deep enough into the muscle without injuring a vein or nerve. This type is used in administering either large quantities of medicine or oily substances, because these would produce too strong a reaction in the superficial tissues. The injection should preferably

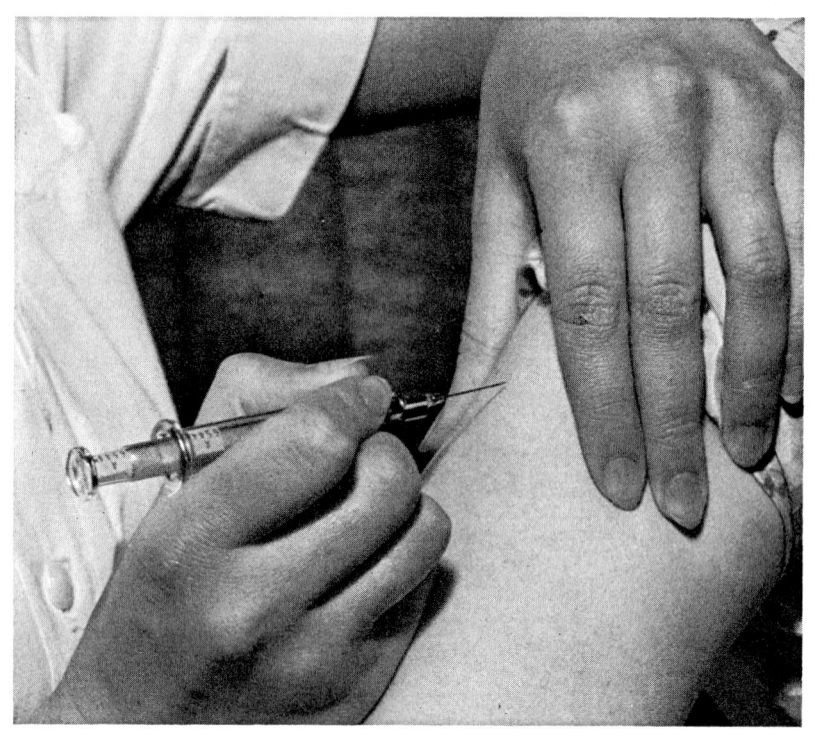

Fig. 7-1. Giving an injection.

be given in the upper part of the buttocks, so that any reaction that occurs will not interfere with sitting down. The injection is made in a vertical direction. The skin is stretched between the thumb and the index finger. The needle should be at least 1½ inches long. If any blood shows in the syringe, the needle has penetrated a vein and must be withdrawn at once.

Intradermal Injection. This is given when a reaction in the skin is desired, as in an allergy test. Short, thin needles are necessary, and only a minute dosage can be administered in this way. The technique requires careful training.

Intravenous Injection. When a substance is introduced into a vein, it enters the blood stream immediately and acts rapidly. Intravenous injections are used for (blood) transfusions and parenteral feeding. Only watery solutions can be injected in this manner. Oily medications could lead to fatal occlusion of blood vessels.

Intravenous injections may be given by a physician only, according to the medical practice act in most states. There are two reasons for this. First, there is always the danger of air entering the blood stream, and this might prove fatal. Second, it is important to see that the needle is actually in the vein. If the needle has perforated the vein and the opening of the needle is in the surrounding tissue, a severe reaction may follow.

Intra-articular Injection. This is a new technique of injection. It is used in therapy for cases in which medication is to be introduced directly into the joint to treat inflammation (arthritis) or to produce anesthesia.

Injection into a Fracture. For the reduction of fractures and also for dislocations, local anesthesia is produced by injecting an anesthetic agent into the fracture. This method of injection was devised by Lorenz Böhler. He emphasized that for this procedure everything must be absolutely sterile, as the danger of infection is always present with a fracture.

The skin is painted with iodine, the needle inserted into the bone, and the anesthetic solution (Novocain) injected. The fracture can then be set without pain; no general anesthesia is necessary.

The patient must be watched very carefully so that he does not make any motion. Because of the absence of pain, he may forget his injury and use the fractured part, thereby causing further injury.

Lumbar Puncture. The lumbar puncture is made for the purpose of withdrawing spinal fluid for examination or of injecting anesthetics in the case of operations (spinal anesthesia). The epidural injection (*epidura*—"around the outer membrane of the spinal cord") has been used in the treatment of the sciatic syndrome. This injection is given into the lowest part of the sacrum. Injections into the spine are given by physicians, usually in the hospital, where the patient can remain in bed. They are mentioned here merely for the assistant's information.

Giving Injections

Materials. Whenever an injection is to be given, a tray is prepared with the equipment and the materials to be administered. Substances for injection are of practically the same variety as those given orally. They may be obtained ready for use or in powder or tablet form to be prepared as needed.

In prepared form, ready to use, solutions for injections come in vials or ampuls that keep the material sterile. Ampuls are the more popular, as they contain the exact amount of medication to be injected. The ampul has a very thin neck, which is broken off with a knife or file (see Fig. 7–2). New-style ampuls are made so that the stem can be broken off easily without using a file. The needle of the syringe is inserted into the ampul, which is held in one hand, and the fluid is drawn into the syringe.

Vials containing injection material have a rubber, self-sealing stopper, which is punctured by the needle so that the desired amount may be withdrawn. Fig. 7–3 illustrates the way in which a syringe is filled from a vial.

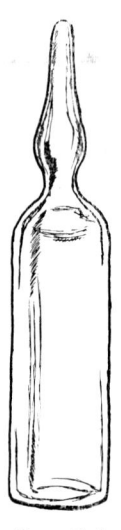

Fig. 7–2. Ampul.

If the solution is prepared by the assistant, the powder or tablet is mixed with sterile distilled water or sterile saline solution in a sterile container. The desired amount is then drawn into the syringe.

The equipment needed includes:

1. Small tray
2. Sterilized Luer syringes
3. Sterilized hypodermic needles, which come in different thicknesses and lengths

TECHNIQUES OF GIVING INJECTIONS

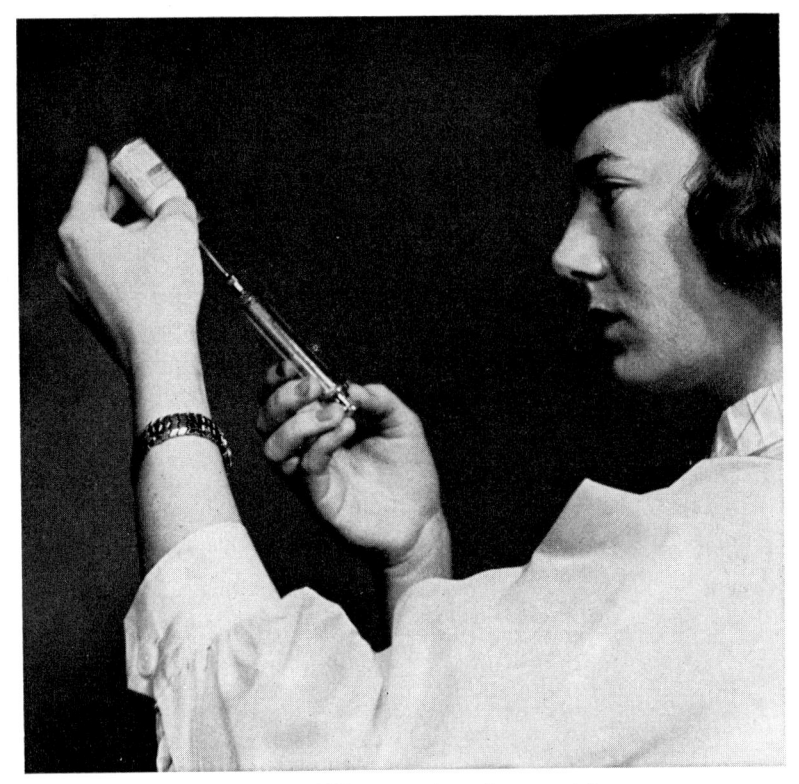

FIG. 7-3. Filling a syringe from a vial.

4. Sterile forceps in antiseptic solution
5. Sterile sponges or sterile cotton swabs
6. Antiseptic solution (alcohol, iodine)
7. Bottle, vial, ampul, with file, or container of solution (to repeat, a solution prepared before use must be absolutely sterile!)

General Procedure. The following steps are necessary in all types of injections:

1. Check the serial numbers on the barrel and the plunger of the syringe to make sure they correspond.
2. Examine the needles to make sure that they are not bent, hooked, or clogged.

3. Boil the syringe and needle for 10 to 15 minutes, unless they have been in a sterile pack.

4. Remove the syringe from the sterilizer with sterile forceps and place on a sterile towel or gauze.

5. Pick up the barrel with forceps and place it in your left hand.

6. Pick up the plunger with forceps and insert into the barrel.

7. Pick up the needle with forceps by the square part (the hub) and insert it into the syringe tip. Be sure that no part except the outside of the barrel, which you are holding in your left hand, is contaminated.

8. Rest the syringe on sterile gauze or cotton.

9. If an ampul is used:

   a. Wipe the neck with an alcohol sponge or cotton swab.

   b. Collect all the drug by tapping the tip until the liquid goes down.

   c. File and break the tip at the neck.

   d. Draw the liquid into the syringe through the needle.

   If a rubber-tipped vial is used:

   a. Wipe the top of the vial with cotton moistened in alcohol.

   b. Push the plunger partly down.

   c. Insert the needle through the rubber stopper into the solution.

   d. Push the plunger all the way down.

   e. Withdraw the solution by pulling back the plunger slowly until the required amount is reached on the scales on the barrel.

10. Place the needle in a sterile cotton or sterile gauze sponge dipped in 70 per cent alcohol.

11. Place the needle on the tray.

12. If this is a first injection, explain the procedure to the patient.

13. Wipe the injection site with alcohol, iodine, or whatever antiseptic the doctor likes to use.

14. Holding the syringe with the needle pointing upward, expel the air from it.

15. With the left hand, grasp the arm or thigh, on either side of the puncture site, making a cushion of the tissue, or press hard.

16. Holding the point of needle near the skin and the syringe at a 60° angle, introduce the needle with a quick motion.

17. Withdraw the plunger slightly to make sure the needle is not in a blood vessel.

18. Inject the solution by pushing the plunger down slowly until the syringe is empty.

19. Remove the needle quickly; press over the area of injection.

20. Massage the area gently with a sterile cotton ball, a gauze pad, or the hand, to lessen pain and prevent swelling.

Special Procedures. In preparing the patient for an intravenous injection, or for withdrawal of blood from a vein, the following procedure is followed:

1. Apply a tourniquet on the upper arm, just above the elbow.
2. Tell the patient to rest his arm on a table in as comfortable a position as possible.
3. Ask him to flex the arm several times, to enlarge the vein below the tourniquet.
4. Cleanse the skin in the bend of the elbow thoroughly with alcohol, ether, or any other antiseptic.
5. After withdrawing the needle, place a sterile gauze dressing over the puncture and instruct the patient to bend the elbow and hold it in that position for several minutes.

For an injection into a joint, or paracentesis (puncture, tapping), as it is commonly referred to, the following materials—in addition to those enumerated above—are necessary:

1. A 5-cc. syringe for an anesthetic that is administered prior to the injection itself
2. A 20-cc. syringe for aspiration (withdrawal) of joint fluid
3. Prepared sterile gauze dressings
4. Elastic bandage
5. Culture tubes
6. Graduated glass container for measuring synovial fluid withdrawn

Figures 7-4 and 7-5 show, respectively, an injection into the shoulder joint and one into the knee joint. After the needle is withdrawn, a dressing is placed on the punctured site. An elastic bandage may be applied to give support to the affected joint.

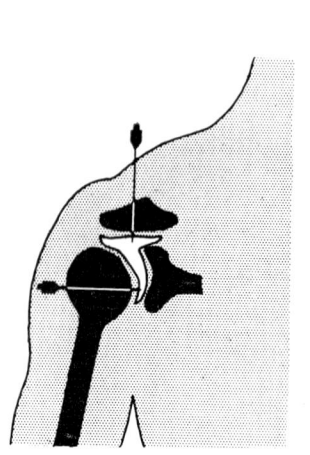

FIG. 7-4. Injection into the shoulder joint. (*Merck, Sharp & Dohme International Division.*)

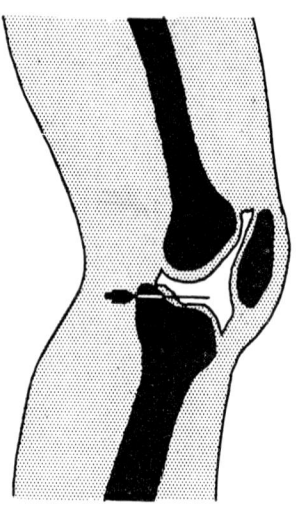

FIG. 7-5. Injection into the knee joint. (*Merck, Sharp & Dohme International Division.*)

Care of Syringes and Needles

Syringes. Syringes come in various sizes, from 2 cc. upward. If 2 cc. of a substance is to be injected, for instance, and a 2-cc. syringe is used, the syringe obviously will be completely filled. But if the capacity of the syringe is greater than the required dosage, the amount taken into the syringe must be gauged by the scale engraved on the barrel of the syringe. Very large metal syringes without scales are used for irrigations, of the ear for example.

Syringes are delicate instruments and must be handled with care. Breakage can be kept to a minimum if certain safety precautions are observed:

1. Each barrel and each plunger is marked with a serial number; therefore, when assembling a syringe, check this number to see that

the number of the plunger corresponds to the number of the barrel. Even a slight difference in size may cause trouble.

2. Before boiling a syringe, always separate the barrel and the plunger.

3. Place the parts into cold water in the sterilizer and heat them up gradually.

4. After the syringe has been used, flush it several times with warm water. If there is blood in the syringe, flush with cold water until syringe is clean.

5. Separate the barrel and plunger and wash the syringe in soapy water (a detergent, if an oily substance has been used) or in a special cleaning solution. Use a regular bottle brush and scrub off any deposits.

6. To remove stains and deposits that cannot be washed off, use a 10 per cent solution of nitric acid. Dip a cotton applicator into the solution and swab the inside. Rinse after swabbing.

7. Hold all parts under running water to remove soap or cleaning solution, and then rinse in alcohol or distilled water.

8. Either sterilize or store the syringes, leaving barrel and plunger separate.

Sometimes the plunger gets stuck in the barrel. To separate these parts, use a special device called a syringe opener (see Fig. 7-6). Or boil the syringe in a solution of 25 per cent glycerin, 75 per cent water for 15 minutes and rotate the plunger while the syringe is still hot. If the syringe cannot be separated, allow it to stand in ether for about half an hour.

Excessive boiling or leaving a syringe immersed too long in an antiseptic solution can shorten the life of the syringe.

Nylon Syringes. Recently syringes made of nylon have come on the market. The advantages of these syringes, as stated by the manufacturers, are that they are unbreakable; they do not affect pH of serum [1] when withdrawing blood; the pistons and barrels of different syringes are interchangeable; and the piston never sticks in the barrel. Nylon syringes may be sterilized by any accepted method,

[1] pH is the symbol representing the state of acidity or alkalinity of a substance.

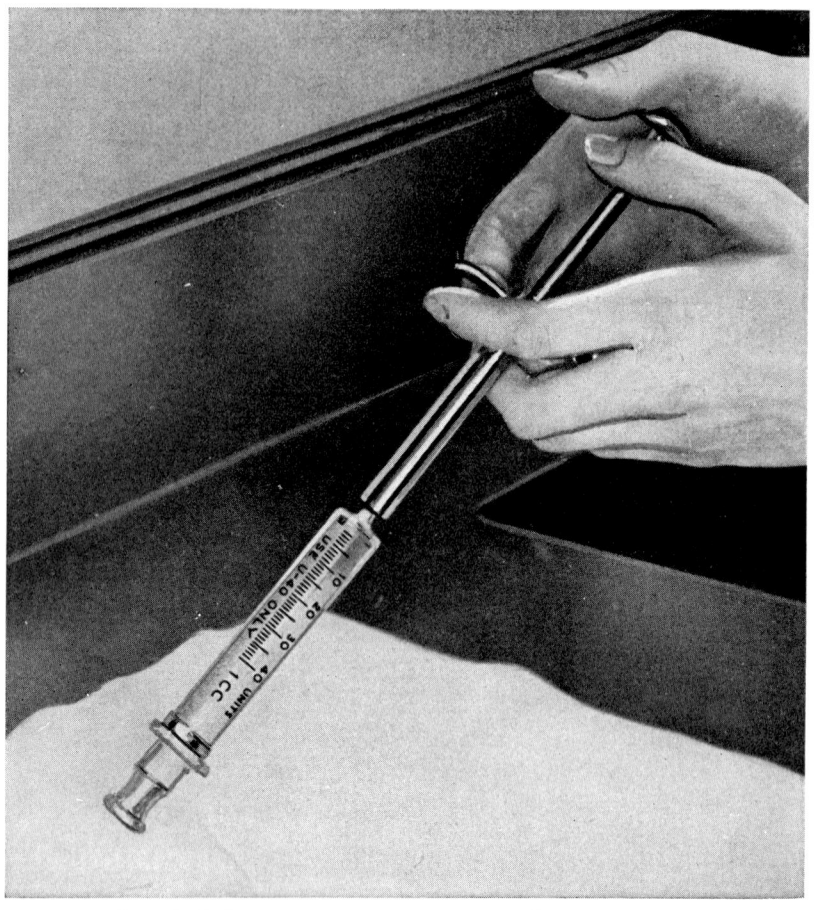

FIG. 7-6. Syringe opener. (*Becton, Dickinson & Co.*)

though instructions should be followed as to the permissible amount of pressure in the autoclave or the proper length of immersion in a germicidal solution.

In clinic practice, where time is of the essence, sufficient care cannot be given to syringes, and breakage is usually heavy. Unbreakable nylon syringes may therefore prove especially advantageous in these circumstances.

Needles. Since needles penetrate into the patient's tissues, they must be especially cared for, lest they cause pain, infection, or injury. Different sizes of needles are required for different types of

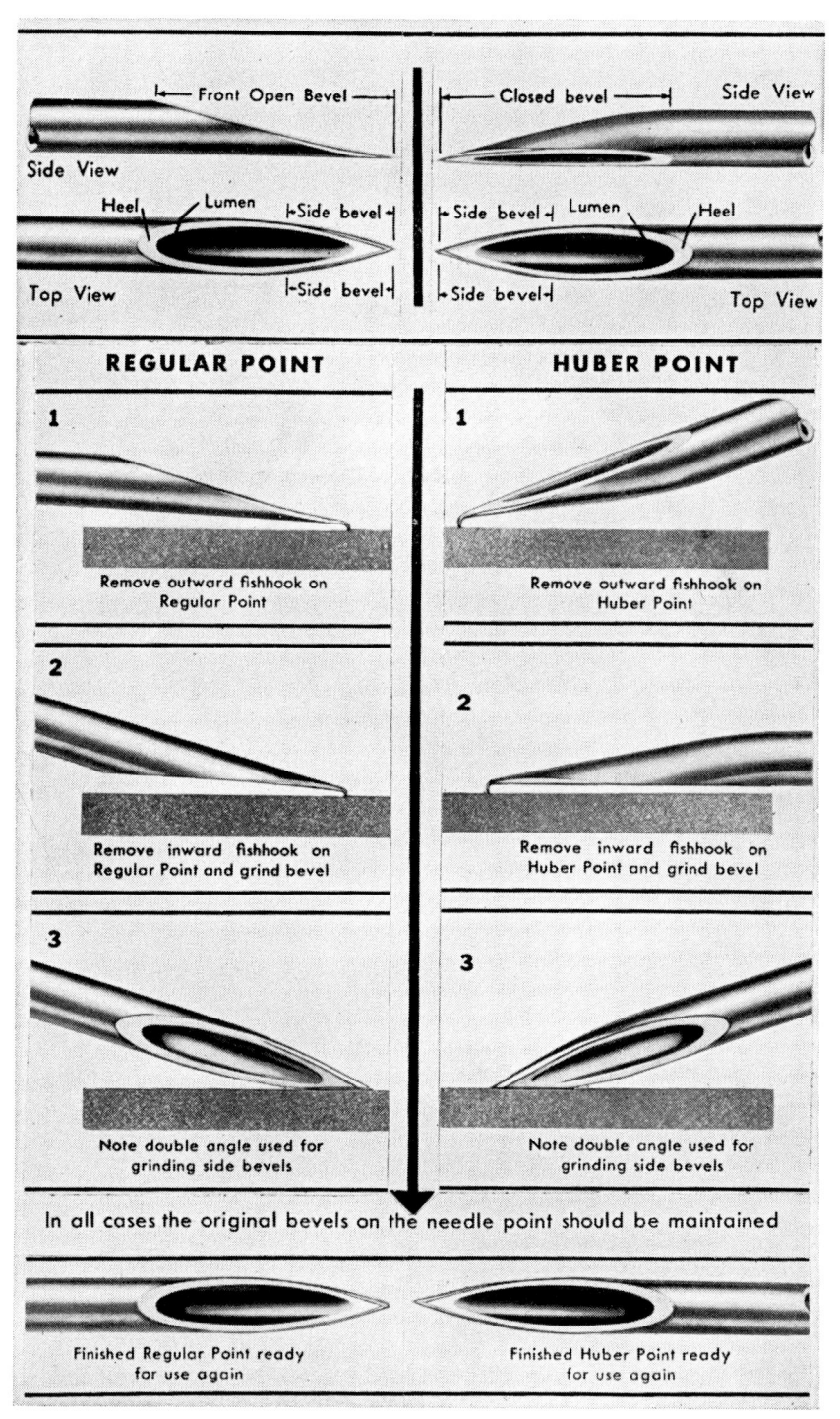

FIG. 7-7. Needle-sharpening technique. (*Becton, Dickinson & Co.*)

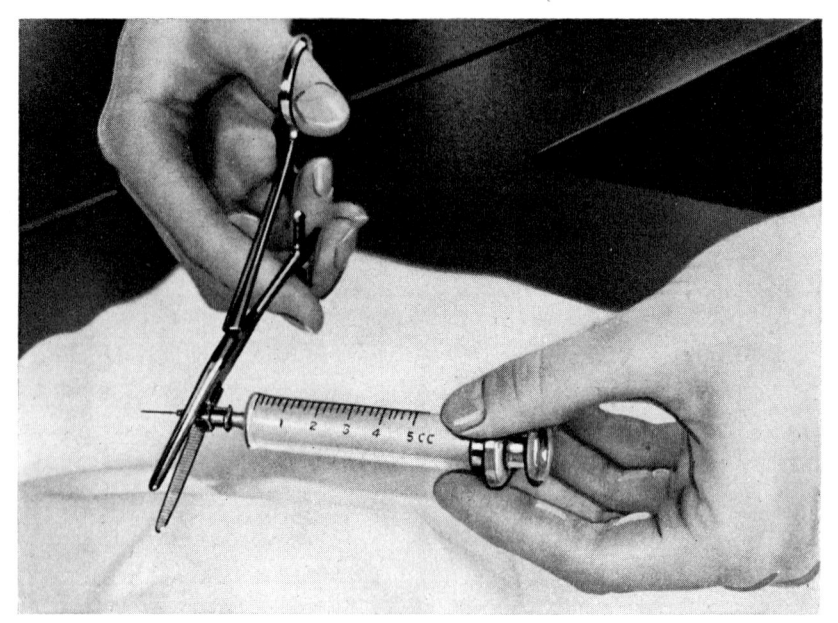

Fig. 7-8. Removing needle stuck in a syringe. (*Becton, Dickinson & Co.*)

injection. Needles vary in length and in thickness (gauge). Length is determined by measuring from the hub (which is not included) to the tip. Thickness, that is, the diameter of the needle, is expressed by gauge numbers ranging from 13 to 27. The higher the number, the thinner the needle.

1. After needles have been used, rinse them under running water —immediately, if possible.
2. Insert a stylet or thin wire to keep the cannula open.
3. Clean the inside of the hub with a cotton applicator.
4. Attach the syringe and flush a cleaning solution through the needle.
5. Inspect for defects.

As needles may become bent or develop fishhooks on the tip, they must be examined carefully before reuse, preferably under a magnifying glass. If the slightest imperfection is noted, they must be sharpened on an oilstone (see Fig. 7-7). Becton, Dickinson &

Company recommend the use of a light mineral oil on the stone to hasten sharpening and give a smoother finish.

To remove a needle stuck in a syringe, soak the syringe for 15 minutes in a cleaning solution; then grasp the hub of the needle firmly with pliers and rotate the syringe (not the pliers) until the needle loosens (see Fig. 7–8).

The technique of sterilizing syringes and needles is discussed in Chapter 3, Protection through Sterilization.

BIBLIOGRAPHY

Böhler, Lorenz: "The Treatment of Fractures," 5th English ed., Grune & Stratton, Inc., New York, 1956, vol. I.

8

Surgery in the Office

Only so-called "minor" surgery is performed in the doctor's office and is therefore of concern to the medical office assistant. Minor surgical operations include procedures such as the lancing of a boil, removal of a wart, and suture of an open wound. Occasionally a patient who has had an operation in the hospital comes to the surgeon's office to have the dressing changed.

Assisting in any form of surgery is a highly responsible job, and the doctor's aide must be familiar with and strictly observe surgical technique from beginning to end.

Preparation of the Patient

Each doctor has his own particular method of preparing a patient for minor surgery. Before surgery, the patient is bound to be tense, nervous, and apprehensive. As the assistant is with him before the operation, she can do much, just by her general attitude, to calm him and help prepare him mentally for the operation.

An understanding of the patient's personality will be of great help to the assistant in dealing with him. Some patients must be reassured and protected from too much knowledge, while others cooperate much better if told the truth as to what is to be done, how long the procedure will take, whether it will hurt and, if so, whether briefly or steadily. The assistant greatly facilitates the doctor's task if she can make the patient relax and face the ordeal without fear or dread.

When the patient arrives at the office, everything should be in readiness for him. The less time he has to wait, the better it is for all concerned. The best procedure is to take him into the operating room at once—or into the dressing room to disrobe, depending on the type of operation. He may be given a sedative as soon as he comes in. The principles of draping described in Chapter 4, Helping with Examinations, apply also for surgical procedures.

Office Anesthesia

For minor surgical operations and for certain painful treatments, some type of anesthesia is required. Today patients do not expect to suffer pain under the ministrations of the doctor. It is difficult to realize that anesthesia was discovered only a little over a hundred years ago and that it has been used generally for barely seventy-five years. Before the discovery of anesthesia, surgical operations, even amputations, were done with the patient almost fully conscious and sensitive to pain. Alcohol and other drugs were, of course, administered to deaden sensation, but complete, controlled unconsciousness was not produced until the discovery of ether and its properties. In 1842, Crawford W. Long, a country physician in Georgia, was able to produce general anesthesia. He did not publish his results, however, and in 1846, W. T. G. Morton, quite independently of Long's discovery, used ether in the Massachusetts General Hospital. A long controversy over the priority of the discovery followed. The term *anesthesia* was suggested by Oliver Wendell Holmes.

Anesthesia refers to loss of the sensation of touch or pain with or without loss of consciousness, while the term *narcosis* means deep unconsciousness produced by a drug. The essential characteristics of an anesthetic agent are (1) that it produces complete unconsciousness or dulling of consciousness, if general; or complete loss of sensation in the part anesthetized, if local; (2) that this process is reversible; and (3) that consciousness or sensation returns as soon as the administration of the drug is stopped or the effect has worn off.

General Anesthesia. If deep, prolonged general anesthesia is necessary, the patient must be hospitalized, for there is always the danger that the subject may stop breathing, and the heart may stop. Also, it frequently happens that the patient vomits afterward. Except in emergencies, only a trained anesthetist may administer a general anesthetic.

For certain procedures in the doctor's office a dulling of consciousness or a short loss of consciousness may be desired. In the dentist's office, "laughing gas" (nitrous oxide) is often used for extractions. In the doctor's office this has not been found practicable. However, other forms of inhalation anesthesia have recently been introduced and have been found suitable in many cases.

For this type of anesthesia, the patient is given an inhaler filled with a volatile liquid, which he holds to his mouth and nose. The drug produces insensitivity to pain, and the amount inhaled is regulated by the patient himself. If loss of consciousness occurs, the patient automatically stops inhaling, and consciousness returns within half a minute or so. One such inhaler, the Duke inhaler, is illustrated in Fig. 8–1. The container is filled with the drug, connected to the mask, tested, and handed to the patient. The information supplied with this apparatus includes detailed instructions on filling it, explaining its use to the patient, and caring for it after use. The manufacturers emphasize especially that only the patient himself should hold this inhaler over his face. The only drug that should be used with this inhaler is an analgesic, that is, an agent for relief of pain and not an anesthetic.

Patients who are to be given a general anesthetic of any kind should be instructed not to eat or drink anything prior to coming to the doctor's office, as nausea or vomiting may occur.

Local Anesthesia. For most procedures in the doctor's office local anesthesia is used. The discoverer of local anesthesia, Carl Ludwig Schleich, a German physician, first proposed its use in 1894, when he injected cocaine under the skin and was thereby able to render the area completely insensate. When Schleich read a paper about his discovery before a distinguished audience of physicians, he was denounced as a liar and a cheat. Today infiltration anesthesia, as this type is called, is universally accepted as effective, although it is sometimes supplemented by block anesthesia, that is, injection of the anesthetic solution into the nerve trunk to cut off conductivity.

SURGERY IN THE OFFICE 111

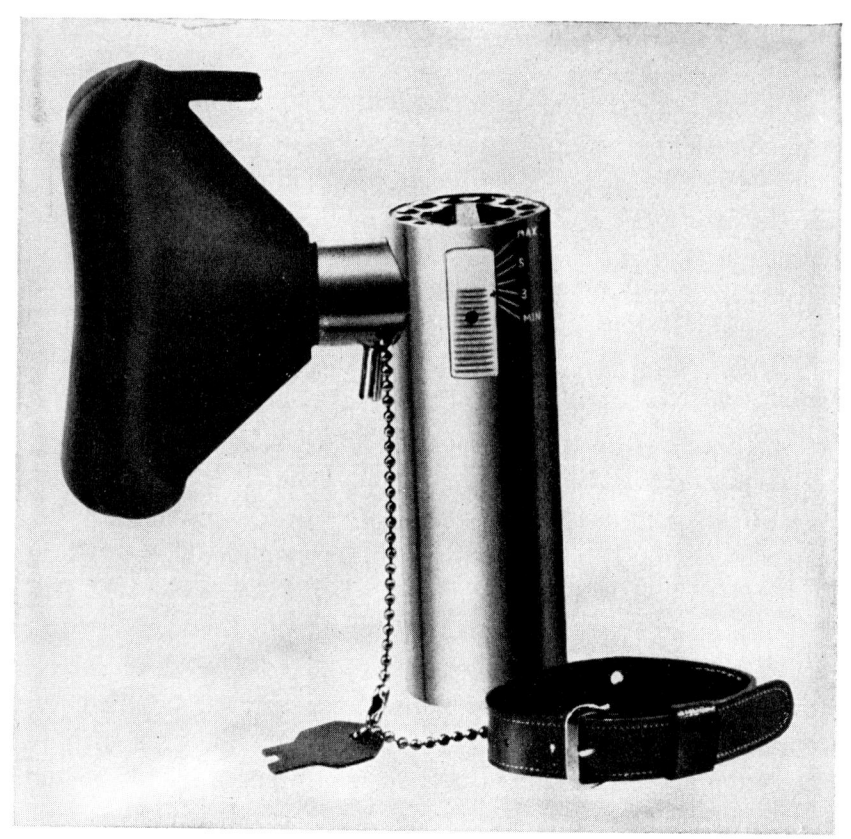

Fig. 8-1. Duke inhaler. (*Ayerst Laboratories.*)

Cocaine is now used only rarely; many other substances are available, such as Novocain or procaine, for instance.

The type of local anesthesia to be selected in each individual case depends on the severity and the extent of the procedure. If only a superficial surgical incision is to be made, a surface anesthesia may be sufficient. If deep tissues are involved, conductive anesthesia is required. The different types of local anesthesia are produced as follows:

1. *Topical anesthesia.* This is produced by treating small parts of the skin or mucous membranes with a drug that, when painted or sprayed on, freezes the tissue and deadens sensation. This type of

anesthesia is short-lived, as sensation returns as soon as the skin becomes warm again.

For topical anesthesia, the region of the skin to be anesthetized is washed with tincture of green soap and dried with a sterile towel or gauze. The drug is applied with cotton or sprayed on. If needed in the throat or nose, it is sprayed on. The tissue becomes anesthetic as soon as it is frozen. This may take a couple of minutes. As the effect passes quickly, all preparations must be completed beforehand, and the work must be done swiftly.

2. *Infiltration anesthesia.* The anesthetic is injected under the skin at the site to be operated on, so that all nerve endings are anesthetized. A thin needle should be used. The rules for giving injections, described in Chapter 7, apply here.

3. *Block or conductive anesthesia.* The drug is injected into the nerve trunk above the area where the procedure will take place, and sensation in the distribution of this nerve is thus blocked. This loss of sensation lasts a fairly long time.

Occasionally a patient faints after the administration of an anesthetic. This may be caused by emotional factors or by an allergic condition. Lowering the patient's head usually restores consciousness promptly. Some patients are allergic to anesthetic drugs and may react with respiratory or cardiac symptoms. It is therefore advisable to make a skin test before injecting the drug. Preparations for emergencies should be completed beforehand; that is, sterile syringes and needles, as well as medications (vasodepressor, Adrenalin, barbiturates, antihistamines), should be in readiness. Artificial respiration may even have to be administered.

In preparing the patient for anesthesia, the assistant should find out whether he has a history of allergic reactions to any drug, whether he has any cardiac involvement, and whether he has ever had any type of anesthesia. This information should be included in the patient's medical history.

The Operating Room

When the doctor is scheduled to perform any kind of minor surgery in the office, the assistant is responsible for preparing every-

SURGERY IN THE OFFICE

thing for him. The operating room, obviously, must be spotlessly clean, well ventilated, and well lighted. Draping sheets, if needed, should be laid out; the doctor's gown, cap, mask, and sterile rubber gloves, in readiness. The instrument tray should be set with instruments, properly sterilized and in sterile wrappings, and sterile pickup forceps.

Just what instruments and materials the doctor will need depends, of course, on the procedure involved. Also, each doctor has a preference for certain instruments. Below is a check list of articles used in minor surgery, though certainly not all are needed in any one operation. The assistant should make up a similar list for her own use and check it each time surgery is scheduled. The following articles might be included:

1. Gloves
2. Cap and mask
3. Syringes and needles
4. Anesthetic solution
5. Pickup forceps and container
6. Scalpel
7. Knife blades
8. Hemostatic forceps, straight and curved
9. Dressing jars
10. Utility jars for swab sticks, tongue depressors, cotton and alcohol sponges
11. Instrument-sterilizing jar
12. Knife blade sterilizing jar
13. Cotton
14. Dressings
15. Bandages
16. Scissors, curved and straight, and bandage
17. Retractors
18. Skin hooks
19. Forceps, thumb and dressing
20. Probes with eyes
21. Grooved director
22. Needle holder
23. Surgical needles
24. Sutures
25. Towel forceps
26. Curet
27. Specula, vaginal
28. Splints
29. Adhesive tape
30. Basins
31. Towels, sheets, pillowcases, gowns
32. Tissues
33. Glass slides
34. Biopsy specimen jars
35. Culture tubes
36. Rectal diagnostic and treatment set
37. Rectal biopsy forceps
38. Rubber dam for drains
39. Catheter

Some of these instruments are illustrated in Fig. 8–2, and a tray with a simple setup for dressing a wound is shown in Fig. 8–3.

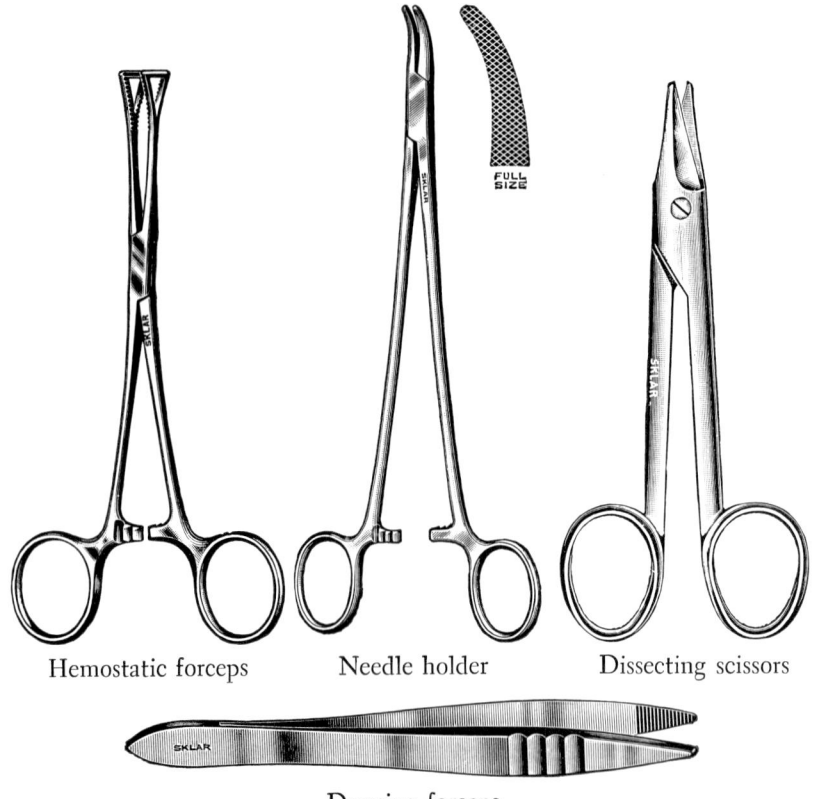

Hemostatic forceps   Needle holder   Dissecting scissors

Dressing forceps

Fig. 8-2. Surgical instruments. (*J. Sklar Mfg. Co.*)

The Assistant's Role

Before the doctor starts to work, the patient should be made comfortable, whether he is sitting in a chair or lying prone on the operating table. Clothing should be removed, pushed back, or covered with a towel or rubber sheet, depending on the area involved. It may be necessary to shave the area where the doctor will operate.

At the beginning of the operation, the assistant opens the instrument pack and sterile towels. The first step will probably be the injection to produce local anesthesia. During the surgical procedure the assistant hands the doctor the instruments he needs. When handling instruments or assisting in an operation, she should wear sterile rubber gloves. For smooth procedure during the operation,

SURGERY IN THE OFFICE

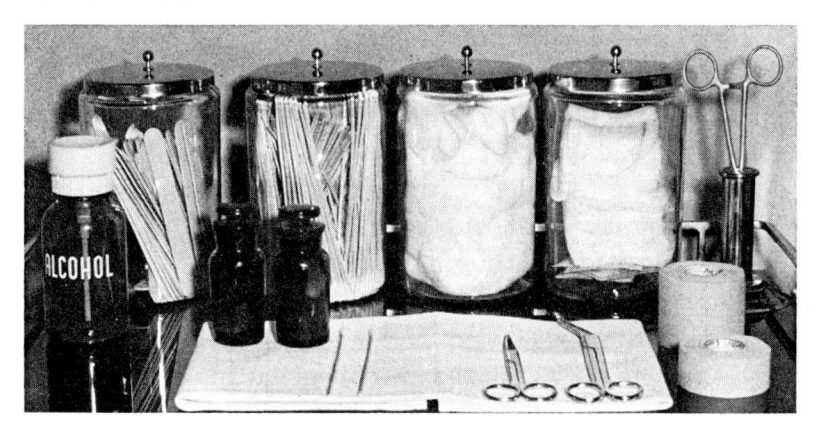

FIG. 8–3. Dressing tray. (*Courtesy of Dr. Earl C. Shaw.*)

the assistant should know beforehand not only the instruments the doctor will need but the order and manner in which he wishes to have them given to him. She should hand them to the doctor in such a way that he can grasp them quickly. Basins for discharge, blood, or discarded dressings must be held close to the area involved. There should be a basin on the tray or near the operating table for soiled instruments. Figure 8–4 shows the assistant helping the doctor during an office surgical operation.

It is important not to cause any delay by fumbling or by having to look for something the doctor asks for. At the risk of being repetitious, it must be emphasized that the assistant should be thoroughly familiar with the procedure, certain of each successive step and of the instruments, medications, dressings, drainage tubes, syringes, etc., that the doctor will need.

Instruments that are soiled should be put out of sight of the patient. Care must be taken that they do not touch anything on the dressing table and contaminate other instruments or materials. Paper bags or cardboard containers are the most practical and easily disposable receptacles for soiled dressings.

Count the instruments immediately after use, to make sure that none is disposed of with soiled linen or dressings. Place the instruments in a basin of cold, 2 per cent Lysol solution and clean them as soon as possible, in this way:

1. Pour off the Lysol solution.
2. Cover the instruments with cold water.
3. Clean them thoroughly with cold running water, making sure that all blood and discharges are removed.
4. Scrub them thoroughly with a mild abrasive and a soft cloth or a brush, on a wooden board specially used for this purpose.
5. Rinse them thoroughly under warm running water. Be sure that all cleaning powder is removed.
6. Dry them thoroughly.
7. Either return them to the instrument cabinet for later use or prepare them for sterilization.

Place basins, rubber gloves, and any other washable materials in soapy water until there is time to attend to them. Then, tidy up the operating room, dispose of all soiled linen, return medications to their proper place, and prepare the room for the next patient. No

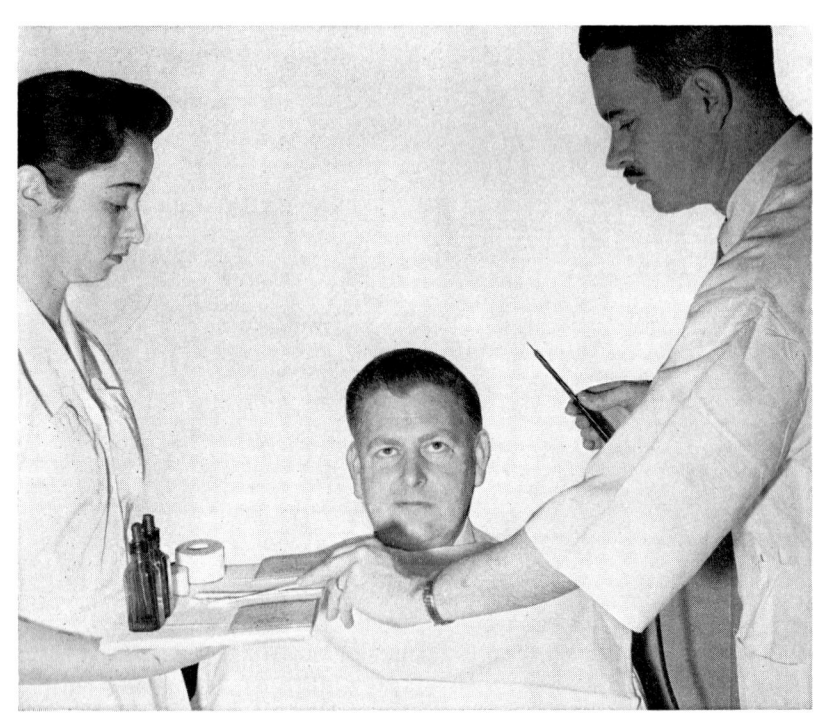

FIG. 8-4. Assisting at an office operation. (*Courtesy of Dr. Earl C. Shaw.*)

sign of a previous operation should be in evidence when the new patient enters.

Dressings

After an operative procedure, the wound is dressed; the patient will probably return to the office several times to have the dressing changed. The type of dressing naturally varies according to the type of wound—a burn, a cut, a boil that has been lanced, to name only a few. If the wound is clean, a dry dressing is used; if it is draining, a wet dressing may be applied, and a sterile rubber tube may be inserted. After it is cleaned, an open wound is covered with gauze. A surgical wound is covered with gauze only, while a burn or an infection may be covered with ointment or powder. Each doctor has his own preference for a particular type of dressing in each individual case. But the assistant must prepare the dressings for him; have everything assembled before the patient enters the treatment room; assist the doctor in the procedure; and in some simple cases, or in the doctor's absence, even change the dressing herself.

In addition to the dressing materials, the dressing tray must contain pickup forceps, dressing forceps, adhesive tape, and medications. The assistant hands the dressing materials and instruments to the physician in such a way that no part that may come into contact with the wound is contaminated. If the dressing is being changed, the assistant should hold a basin near the doctor so that he may drop the discarded dressing into it.

Dressings for open wounds are made of many different materials. Formerly, cotton and sometimes silk were used; nowadays various synthetic, wood, and paper fibers are also used. Gauze, however, is still the type of dressing preferred by most surgeons.

Ready-made dressings may be purchased in many different sizes, shapes, and thicknesses, and they are available in sterile containers. Such dressings, however, are quite expensive and, in an office where many are used, might prove too costly to be practical. It is therefore wiser to buy gauze by the yard and make one's own dressings. Gauze can be cut into squares or strips and folded into the desired size and thickness; it is very important that all raw edges be turned inward, as loose threads may get into the wound. After they are made, dressings are enclosed in muslin, towels, or paper wrappings to be autoclaved.

Small dressings may be held in place by adhesive tape. Ordinary adhesive comes on a spool and may be cut to the desired size, but the newer plastic adhesives come in various sizes and shapes (round, oblong, square). If these are used, an assortment of the various types should be on the tray, as the doctor may not know beforehand which one will be best. Ordinary or plastic adhesive tape attached to a gauze dressing and enclosed in a sterile container may be bought at any drugstore. For the face, hands, and arms, and for women's legs, these dressings come in flesh color. To apply such a dressing, open the paper container by pulling the string; with each hand, grasp one edge of the crinoline covering and pull the edges apart; apply the gauze part to the wound. When applied in this manner, the dressing remains sterile (see Fig. 8–5).

Absorbent cotton should not be placed directly on a wound, but may be used as padding between the gauze and the bandage or a splint. It may also be used for cleaning a wound with antiseptic or

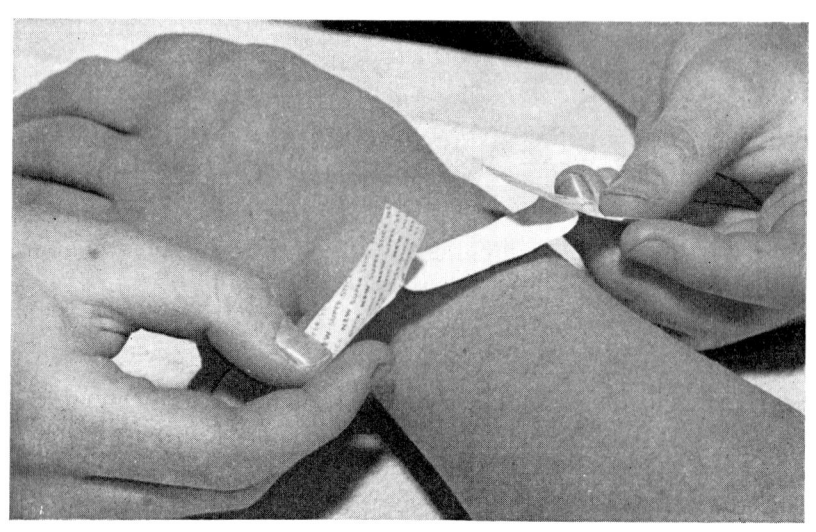

Fig. 8–5. Applying sterile adhesive dressing.

for cleaning and sterilizing the skin before an injection. Cotton therefore belongs on the dressing tray.

Removal of Dressings. A dressing that has been secured with adhesive tape often presents a problem. When the tape is pulled off, it should be done as quickly as possible, to minimize the pain. The skin should be pulled away from the tape, not the tape from the skin. Also, the tape should be removed toward the wound. If the area around the wound has been shaved, taking off the tape will be less painful. The tape may be loosened with benzin or one of the specially manufactured removers. A cotton ball soaked in benzin or remover is used for this, so a small glass or bowl to pour the liquid in should also be on the dressing tray. The old dressing is picked up with forceps and dropped into a basin, paper bag, or airtight cardboard container for later disposal.

Bandages

Bandages are used for several purposes:

1. To hold a dressing or a splint in place
2. To immobilize a part
3. To support or protect an injured part
4. To apply pressure in order to control bleeding or swelling

In some offices applying bandages is an important part of the assistant's work. A great variety of types of bandage and ways of bandaging exist. For the medical assistant, however, only three basic types are of importance: (1) roller bandage, (2) triangular bandage, and (3) cravat bandage.

Roller Bandage. The roller bandage is a long strip of material. It comes in widths of ½, 1, 2, and 3 in. and in lengths from 1 to 10 yd. It may be made of gauze or of elastic material. The latter may be muslin, which gives because of the way it is woven, or rubberized material, which actually stretches. The reason for using elastic bandages is that they stretch under pressure, which is important in the case of swelling, for instance. Elastic bandages may be obtained in flesh color. Some bandages are also medicated.

The roller bandage may be applied in different ways: circular, spiral ascending and descending, spiral reverse, figure-of-eight, monocular (eye), and melon (head). Figures 8–6 to 8–8 illustrate some of the standard forms of bandaging.

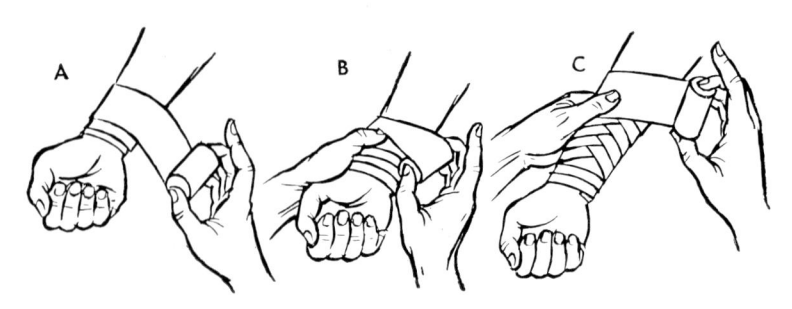

Fig. 8–6. Spiral reverse bandage for forearm. (*From American National Red Cross, "First Aid Textbook," 4th ed., Doubleday & Company, Inc., New York, 1957.*)

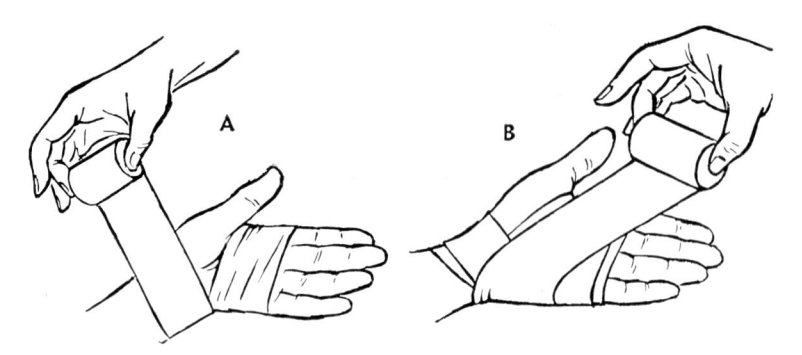

Fig. 8–7. Figure-of-eight bandage for the hand and wrist. (*From American National Red Cross, "First Aid Textbook," 4th ed., Doubleday & Company, Inc., New York, 1957.*)

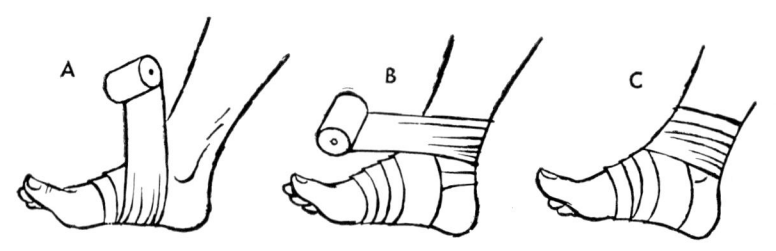

Fig. 8–8. Figure-of-eight bandage for the ankle. (*From American National Red Cross, "First Aid Textbook," 4th ed., Doubleday & Company, Inc., New York, 1957.*)

Application of the roller bandage is always started with the *inside* of the bandage facing the operator. The bandage is wrapped around the starting point two or three times, in order to anchor it firmly. It should be applied smoothly and firmly, but under no circumstances should it feel uncomfortable to the patient. In fact, the bandage should feel like a support of the injured part. The bandage is wrapped back and forth over the injured part, to ensure even distribution.

In a circular bandage, the layers should overlap slightly and be equally distant from one another. In the spiral reverse bandage, the bandage is reversed and folded back at each turn, so that the outside of the bandage faces the operator on alternate turns.

Two skin surfaces should never touch each other under a bandage. If two fingers are to be bandaged, for instance, cotton or gauze should be placed between them.

The end of the bandage is fastened with a safety pin or one of the special clamps used for this purpose. It should not, however, be fastened so that the patient may lie on the pin or clamp. Tying a bandage is sometimes indicated; that is, the last quarter yard of the bandage is cut in the middle and the ends tied around the arm, leg, or finger. This is a good emergency measure, though it does not look very neat and the ends are likely to ravel.

Roller bandages can be washed and used over again. It is important to wind them as tightly as possible in rolling them up, for a loosely rolled bandage cannot be properly applied.

A supply of bandages in assorted widths should always be kept on hand, if the practice of the doctor requires their use.

Triangular Bandage. The triangular bandage consists of a triangular-shaped piece of muslin. A square piece of material folded diagonally in half will, of course, produce a triangular piece. The triangular bandage is used principally as a sling to support an arm, chin, or jaw. It may also be used to hold a dressing in place on the scalp or forehead, by placing the widest part on the forehead, close to the eyebrows, and tying the ends over the forehead (see Fig. 8-9). Large dressings on the chest or back may also be covered with a triangular bandage.

122   The Medical Assistant

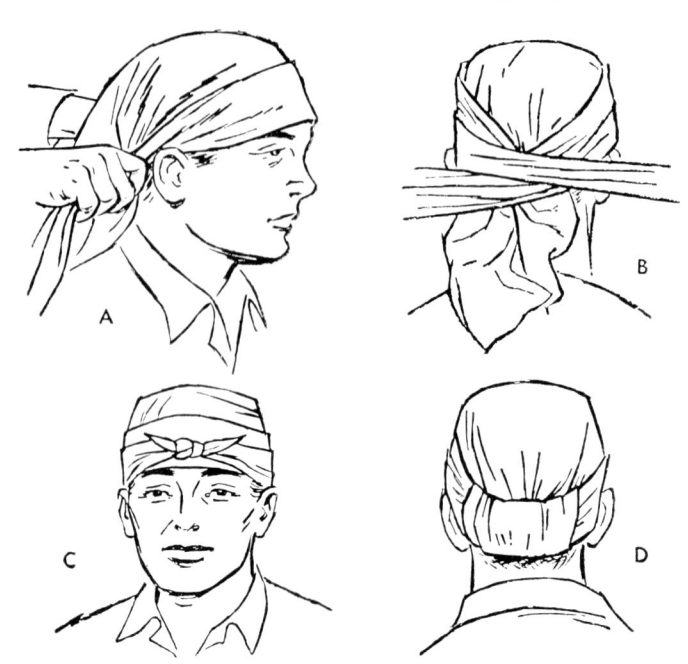

FIG. 8-9. Triangular bandage for the head. (*From American National Red Cross, "First Aid Textbook," 4th ed., Doubleday & Company, Inc., New York, 1957.*)

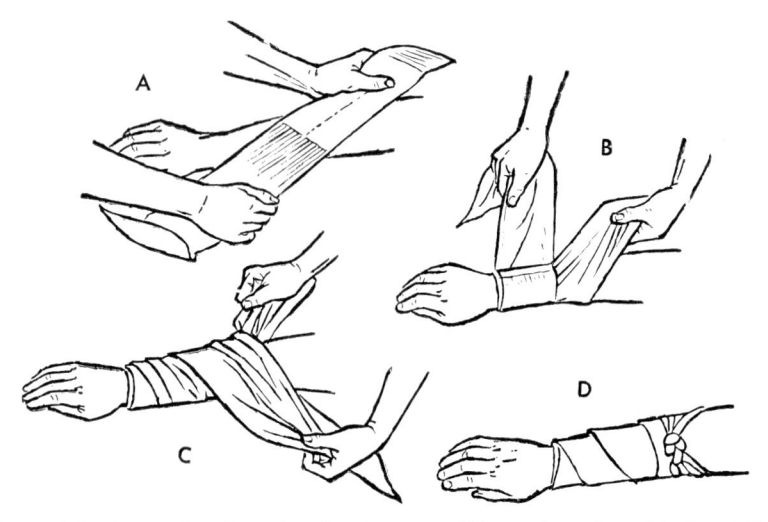

FIG. 8-10. Cravat bandage for the forearm. (*From American National Red Cross, "First Aid Textbook," 4th ed., Doubleday & Company, Inc., New York, 1957.*)

Cravat Bandage. By folding a triangular bandage in the following manner, a narrow strip bandage, called a cravat bandage, is made:

1. Fold over the long side about an inch and a half.
2. Fold the point down and tuck under the fold.
3. Fold from above to the bottom fold.

This will make a narrow bandage, about 2 in. wide, but the width may be varied as desired. Such a bandage is extremely useful for many purposes. It may serve as a tourniquet, to hold a dressing in place, or as a support. Its use on the arm is illustrated in Fig. 8–10.

Detailed descriptions and illustrations of many types of bandage are given in every book on first aid and are therefore not duplicated here.

BIBLIOGRAPHY

Christopher, Frederick: "Minor Surgery," 7th ed., W. B. Saunders Company, Philadelphia, 1956.

9

Application of Physical Therapy

Physical therapy, or physical medicine, as it is now called, means the treatment of diseases by physical means, such as water, electricity, heat, light, and mechanical forces—in contradistinction to medicinal therapy. In physical therapy, electrical treatment, light, heat, and mechanical stimulation are applied by a great variety of apparatus and machines. It is in these forms of treatment that the medical office assistant is most directly involved and of special help to the doctor.

Generally speaking, only a physiatrist, that is, a physician who specializes in physical medicine, will use the entire group of modalities in his office, and he probably will have a registered physical therapist to apply the treatments. In most doctors' offices, however, a few of these methods are used, and the administration of the treatments is usually delegated to the assistant. It must be pointed out here that in a few states the medical practice act forbids anyone but a physician or a registered physiotherapist to apply such treatments; but even in these states, although the doctor must start the treatment, the office assistant often remains with the patient and watches him during the treatment. Some acquaintance with each modality is therefore a requirement for the well-trained medical office assistant.

To understand the purpose and the effect of physical therapy, one must realize that the various modalities do not "cure" any disease. By these methods it is possible to influence the pathological physiological processes and improve circulation, thereby relieving pain, preventing stiffness of joints, improving motion, and promoting the healing of wounds. Physical therapy increases the blood and lymph circulation by application of heat and mechanical stimulation; it decreases it by cold applications. By stimulating weak muscles, it increases the circulation in them and thus strengthens them. Heat relaxes stiff tissues and encourages mobility of joints. The only chemical action definitely known is that of ultraviolet rays and the galvanic current.

Ultraviolet Light

Ultraviolet rays are the rays beyond the violet rays of the spectrum. They are a natural component of sunlight but produce very little heat; the very short rays, none at all. Their action includes the following:

1. They destroy or inhibit the growth of bacteria. For this reason they are used in operating rooms, for instance.
2. They cause erythema (redness) and tanning, whether natural sunlight or an artificial source of the rays is used.
3. They activate the formation of vitamin D, which controls the calcium metabolism, by improving the process whereby calcium is absorbed from the intestines and deposited in the bones.

Ultraviolet rays are used in a number of skin diseases, although evaluations of their usefulness have varied widely. They have been found helpful in rickets and in tuberculous skin lesions. They have sometimes been recommended to help prevent colds, or at least decrease susceptibility to colds, but claims made in this regard have not been proved. Both relaxation and stimulation have been frequently reported among subjective reactions to ultraviolet radiation.

There are various apparatus that supply ultraviolet rays. At present the lamp most commonly used is the quartz lamp, which is often referred to as "artificial sunlight." The lamp used for skin diseases is called a cold quartz lamp, because it produces no heat rays.

The intensity of the erythema produced depends on (1) the strength of the lamp, (2) the distance of the lamp from the patient, (3) the duration of exposure, and (4) the sensitivity of the patient. Dark-skinned people (those having more pigment in their skin) can take much more exposure than light-skinned people, especially those who are very fair and who freckle easily. An ultraviolet lamp is illustrated in Fig. 9–1.

To determine the sensitivity of a patient, the following method is recommended.[1] Cut about six holes in a piece of cardboard. Place the cardboard on the patient's arm and place the patient under the lamp. Cover the holes with paper. Expose the first hole for 1 minute; then expose the second hole; then the third, fourth, fifth, and sixth, at 1-minute intervals, so that the first hole is exposed 6 minutes and the last, 1 minute. The holes that fail to show a reaction determine the suberythema dose. The effect should be observed after 6 hours. For an illustration of this technique, see Fig. 9–2.

Erythema is classified into suberythema (no redness), erythema (redness), second degree (blister), third degree (burn), and fourth degree (deep burn). It must be remembered that redness develops several hours after exposure.

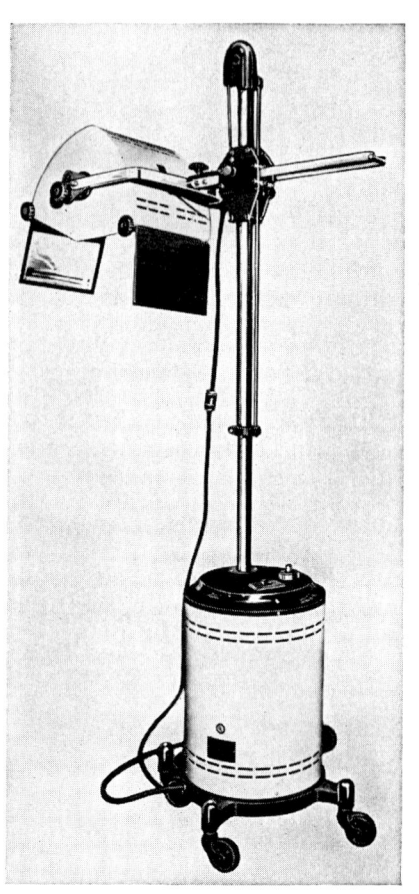

Fig. 9–1. Ultraviolet lamp. (*Hanovia Chemical & Mfg. Co.*)

In general, the treatment is given for ½ to 1 minute the first time, with the lamp 3 ft. away; then the time is increased by ½ or 1 minute each day. The strength of the light source must be taken into consideration. Some lamps are so constructed that they are

[1] Heinrich F. Wolf, "The Practice of Physical Medicine," Wilcox & Follett Company, Chicago, 1947.

APPLICATION OF PHYSICAL THERAPY 127

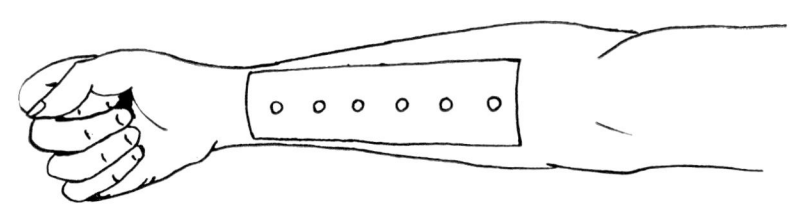

FIG. 9-2. Device to determine a patient's sensitivity to light from a given source.

shut off automatically by a clock. If the lamp is not equipped with such a clock, the treatment *must be* stopped should the attendant have to leave the patient (to answer the telephone, for instance); otherwise, severe burns may occur.

Only the part to be treated should be exposed. If the whole body is to be treated, the genital regions and the breasts of women should always be covered. Both the patient and the operator should protect their eyes by wearing dark goggles, to prevent conjunctivitis.

Heat

Superficial heat is produced by lamps, infrared radiation, and the microtherm (a heat generator of smaller wavelength than infrared). Infrared radiation represents the rays with a lower frequency than those of the red end of the spectrum. They are heat or thermal rays.

Application of heat is permissible only if the blood circulation in the treated part is increased by the treatment and the tissues which are under the influence of heat are cooled by the circulating blood. If the arteries are occluded (arteriosclerosis) and the blood supply is reduced, the cooling is inadequate, and burns will develop. It is therefore very important not to use too much heat, especially in the feet and legs, where the circulation may be poor.

Heat lamps must be kept at the correct distance, from 2 to 4 ft. as a rule. The stronger the heat, the farther away the apparatus must be. The duration of treatment is about 15 to 20 minutes. There is no particular difference in the action of the various infrared apparatus.

Heat may also be applied by a hot-water bag made of rubber, metal, or glass. Electric heating pads, as well as electric blankets, are used because of their simplicity and cleanliness. This is the method of choice when dry heat is to be applied in the patient's home.

Poultices. Poultices have been used from time immemorial to apply strong heat to a small surface. Linseed poultices were extremely popular until a short time ago. To make this type of poultice, linseed is heated with a little water in a double boiler and placed on a towel or a cloth; the poultice is then applied to the affected part. Such poultices keep hot for an hour, but care must be taken that they are not too hot when first applied. They should be tested with the back of the hand.

In recent years ready-made poultices of various sorts have been available commercially. They are placed in hot water and then applied. They keep their heat for many hours, and when they cool off, they can be heated over again.

Galvanic, Sinusoidal, and Faradic Currents

These three modalities all represent currents of low voltage and are generally supplied by one apparatus. On such an apparatus, each modality is clearly marked, so that one may choose the one desired, galvanic, faradic, or sinusoidal—continuous or interrupted.

The sinusoidal and faradic currents, which are alternating currents, are used mainly for the stimulation of weak muscles whose nerve supply is normal. Both currents have the same physiological effect. They cause contractions, which in turn, increase the blood supply of the muscle and thus help the muscle gain strength. They are ineffective if the muscle does not contract.

Galvanic current, which is a direct current, is used for stimulating muscles whose nerve supply has been disturbed or lost completely. Such muscles do not contract when stimulated by faradic or sinusoidal currents, but they do react to galvanic current.

To stimulate muscles, the current must be interrupted. This is done by an interrupter built into the apparatus or by a hand interrupter. A hand interrupter is illustrated in Fig. 9–3. The button electrode must be soaked thoroughly in a salt solution. All three currents must be applied with electrodes padded with cotton that

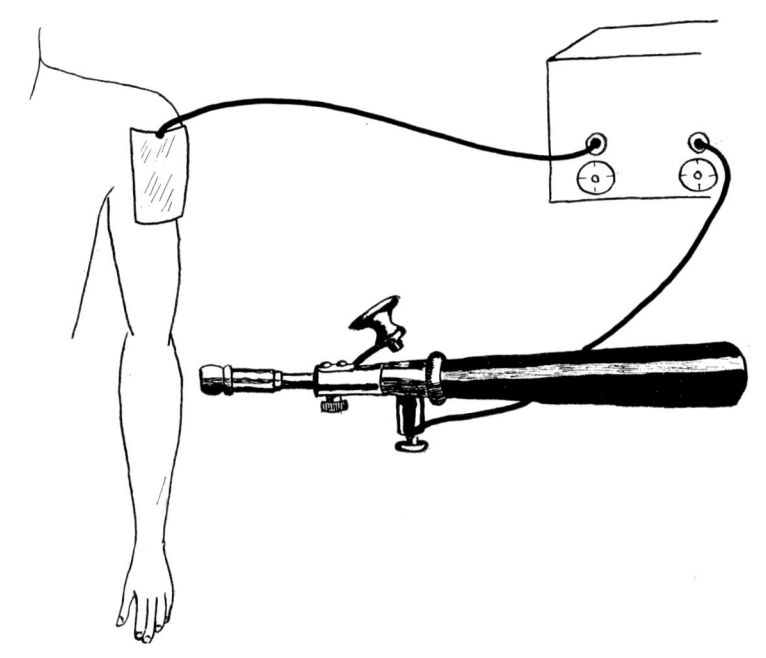

FIG. 9-3. Hand interrupter.

has been soaked in salt water; otherwise, severe wounds may result.

The constant galvanic current is used to carry substances such as histamine or penicillin from an electrode into the body. For application of the constant current, a large (indifferent) padded electrode is placed on the body where it is most convenient, and a small (active) electrode on the place to be treated. The active electrode is soaked with the substance to be introduced into the body. The positive (+) and the negative (−) poles are indicated very distinctly on the apparatus. The active electrode is connected with the positive pole in this treatment. The current must be started from zero and increased very gradually. The gadget regulating the current is called the rheostat.

Diathermy

The most frequently used modality in both general and specialized practice is the diathermy apparatus. Diathermy creates heat *within* the tissues by changing electrical energy into heat. Only so-called short-wave diathermy on three prescribed wavelengths is now permitted to be used, according to the rules of the Federal Communications Commission. The reason for this is that the old-time long-wave diathermy machines interfered with radio transmission.

When the current is turned on in a diathermy machine, an electric field is formed between two electrodes, and any part of the body placed within this field is heated up. If the electrodes are in order and not too much energy is used, there is no danger in the application, *provided that no metal parts, such as rings, hairpins, buckles, or garters, are within the field.* The assistant must make sure that the patient has removed any metal object within the field from his person. Severe burns may occur if this warning is not heeded, as the metal will become heated. The patient must lie on a wooden bed or sit on a wooden chair.

Diathermy relaxes the tissues and therefore dilates the blood vessels, thus improving the circulation. It has been found that very mild applications of short-wave diathermy dilate only the blood and lymph capillaries and not the arteries, with the result that an edema (swelling) is drained, and pain and swelling decrease or disappear. Higher temperatures increase the arterial blood supply by dilating the arteries. This leads to higher pressure in the affected region and interference with the capillary circulation. In other words, the local inflow of blood is greater than the outflow, and increased edema, pain, and inflammation result.

However, Heinrich F. Wolf states: [1] "This seems important only if we have to deal with edematous tissue. In tissues with normal circulation, and where no edema exists, even stronger currents do not increase the volume, as the capillaries can take care of the additional blood supply, following the dilatation of the arteries." Mild short waves are therefore recommended for all acute inflammatory conditions because these conditions are almost always accompanied by swelling. For chronic conditions, on the other hand, where the problem is to improve the circulation, higher intensities are indicated.

[1] Wolf, *op. cit.*, p. 185.

APPLICATION OF PHYSICAL THERAPY 131

Technique. Short-wave diathermy is applied by means of electrodes of various sorts: (1) air-spaced electrodes (plastic disks attached by movable arms to the apparatus), which can be applied to each side of the head, shoulder, or whatever part is to be treated (see Fig. 9–4); (2) contour electrodes (Fig. 9–5); (3) flexible inductance applicators (Fig. 9–6); (4) inductance cable, made of rubber cable, which may be coiled around the part to be treated or

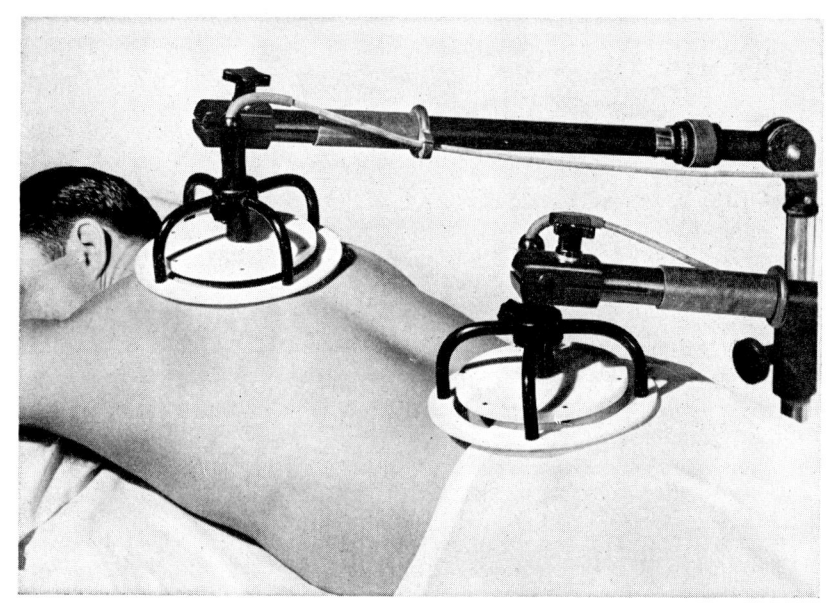

FIG. 9–4. Application of short-wave diathermy, using air-spaced electrodes. (*The Burdick Corporation.*)

used in pancake form but must be applied over a towel (see Fig. 9–7).

Before the treatment is started, the assistant should make sure that the machine is plugged in, that the electrodes to be used are in readiness, and that a chair, bed, or table is provided so that the patient will be completely comfortable during the treatment.

The electrodes are put in place *before* the current is turned on. The strength of the current is controlled by several dials similar to those on a radio. In fact, if one remembers that the construction of a diathermy machine is essentially the same as that of a radio,

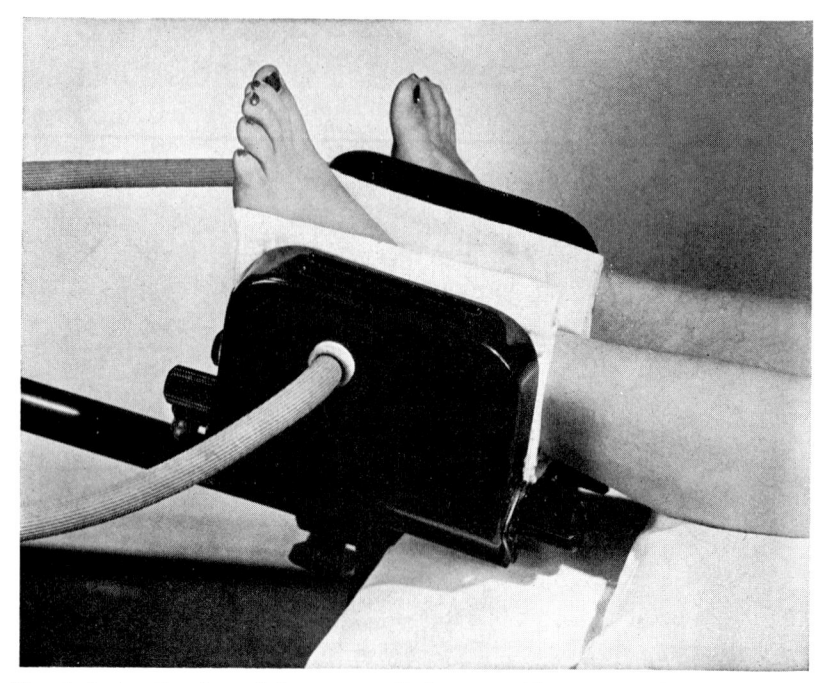

FIG. 9-5. Application of short-wave diathermy with contour electrodes. (*The Burdick Corporation.*)

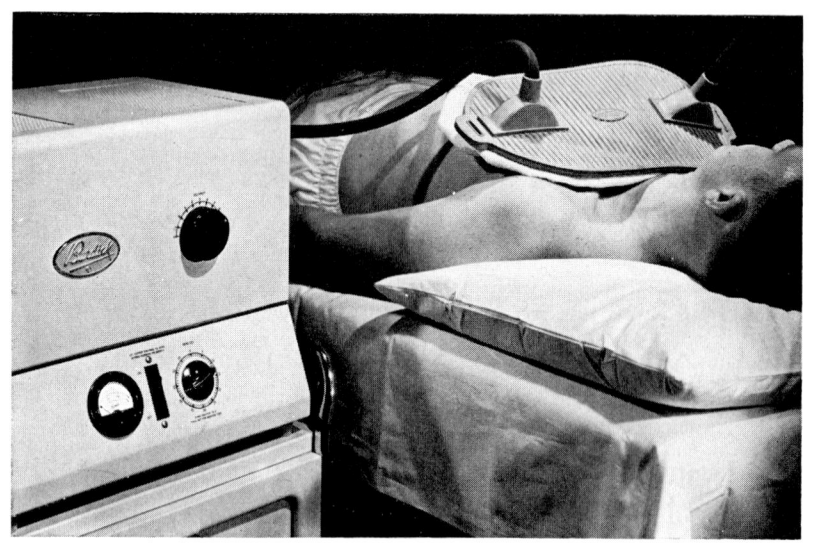

FIG. 9-6. Application of short-wave diathermy with flexible inductance applicators. (*The Burdick Corporation.*)

APPLICATION OF PHYSICAL THERAPY 133

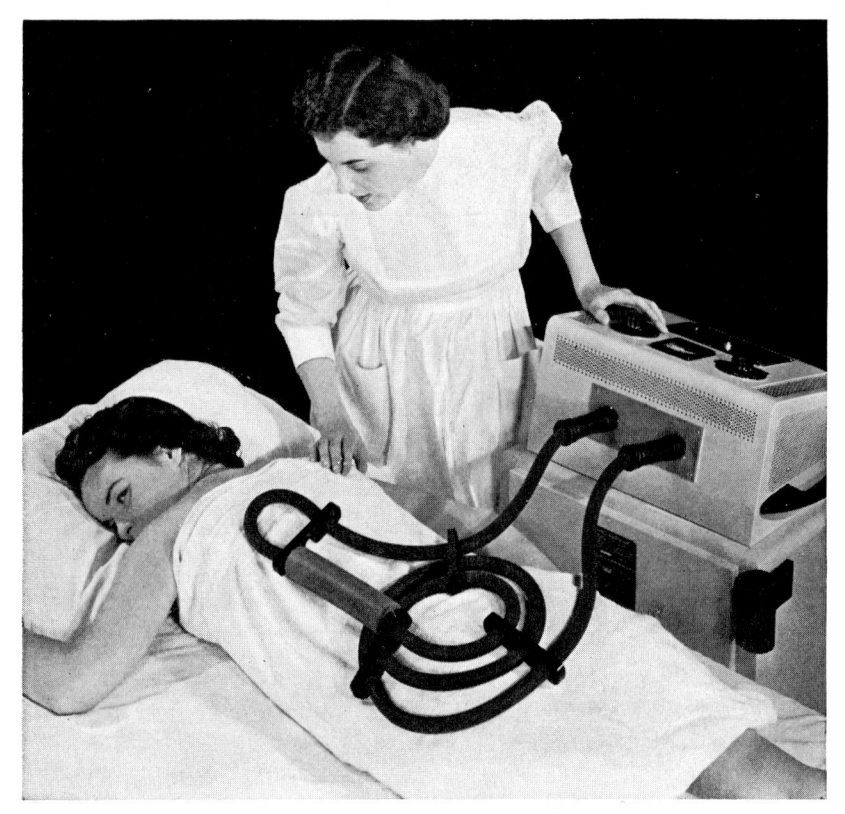

Fig. 9-7. Application of short-wave diathermy with inductance cable. (*The Burdick Corporation.*)

it is easy to understand its operation: (1) move a switch to turn on the current; (2) then tune in the machine by manipulating a dial until the needle stands at its highest point; (3) finally, regulate the other dial to provide the power wanted. (The dials differ somewhat in the different brands of apparatus.) The power must be increased *very gradually*. The two electric cords connected with the electrodes must never touch one another. Duration of the treatment is usually 15 to 20 minutes.

If mild short waves are used, the patient should barely feel the heat. With more intensive treatment, he should have a comfortable feeling of warmth. If the patient complains that the treatment is too hot, the treatment must be stopped immediately. It is advisable to explain this to the patient beforehand, as many patients will endure uncomfortable heat because they believe this to be necessary and do not want to appear too sensitive. If diathermy is applied over a bone, for instance the wrist, and the current is too strong, the patient feels a severe dull ache in the bone. This disappears immediately if the current is reduced in strength. Every machine should have a cutoff switch, and this should be shown to the patient, so that he can turn off the current immediately if he feels too hot.

Ultrasonic Therapy

One of the newest modalities in physical medicine is the ultrasonic generator, which produces a frequency of 1,000,000 vibrations per second. The ultrasonic waves (waves that are faster than sound waves) penetrate deeply into the tissues—in fact they can penetrate into and through a bone. They produce heat when the applicator is held steadily in one place, but they are rarely used for this purpose, because there are better and less dangerous means of producing heat. The vibrations, however, constitute a massage in the deep tissues, and they are therefore used in the treatment of deep-lying pain or of scars, where they loosen the tissue.

Ultrasound is applied by means of an applicator in the shape of a mace with a sound head of about 2 in. in diameter. Water or oil must be spread on the part to be treated, to protect the skin. The sound head is moved steadily up and down and in a rotary motion over the skin. If the applicator is not moved, internal burns and destruction of tissue may result. For the technique of application, refer to Fig. 9–8, but remember that the applicator must be moved. Duration of treatment is usually about 10 minutes.

Another technique for applying ultrasound on a hand or a foot is to place the hand or the foot into a basin of water, immerse the applicator to within about an inch of the hand or foot, and move it up and down in a rotary motion.

Massage

Massage is probably the oldest form of physical therapy. The person who instinctively rubs the place where he has hurt himself,

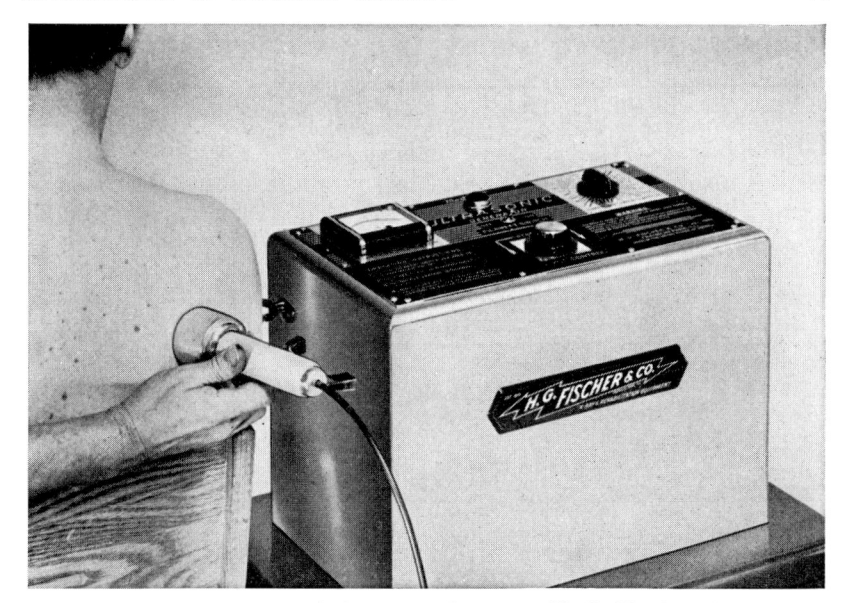

FIG. 9-8. Application of ultrasonic therapy. (*H. G. Fischer & Co.*)

the mother who strokes the spot where her child has injured himself—both practice the very type of massage that is used in a doctor's office, that is, medical massage.

There are several types of massage:

1. Effleurage—stroking
2. Friction—stroking or rubbing deeper tissue
3. Petrissage—rolling or kneading
4. Tapotement—tapping or beating the body with the fingers or the sides of the hands
5. Vibration—quick tapping, alternating all finger tips

The so-called Swedish and reducing types of massage are not practiced in a doctor's office.

The type of massage most frequently used in a doctor's office is effleurage. Though special training is needed for the other types, this is easy to apply. In effleurage, the hands must be completely relaxed. The best way to describe the procedure is to say that it is the sort of stroking used in a caress, with the difference that more pressure is exerted. The motion originates from the shoulder; the fingers must remain relaxed. The basic position of the hands is shown in Fig. 9-9.

The purpose of massage is first of all as an aid to circulation, inasmuch as the venous blood is carried toward the heart. Secondly, there is a subsidiary effect in that waste products, such as blood in the tissues after an injury, are removed and forced into the blood and lymph stream, while fresh blood, which aids the healing process, is brought to the injured part. This principle is illustrated by the

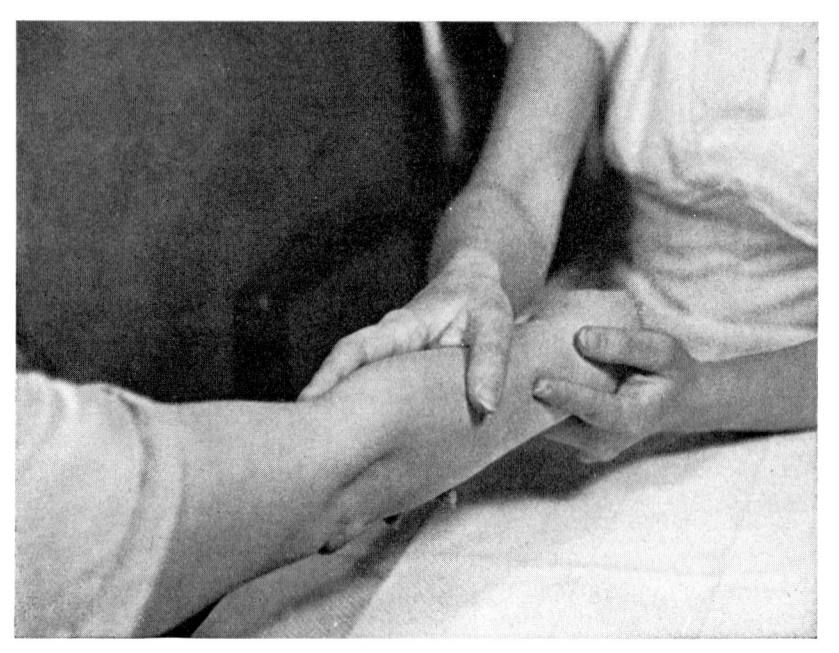

Fig. 9-9. Basic position of hands for massage.

following well-known example: If a person sustains an insect bite or sting, the site of the bite, where the poison was injected, becomes red and swollen and painful. If this spot is massaged immediately, the poison is carried into the blood stream, where it is diluted and becomes harmless, so that no swelling results.

Pathological conditions of the joints are often greatly relieved by massage. Again the physiological reason is the same: increased blood circulation brings fresh blood to the affected tissues, carries off debris (wreckage), and aids in restoring motion and in recovery. It also relaxes the muscles, and this benefits motion and reduces pain.

Frequently after an injection, soreness and swelling occur. This can be greatly relieved by massaging the sore part. When an injection of a very irritating substance or a very large amount has been given, massage should be applied immediately after the injection to prevent swelling. One might say that any injury is benefited by massage, provided that the skin is intact. Almost everybody is familiar with the soothing, relaxing effect of massage; and it is therefore easy to understand that massage will benefit sore muscles, swollen joints, and painful swellings.

There are, however, a number of conditions in which massage is strictly contraindicated. They are listed here for the guidance of the medical office assistant:

1. Any skin infection or rash
2. Suppurative (pus-forming) processes or infections
3. Open wounds or cuts
4. Malignant tumors
5. Hyperesthesia (excessive sensibility) of the skin

When applying massage, the operator, as well as the patient, should be completely comfortable; otherwise, the operator would quickly feel a strain and her arms would become tense. Her hands should always be warm, so as not to be unpleasant to the patient. Warm hands relax more easily too. Holding the hands under hot water for a few minutes will warm them quickly if they are too cold to apply massage. If the hands are moist, a lubricant should be used. Talcum powder effects better and smoother gliding. Massage should *never hurt*, or it will harm rather than help the patient.

Exercises

Therapeutic exercises are currently used a great deal in the rehabilitation of a variety of conditions. Calisthenics is one type; underwater exercises, another. These are given in hospitals only, under the supervision of a specially trained technician.

In a doctor's office, exercises may be given to restore motion after a joint fracture or an injury; after immobilization resulting in stiff joints; or, especially in the office of an orthopedist, after poliomyelitis. Such exercises consist of passive and active exercises, in which the operator moves the patient's extremity, makes the patient move it by himself, or makes him move it against resistance. There may be special apparatus in the office for the patient to operate. The doctor prescribes and demonstrates these exercises, but the assistant supervises them or works with the patient. As exercises are most frequently carried on in the office of orthopedists, they are discussed in Chapter 13 under Orthopedics.

Hydrotherapy

One important phase of physical therapy is the use of water. This may be in the form of whirlpool baths, hot or cold showers, hot or cold wet compresses, baths, or wet packs. All these are given mostly in the hospital or the patient's home, and rarely come within the duties of the medical office assistant. They are mentioned here only for the sake of completeness in enumerating the various physical therapy modalities.

One exception, however, may be wet dressings, as there may be occasions when the doctor will tell the patient to use a wet dressing —for instance, in the case of a sore throat, a bruise, or a sprain. If the patient does not know how to apply a wet dressing, he may ask the assistant about the procedure, and she should be able to explain it to him.

A large handkerchief or a towel should be dipped into cold water and wrung out to prevent dripping, but it should still be quite moist. (Burow's solution might be added to the water in 1:10 strength.) The towel is put over the part to be treated and then completely covered with either a rubber sheet, plastic material, or wax paper. A bandage is applied over this—if possible, a woolen covering. Such dressings should be changed every 6 to 8 hours. Wet dressings should never be used if eczema is present.

It might also be mentioned that a cold wet dressing (a wet towel into which an ice cube has been placed) reduces bleeding, as well as swelling, in fresh injuries. Immediate application of ice to a part that has come into contact with a hot object will prevent blistering.

Electrosurgery

The use of an electric current for minor surgery is another form of physical therapy. The electric current destroys or cuts tissues. Its advantage is the fact that the wound is automatically sterilized (cauterized) and self-sealed by the cutting current.

Electrosurgery is divided into:

1. The cutting current
2. Fulguration
3. Desiccation

The *cutting current* is used for the excision of small growths, such as warts or superficial blemishes; for biopsies; and for coagulation. *Fulguration* is essentially a searing of the tissue. Its use is considered limited. *Desiccation* is used for very small areas, to remove minute ulcerations (warts). As the actual contact with the tissues is longer in desiccation than in coagulation, the power employed must therefore be lower.

The instruments that are used in electrosurgery are a knife, a wire loop, or specially designed cutting electrode tips. They are attached to the machine by electric cords, like any other electrode. The instruments may be used with an ordinary diathermy machine, or they may be attached to a special electrosurgical unit. One such unit, which is especially popular, is the Hyfrecator, which is used by doctors in various specialties.

Whenever the doctor uses electrosurgery, the assistant's tasks are similar to those mentioned in Chapter 8 on Surgery in the Office. In addition, it is her responsibility to keep all the physical therapy equipment clean and see that it is in good working order. It is hardly ever necessary to sterilize any part of these apparatus, but they must be wiped clean after use. The machines must be dusted and occasionally polished. If the apparatus is not working properly, a repairman must be called in. Whenever the electric cords begin to show signs of wear, they should be changed; for frayed cords are not only unsightly but dangerous, in that they may cause a short circuit.

10

Preparations for X-rays

The practice of radiology, that is, the application of x-rays or roentgen rays (so called after their discoverer, Wilhelm Konrad Roentgen), is a distinct medical specialty. Radiologists limit their practice to the taking of radiographs, or x-ray pictures, as they are popularly called; their interpretation; and x-ray treatment. But many physicians in other specialties also have an x-ray machine in their office, in order to take x-rays pertinent to their specialty. If x-rays are taken while the patient is in the office for an examination or for treatment, a great deal of time is saved. Also, the patient is less inconvenienced if he does not have to visit another doctor's office just to have x-rays taken. X-ray therapy is usually given by radiologists.

The x-ray technician who works for a radiologist (or in an x-ray department of a hospital) must have a thorough knowledge of anatomy, for he is called upon to take x-rays of every part of the body. He must also be thoroughly familiar with the fundamentals of electricity and the application of these fundamentals to the operation of x-ray equipment, so that he will be able to operate any type of machine he may encounter. A physician who is not a radiologist but who has an x-ray machine will of course prefer a medical office assistant who has had training in x-ray technique. Only a few such fully trained assistants are available, however, and most doctors must therefore train their own aides. Under these circumstances the doctor will teach his assistant how to operate his machine, how to develop films, and how to position the patient for the particular procedures needed in his specialty. It is also necessary for the assistant to learn some general rules regarding protection, preparation of the patient, and record keeping. This chapter is concerned with the latter duties and is written for the guidance of an assistant who is learning to be an x-ray technician while on the job.

Danger of X-rays

First of all, the assistant should keep in mind the fact that x-rays constitute a potential danger and that she must at all times take proper precautions so as not to expose herself to the rays. The unit used for determining x-ray dosage is the *roentgen*. According to the International X-ray and Radium Protection Committee, the safe allowable exposure to x-rays for a person of normal health is about 3/10 of a roentgen a week. X-rays penetrate deeply, and continued exposure could result in destruction of tissues.

Each x-ray machine is equipped with a lead screen behind which the technician stands while taking the x-ray. As the time of exposure is so short—actually a fraction of a second—the tendency is to become careless. But frequent exposure can in time have a deleterious effect. Also, rays scatter and may bombard the operator during exposure. The following simple test is recommended as a means of determining how much radiation is absorbed. The operator clips a dental film to the pocket of her uniform and after a week has the film developed. If the results show that it has been exposed, she must take greater care. A small package of dental films may be ordered from the supplier of the x-ray films, and the test made at least once monthly to guard against careless exposure.

Most x-ray machines are also equipped with a fluoroscopy screen. This apparatus, which permits visual examination of deep tissues by means of roentgen rays, is handled exclusively by the physician. If the aide is asked to assist him—by supporting the patient, for instance—she must wear a lead apron.

Attitude toward the Patient

It is the assistant's duty to take the patient to the x-ray room and prepare him for the procedure. It must be remembered that most patients are rather fearful of x-rays. They are afraid of the machine, of the danger about which they may have heard, of the discomfort involved, and of the diagnosis that will be made as the result of the x-rays. The assistant must be friendly, cheerful, and reassuring. While the x-ray procedure may be a routine matter to her, she must remember that to the patient it is a major event and not a pleasant one. She must show that she respects and understands his attitude.

As she comes into very close contact with the patient while helping him onto the table or adjusting his position for the x-rays, there must be no trace of any odor about her, such as from smoking, heavy perfume, or perspiration. If the assistant wears an apron in the darkroom while developing the films and this has become stained, something that is unavoidable, she should take it off before working with the patient. A laboratory coat or an apron with large, dark stains can be most repellent and may actually cause some sensitive patients to become ill.

A word of caution: It is against the law in almost every state for anyone but the physician to make a diagnosis from x-rays. The patient is usually anxious to find out what is the matter with him and will often inquire from the technician about the results of the x-rays. She must tactfully decline to give this information, even when she herself can easily read the film. Nor should she discuss interpretation of films with other patients or show films of one patient to another.

Preparation of the Patient

General Rules. Certain preparations are necessary for every patient who is going to have radiographs taken. Clothing must be removed from the part to be x-rayed. For an x-ray of the foot or leg, it is only necessary, of course, to take off the shoe and stocking. For an x-ray of any part of the trunk, all clothing should be removed. Usually a special dressing room is provided. If the patient has to undress in the x-ray room, the assistant should leave the room for a while to give the patient some privacy.

If the patient has to undress entirely, an examination gown is given him. Although the examination gown is loose and shapeless, it should be long enough and wide enough to cover the patient properly, yet not so large that the patient has difficulty managing it.

The patient's modesty must be taken into consideration at all times. The laundry should be instructed not to starch these gowns, not only because starched gowns are uncomfortable, but also because they may throw a shadow on the film. It is important to explain to the patient just what garments to remove and how to put on the examination gown. In some offices, crepe-paper slippers are provided.

No metal parts should be in the field of the roentgen rays. Patients, therefore, must remove all jewelry, tie clasps, belt buckles, girdles with metal garter fasteners. A woman should be instructed to place all her jewelry in her handbag and take this with her into the x-ray room. If part of the head is to be x-rayed, dentures must be taken out, and eyeglasses, hairpins, or earrings removed. Tissues should be given to the patient so that he may wrap his dentures in them. Bandages, dressings, or splints may not be removed without the express order of the physician.

Patients coming for x-rays are often injured, handicapped, or in pain. They may need help in getting to the x-ray room and getting on and off the x-ray table. A definite technique is required for an operator to lift a patient without strain. The body should be flexed at the hips, as this gives the operator more strength and puts less strain on the back muscles than if the back were bent. A footstool should be in front of the x-ray table, as the table is usually higher than most persons can reach comfortably.

Always explain to the patient what is going to be done and what is expected of him. Ask him courteously to lie still, to move up or down, to flex his leg, or to do whatever may be necessary. Always remember that he may be excited and therefore not concentrating on your remarks. Do not become impatient if he carries out your instructions incorrectly.

The assistant should show concern for the patient's comfort. Whenever possible, a small pillow should be placed under the head. The x-ray room and the dressing room should be comfortably warm and free from drafts. A blanket should be within easy reach to cover the patient if he complains of being cold or if he must wait a few moments between having radiographs taken. All adjustments on the machine should be made before the patient is placed on the table, as the table is hard and most uncomfortable.

Fracture injuries are probably the cases most frequently x-rayed. Patients with fractures generally have severe pain and must be handled with great care. One of the most important functions of the assistant in placing the injured part on the table is to relax completely and follow the movements of the patient; that is, she should place both hands under the injured part, tell the patient how the part should be placed, and then follow his movements with her hands and arms under the injured part. Her own movements must be slow and steady so as not to jar the patient. This of course holds true for any painful part, not only for fractures.

The patient may have to be turned on his side, and this may present a problem if he is in pain, handicapped, or very heavy. It is advisable to place such a patient on a sheet or blanket. When he is to be turned, grasp both ends of the sheet on the side opposite the one toward which the patient is to be turned. Pull the sheet or blanket toward you to start the patient turning, and then push him gently in the desired direction.

If the patient is ill or in pain, he may feel faint when getting up from the x-ray table; therefore, spirits of ammonia and a basin, in case the patient has to vomit, should be on hand.

Special X-ray Examinations. In addition to viewing the bones of the body, it is possible, by x-ray examination, to observe the outline of internal organs and to determine certain physiological functions. This is done by means of materials that are visible on x-ray films. They are called contrast media and are administered to the patient internally. Preparing a patient for these special procedures requires specific knowledge and careful attention to all the details involved.

First of all, the assistant must be familiar with the different materials that are used in these procedures. They may be given orally or by intravenous injection. It will be her task to prepare them and, when they are given orally, to administer them. It is therefore necessary for her to know beforehand just what the doctor is planning to do in each case. Some of the procedures that are carried out routinely in doctors' offices are briefly discussed here. The setup for these procedures follows the principles set forth in the preceding chapters on examinations and injections. Special instruments that the doctor uses may be added.

Gastrointestinal Series. This is an examination of the digestive tract by means of fluoroscopy and radiographs. An opaque material, usually barium sulfate, is taken orally by the patient. This material shows up on x-ray films and thus makes the digestive tract clearly distinguishable.

The preparation of the patient begins before he comes to the office. The assistant must explain the procedure to him when making his appointment. If the patient understands what is to be done and the reason for it, he will cooperate much better. He should be instructed not to eat or drink anything after the midnight preceding the appointment, not even medications that he may be taking regularly.

Appointments for a gastrointestinal series should always be made for early morning, as soon as the office opens. The barium sulfate is prepared according to directions and given to the patient to drink. It may be mixed with plain water or with buttermilk. Some ready-made barium preparations are chocolate-flavored and therefore more palatable. When the patient has swallowed the mixture, a fluoroscopic examination of the patient is done by the doctor and x-rays are taken.

After the x-rays have been taken, the patient may dress and leave, but he must return 3 to 5 hours later for another roentgenogram. The purpose of this is to determine how quickly the stomach empties and to observe how far the barium has advanced in the intestinal tract. The patient may not eat anything during the 3- to 5-hour period, as food would interfere with the test. After the second group of x-rays has been taken, the patient may eat whatever food the doctor permits. When making the appointment with the patient, the assistant should mention this second visit to him, so that he may arrange for the time.

Frequently another examination is made 24 hours later to determine the condition of the large bowel. If the barium meal, which by this time should have advanced into the large bowel, does not fill it sufficiently, a barium enema is given. Before this is administered, a cleansing enema of a soap solution should be given to evacuate the colon of all fecal matter. The patient should have no breakfast before this examination, as the doctor often wishes to have another x-ray taken of the stomach at that time.

Cholecystography. This is radiography of the gallbladder after it has been made visible by opaque material. For this procedure the patient is instructed to have a light, fat-free meal the evening before, consisting mainly of fruit, salad, and vegetables and prepared without butter or oil. The opaque material, or dye, is taken by the patient after the meal, usually in the form of tablets. Directions for taking them must be carefully followed and should be discussed with the patient. The tablets usually have to be taken a few minutes apart with a little water or fruit juice. Once the tablets have been taken, no food or liquid should be consumed. Occasionally the dye is administered intravenously in the doctor's office.

The x-rays are taken the following morning, about 12 to 14 hours after the medication has been ingested. Following these x-rays, the patient should have a fatty meal. He may either be sent to a restaurant and instructed to eat eggs, ice cream, buttered toast, etc.; or (often more practical) he may be given a commercially prepared meal at the office. Another x-ray is taken about an hour after this meal has been eaten.

Pyelography. This is an x-ray examination of the kidneys. For this examination, a cathartic should be taken the evening before, and an enema in the morning. No food or fluids should be taken after midnight. The contrast medium is given intravenously just before the examination.

Hysterosalpingography. This is discussed in Chapter 12 under Gynecology and Obstetrics.

Other procedures, such as cholangiography, bronchography, myelography, angiography, and visualization of the ventricular system of the brain, are not discussed here, as they are usually carried out at the hospital or in the office of a radiologist.

Administrative Routine

In the office of a doctor who has an x-ray department, certain administrative duties devolve on the medical office assistant. All x-rays that are taken should be entered on the medical history record with the date and the results as determined by the doctor. In the x-ray room itself there should be a record book in which consecutive entries are made for each patient, showing the date and the type and number of x-rays taken. This should be kept as a permanent record for a number of years.

Lead letters and numerals should be available, so that the date and the name of the patient can be marked on each film. Films should be placed in film envelopes and filed strictly alphabetically in metal filing cabinets specially designed for this purpose.

The films are the property of the doctor, even though the patient has paid for them. They may be sent to a hospital or to another doctor for examination, but should always be returned to the office where they were originally taken. If a film is removed from the cabinet, a note to that effect should be filed in place of the film. All films should be filed promptly and not left lying around the office.

An x-ray department requires much in the way of equipment and supplies, and this represents a considerable expense. Equipment should therefore be handled carefully and kept clean and in good repair. Supplies should not be wasted. Above all, the department must look clean and neat in every aspect. Cassettes, hangers, sandbags—all paraphernalia should have their proper place and be returned to place after use. It is most distressing for a patient to enter an x-ray room in which these items are scattered about on every chair and table.

A sufficient supply of films in all sizes should always be on hand. New films should be ordered when only half a box remains. However, as x-ray films, like every other type of photographic film, must be used within a specified time, an excess amount should not be ordered, for the films may become outdated. Experience will tell approximately how many films of each size are being used each month.

The developing and fixer solutions may be ordered from a supply house that will empty the tanks and refill them with fresh solution. These solutions may also be ordered in concentrated form and then mixed by the assistant. The important thing is to renew the supply before the solution loses so much of its strength that x-ray films are spoiled because of it.

BIBLIOGRAPHY

Scoggins, Marcella L. Cunningham: "Preparing Patients for X-ray Examinations," *The American Journal of Nursing*, January, 1957, pp. 76–79.

Sante, L. R.: "Manual of Roentgenological Technique," 18th ed., Edwards Brothers, Inc., Ann Arbor, Mich., 1956.

11

Treatment and Diet

Since time immemorial, both medical and nonmedical persons have been concerned about diet. A host of misunderstandings, misinformation, and downright superstitions abound on this subject. The French have a proverb that says that melons must not be eaten in the summer; in countries where mangoes grow, it is believed they should be eaten in the forenoon only; lobster and ice cream are believed to be harmful if eaten at the same meal.

Soups are supposed to be fattening. Obviously a clear broth is not fattening, though a soup made of cream, eggs, and flour would be. In fact, hot soup dilates the blood vessels in the stomach and, by increasing the blood supply, may aid the glands participating in the digestive process and thereby improve the process itself. The experiments made by the Russian physiologist, Ivan Pavlov, are of importance in this regard. He pointed out how greatly the mind influences the digestive organs. If an individual likes a certain food, the glands of his digestive tract, his salivary glands, and the glands of his stomach function better. Appetizing food "makes our mouth water." We digest food we like better than food we don't like. The Eskimos like blubber. The average American would become nauseated if he had to eat it.

People often maintain that a vegetable diet does not supply enough strength, though the horse, the ox, and the elephant, for instance, are vegetarians. It must be noted, though, that these animals have a relatively longer alimentary tract and therefore can absorb more of the nourishing material. Man's alimentary canal and his teeth make him an omnivorous animal. Not only can he mince food; he can grind it. Carnivorous animals, such as the dog and cat, have teeth for cutting only.

Regardless of individual preferences and aversions, opinions and prejudices, the food we consume affects our health in many ways. A person may eat in bulk all he can consume and yet be undernourished because vital constituents are missing from his diet. This is a comparatively recent discovery. The crews of seafaring expeditions who subsisted on salted meats without fruit and vegetables for long periods of time succumbed to scurvy, which was promptly relieved when the men ate citrus fruits, which contain vitamin C.

In Southern Europe thousands of people have died of pellagra, which today is known to be due to a lack of vitamin B complex. In the refining of wheat, this vitamin, which is contained in the membrane, was lost. Similarly, in the Orient, where polished rice is the staple and often the complete diet, there is a prevalence of beriberi, due to lack of vitamins, especially B_1, which is contained in the hull of the rice kernel.

There are many conditions for which a special diet is indicated and may constitute a part of the treatment or, occasionally, the entire treatment. If one wanted to quibble, he might say that there is no hard and fast line between diet therapy and treatment with medication. For are not vitamins, liver extracts, etc., which are bought at the pharmacy, food? Both food and medicine are chemical compounds; however, when a diet is prescribed by the doctor, this usually means that certain foods must be taken and others omitted and that the quantity of the food is regulated. Even the hour and the time interval when food is to be taken may be specified.

Although dietetics is still an empiric science, there are a few specific rules based on our knowledge of physiology and pathology. Sugars or starches must not be eaten by diabetics unless controlled by insulin or medication. Fatty foods should be avoided by persons suffering from diseases of the liver and gallbladder, because the liver does not secrete bile properly when given too much fat. Salt must be withheld from patients whose condition is due to salt retention. Rough food must be forbidden to patients suffering from stomach ulcers.

No general rules can be established, because controlled diet experiments on human beings are not feasible. In any event, they would not be conclusive, as individuals react differently to different foods. It is for this reason that physicians modify a given diet according to their own preferences.

The doctor prescribes the diet, but it is often the assistant's duty to discuss the details with the patient, answer questions, and explain certain points. Most patients hesitate to ask the doctor about the details of a diet, because they feel that such matters are too trivial for his concern. Sometimes the questions involve such simple matters as the preparation of a food item—how long the food should be cooked, what cooking utensils should be used—and other domestic details that the patient may feel the assistant would be in a better position to explain than the doctor. Naturally the assistant should be able to answer routine questions regarding the diets her doctor-employer prescribes. She can do so intelligently only if she has some basic knowledge about nutrition and diet in general.

Although Hippocrates wrote a book about it over 2,000 years ago, diet as a systematic form of therapy is of comparatively recent origin. Before such treatment could be put on a scientific basis, a science of nutrition had to be established. That is, it was necessary to ascertain the components of foods; to determine what substances are necessary, beneficial, or harmful to health; and to discover which foods contain these substances.

Constituents of Food

It would lead us too far astray to relate the history of nutrition, to analyze the various substances of which our food is composed, or to describe the processes of digestion and metabolism by which an organism utilizes the food ingested. Suffice it to state here that the constituents of food are *proteins, carbohydrates,* and *fats.*

1. *Proteins* are found in meat, fowl, fish, milk, cheese, and eggs. (Plants are poor in proteins.)

2. *Carbohydrates* are starch and sugar. Starch changes into sugar under certain conditions.

3. *Fats* may be either animal or vegetable. Vegetable fats include olive oil, linseed oil, and the oil contained in nuts and avocados.

These three substances, however, while essential for nourishment and therefore called nutrients, are not sufficient to maintain health. Vitamins and minerals are also needed. Not only is the importance of vitamins a recent discovery, but the function of some of them is not yet fully understood, nor is it certain that all the vitamins have been discovered. The following list summarizes our knowledge to date:

1. *Vitamin A* has an important role in the processes of growth, reproduction, and lactation, and acts as an aid in maintaining normal vision, resisting infection, and protecting the skin against infection. Its sources are fish-liver oils, butter, cream, egg yolks, and yellow vegetables and fruits.

2. *Vitamin B* has been found to consist of many different parts, and we therefore speak of the *vitamin B complex*, or of B_1, B_2, etc., when referring to the individual parts. The most important of those isolated so far are thiamin, riboflavin (also called *vitamin G*), niacin, and biotin (also called *vitamin H*), each of which is now obtainable in pure form and may be administered separately.

The vitamin B complex aids in many vital functions, including (in addition to those listed for vitamin A) muscle function, nerve function, metabolism, and digestion. Sources of the vitamin B complex are liver, kidney, sweetbread, heart, spleen, fish, milk, eggs, butter, and brewer's yeast.

3. *Vitamin C* (ascorbic acid) is needed for maintaining cellular health. It is found in citrus fruits, tomatoes, and most vegetables.

4. *Vitamin D* regulates calcium and phosphorus metabolism. Sources are fish-liver oils, salmon, milk, butter, and egg yolks. Direct sunshine activates the formation of this vitamin in the organism.

5. *Vitamin E* functions in a way that is not yet fully understood, but it seems essential in the utilization of vitamins A and D and also appears to have antioxidant properties. Sources are wheat germ and other seed oils and practically all leafy vegetables, though it is present in animal tissues also.

6. *Vitamin K* has a blood-clotting property and therefore constitutes a protection against bleeding. This is its most important known function. Green leafy vegetables are the best sources for this vitamin.

Vitamins A, D, E, and K are fat-soluble; vitamins B and C, water-soluble.

Dietary Requirements

The action of the different vitamins is obviously interrelated, but each one has a specific function, and a deficiency of any one of them will produce specific pathological conditions. As vitamins are now being made synthetically, they can be and are being prescribed by physicians either as a treatment for a specific condition, as a means of maintaining health, or as a preventive measure. Excess intake of vitamins, however, may lead to malfunction; the habit, so much popularized by advertising, of taking large amounts of vitamins without the prescription and supervision of a physician is to be deplored.

In addition to vitamins, the organism requires minerals—calcium, iron, phosphorus, and small amounts of many others. Minerals are contained in all vegetable and animal foods.

It will seem obvious from the above that a normal diet should be well balanced and consist of a variety of foods, so that the individual will obtain all nutrients, vitamins, and minerals necessary to maintain good health. The chart illustrated in Fig. 11-1 shows the seven basic food groups and the amounts suggested for daily consumption.

As an excess, as well as a lack, of any of the items enumerated above may cause malnutrition or other specific diseases, many physicians, when first examining a patient, inquire about his eating habits. It is often necessary for the physician to prescribe a normal, well-balanced diet in order to improve the patient's general condition. Sometimes the diet must be regulated with regard to quantity. The intake of food is judged by the number of calories consumed, as most diet-conscious persons know.

A *calorie* is defined as the amount of energy (heat) required to

154   The Medical Assistant

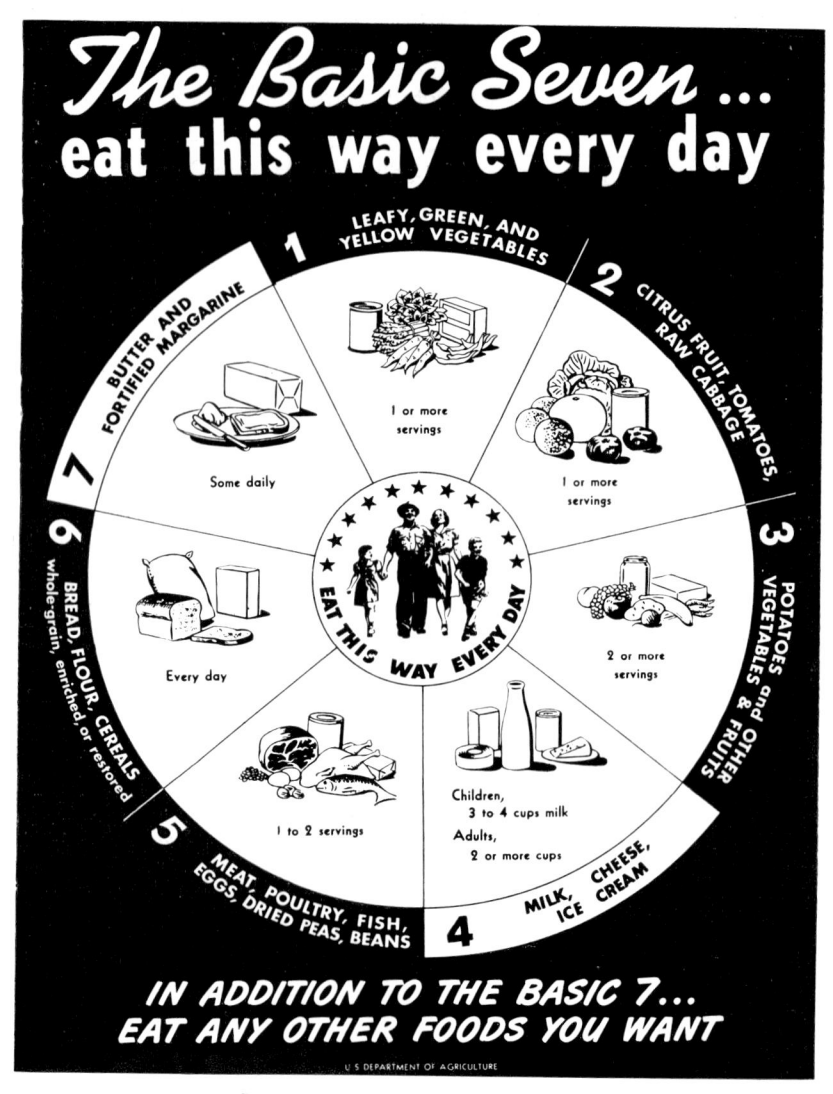

FIG. 11-1. The basic seven foods.

raise the temperature of 1 kg. of water 1° centigrade. It must be remembered that all food is fuel that produces body energy. The calorie content of most foods has been carefully determined. For instance, 1 Gm. of protein equals 4 calories; 1 Gm. of carbohydrates also equals 4 calories; and 1 Gm. of fat equals 9 calories. Most diet books give a list of the accepted calorie requirements of children

TREATMENT AND DIET 155

and adults at different ages, as well as the foods from which these requirements are best obtained. Most physicians find that such tables are useful only as a guide and that allowance must be made for wide individual variations. Certain standard diets have been formulated for different conditions, but each doctor probably will modify such a diet according to his own ideas on the subject.

Various Diets

Some of the most commonly used diets are the following:

1. *Normal, well-balanced diet* is indicated for a patient who has poor dietary habits that impair his health and hinder his recovery from a particular disease.

2. *Soft diet* is indicated for patients who are unable to chew or who require a light diet.

3. *Fluid diet* may be prescribed for a variety of reasons, especially, of course, for patients who cannot swallow or retain solid foods.

4. *Bland diet* is advised for patients with pathological conditions of the gastrointestinal tract that make it essential to avoid irritation of any part. An ulcer is one condition for which a bland diet is commonly prescribed.

5. *High-protein diet* is prescribed for building up strength and is also often recommended for reducing purposes.

6. *Reducing diet* is prescribed, obviously, where loss of weight is one of the main objects of the treatment.

7. *High-carbohydrate diet* is advised for replacing lost body weight.

8. *High-calorie diet* is prescribed in cases of malnutrition.

9. *Salt-free diet* is recommended for many conditions, especially circulatory diseases.

10. *Low-fat diet* is indicated especially in diseases of the liver and gallbladder.

11. *Raw-fruit and -vegetable diet* is recommended for various conditions—often as an introduction to the salt-free diet and also for conditions in which proteins are to be avoided.

12. *Diabetes diet* is a sugar- and starch-free diet prescribed in cases of diabetes.

Prescription of Diet

As the patient would be unable to remember all the details of a diet—the foods he should eat, those he should avoid, the amount to take, and the time to take it—he is given a diet list. Some specialists may have use for only one or two types of diet, while a general practitioner may need a great variety for many different conditions.

In some offices, diet lists are typed, with as many clear carbon copies as the typewriter allows. A copy that is given to a patient should not be so faint and blurred that he may have difficulty in reading it. In an office where many diet lists are needed, much time may be saved if the doctor has a multigraphing machine. And an even better way is to give the lists to a commercial firm that specializes in reproducing typewritten material. The cost is small, and the results are excellent. A neat list that resembles perfectly typed material, printed with the doctor's name, address, and telephone number, is more impressive, from the patient's point of view, than a carbon copy.

There are also organizations that specialize in the production of diet lists. Such a firm may have a list of over forty different diets from which to choose. If the doctor orders a large quantity, the lists will be printed on a reproduction of his own letterhead. In New York, one such firm is the Personal Diet Service; no doubt similar firms exist in other cities. The doctor who needs many varieties of diets may save a great deal of time by using this service. A sample diet list for gallbladder condition is illustrated in Fig. 11–2.

Some manufacturers of medical products supply diet lists, which usually include some particular product of that manufacturer.

Discussing the Diet

When it comes to diet, patients fall into two distinct categories. At one extreme are those who do not consider diet a medical question at all, do not take the doctor's instructions seriously, and interfere with the results of the doctor's treatment. They usually believe quite sincerely that they are following the diet, forgetting or disregarding the lapses and exceptions or the snacks between meals.

Roy Clark, M.D.
353 East 12th Avenue
Centerville, N.Y.

#9 Gall Bladder
(Low Fat, Low Cholesterol Diet)

BREAKFAST

Fruit: Cooked fruit preferred, or fruit juices well diluted.

Cereal: Choice of: farina type cereal, or other COOKED cereal.

Egg: Egg white ALLOWED ONLY.

Beverage: Light tea or coffee or milk (preferably skimmed).

LUNCH

Soup: Vegetable soup ALLOWED ONLY. Meat soups or chicken soup, not allowed.

Vegetables: Cooked vegetables only, such as: carrots, string beans, peas, beets, spinach.
The following vegetables MUST NOT BE EATEN either cooked or uncooked: cucumbers, corn, radishes, asparagus, sauerkraut, onions, green peppers, garlic, cabbage.

Bread: White bread, one day old or toast. NO FRESH BREAD ALLOWED.

Beverage: Light tea, coffee or skimmed milk.

DINNER

Meat: Serving of any lean meat, chicken or turkey. No fried or fatty meats allowed. Meat may be cooked, broiled or baked. No stews or gravies permitted. No duck or goose allowed.

Fish: Baked fresh fish may be taken only once a week. No canned fish such as: salmon, tuna, etc., ALLOWED AT ANY TIME.

Vegetables: Cooked vegetables as above ONLY.

Salad: Lettuce and tomato salad WITHOUT DRESSING. Cottage cheese salad.

Beverage: Light coffee, tea or milk.

Dessert: Choice of: cooked fruits, junket or gelatin dessert (without cream), angel food cake.

– EAT SMALL OR MODERATE SIZE MEALS –

THE FOLLOWING FOODS MUST BE AVOIDED:

All fried and fatty foods.
No eggs except egg white.
No raw vegetables, except lettuce and tomatoes.
No soup except vegetable soup.
No alcoholic drinks, carbonated beverages.
No butter allowed.
Avoid very hot or very cold drinks.

All spicy, salted or canned meats.
No canned fish of any kind.
No raw fruits, except well diluted fruit juices. No gravies allowed.
No condiments or dressings such as: mayonnaise or Russian Dressing.
Avoid the following: asparagus, corn, cucumbers, green peppers, radishes, cabbage, sauerkraut, onions, garlic.

FIG. 11-2. Diet list for gallbladder disease. (*Personal Diet Service, Inc.*)

Patients on a reducing diet are especially likely to neglect the doctor's orders and are inclined to interpret instructions in such a way that they may eat whatever they crave. It is necessary to impress such patients with the importance of following a diet painstakingly.

At the other extreme are those patients who take the diet so literally that they are afraid to vary it even in the slightest detail. One patient, for instance, when told that she could have the white meat of chicken, would not eat the white meat of turkey without first consulting the doctor about it.

The diet list should therefore be as specific as possible, with exact instructions regarding the kind of meat, fish, vegetable, etc., to be eaten or avoided. Reference to just a *type* of food is not sufficient. When, for instance, a diet has specified "fresh-water fish only," it has been found that patients actually did not know whether a certain fish came from the ocean, a stream, or a lake.

Before attempting to explain a diet to a patient, the assistant should study it carefully and familiarize herself thoroughly with the list.

In some diets the manner of preparing the food is also important. Before explaining this to a patient, the assistant should inquire about any preferences the doctor may have in this regard. She should learn enough about the subject so that she can talk to the patient intelligently and convincingly.

Most special diets are monotonous, and patients easily become depressed at having to eat the same type of food day after day, the result being that the diet is often not kept. Sometimes the addition of fresh herbs, or a new combination of permitted foods, or a different way of cooking, baking, broiling, stewing, or braising may stimulate the patient's interest in the food and hence his appetite. There are cookbooks available for almost all of the diets mentioned above. If the assistant keeps a file of some of the recipes and recommends them to the patient, she will certainly earn his gratitude.

Patients seem to object to a saltless diet more than to any other type. Yet experience has shown over and over again that when a person habitually eats food with little or no salt, the palate becomes so accustomed to it that any salty food is distasteful and disagreeable. The explorer Vilhjalmur Stefansson tells the story of his living with the Eskimos for many months and being forced to eat his meat unsalted. He longed for salt constantly, and when the supply ship finally arrived with salt, he eagerly salted his first meal. The following day, completely forgetting that salt was available, he again ate his meals without salt and did not miss it at all.

In an office where diet is an important part of therapy, the assistant may wish to learn more about the entire subject. An excellent presentation can be found in "Nutrition and Diet Therapy," by Fairfax T. Proudfit and Corinne H. Robinson (11th edition, The Macmillan Company, 1955). This book presents a number of recipes for various diets and also has an extensive bibliography, including many books that deal with specific conditions. Diet recipes are included in most of the volumes mentioned.

12

Assisting the Specialist I

Because of the vast amount of knowledge required to practice medicine and the constantly new discoveries in all its fields, many physicians limit their practice to either a certain region of the body or a certain type of treatment. Thus the practice of medicine has become divided into various branches or specialties. The doctor who engages in the practice of any one of these is called a specialist.

In the early days of medicine all physicians were general practitioners, although the term was coined much later. They did not, however, use the knife, as any cutting that was considered necessary was done by the village barber! Only gradually did medical men begin to perform surgical operations, and not until the eighteenth century did surgery attain a position of prestige equal to that of medicine. A reminder of that schism is the existence even today of various organizations of "physicians and surgeons."

Diplomates

As doctors established themselves as specialists in various fields, the need arose for some sort of standard, in addition to the medical degree, by which to judge the specialist's competence in his particular field. Thus a group of specialists, all outstanding in their particular field, set up a board of examiners to determine whether a doctor in that specialty had the necessary qualifications regarding training and experience. The doctor was required to take an examination given by the board and, if he passed, was certified as a diplomate of that specialty.

This practice soon spread, and there are now national certifying boards for many specialized fields of medicine. Their number is steadily growing as new specialties develop by branching out from older specialties. The latter are expanding to such an extent that only a part of each field can be handled by one physician. The new specialties set up their own national boards. As educational and scholastic requirements of these boards are very high, the standing of a doctor who is a diplomate in his specialty is correspondingly high. A directory of all medical specialists who are diplomates is published periodically.

A list of different specialties follows. Those marked with an asterisk are represented by a national certifying board.

Allergy	Pediatrics *
Anesthesiology *	Physical medicine (physiatry) *
Cardiology	Preventive medicine (public health) *
Dermatology and syphilology *	
Endocrinology	Proctology *
Gastroenterology	Radiology *
Gerontology (or geriatrics)	Surgery *
Gynecology and obstetrics *	a. Abdominal surgery
Internal medicine *	b. Cosmetic surgery
Neurology and psychiatry *	c. Neurosurgery *
Ophthalmology *	d. Orthopedic surgery *
Orthopedics	e. Plastic surgery *
Otolaryngology (composed of otology, rhinology, and laryngology) *	f. Psychosurgery
	g. Thoracic surgery *
	Urology *
Pathology *	

A glance at this list will give at least some idea of the great diversity of medical practice. It is easy to understand, then, that the work of the medical office assistant is determined to a large extent by the specialty of the physician for whom she works. The procedures and techniques discussed in the book so far pertain to medical practice in general and are used in the offices of most physicians. In addition, however, there are various examinations, tests, and treatments that are germane to particular specialties. The assistant must be familiar with these special procedures, as well as with the special instruments and apparatus used. Some of these procedures are therefore presented in this chapter under the specialty to which they belong. This does not mean, however, that they are *confined* to this specialty. The assistant should consult the index whenever she wishes to look up a particular procedure.

Allergy

Allergy (meaning an altered reaction) is rightly called the mystery disease, as we still do not know why certain persons react with pathological symptoms to certain foods or substances that others can tolerate without any sign of discomfort. Although allergy is relatively new as a scientific concept, it has been observed for hundreds of years that some persons show abdominal symptoms, skin eruptions, or swelling and reddening of body parts after eating lobster, strawberries, or some other foods. Afflicted persons react with these symptoms each time they consume a particular food, even in minute quantities, while other individuals who have partaken of the same food remain unaffected.

Scientific study of the subject revealed that almost all foods can cause such reactions in some persons. It was also discovered that not only could these reactions, and a variety of others, be caused by food, but they could also be induced by contact with many substances, the most effective ones being plant pollens, feathers, dust, tobacco, and the fur of living or dead animals. Chemicals and dyes used in clothing and cosmetics were traced and found responsible for allergic reactions. Medicines, especially the antibiotic drugs, and even aspirin cause allergic reactions in many persons.

In some individuals an allergy manifests itself from birth—many children cannot tolerate milk, eggs, certain fruits, etc. In others, the allergy develops suddenly and remains fairly constant for the rest of that person's life. One of the striking features of allergy is that even a minute amount of the substance to which the person is allergic will cause a reaction. A person who is allergic to eggs cannot tolerate a cooked dish that contains even one egg.

The diagnosis is often not easy to make, as the symptoms may resemble those of many other conditions. Most patients suffering from allergies are first seen by their own doctor, then by the skin specialist, the nose and throat specialist, the gastrointestinal specialist, and finally the allergist.

The manifestations of allergy are related to the mechanism of immunology. As Dr. Taub states in his book: [1]

> The basic mechanism of the immunologic reaction is as follows. A foreign protein, called the antigen, is injected into an animal. After a suitable time the animal responds with the production of specific proteins which appear in its blood stream and which are capable of neutralizing the antigen. These bodies are called antibodies. When an antigen is brought into contact with a specific antibody, a reaction occurs whose character is dependent upon the nature of the antigen.

Experiments have shown that when a toxin (a protein) is injected into animals in sublethal doses, the animal produces antibodies capable of neutralizing specific toxin. In other words, the animal becomes immunized against the effects of the particular poisonous substance. Moreover, serum taken from such an animal and injected into a human being confers the same immunity on the human being. These findings led to the serum treatment now used in a variety of diseases, diphtheria being the most outstanding example.

It was found, however, that if the same protein is injected a second time, after a certain interval, a severe reaction follows. This is called anaphylaxis (in the case of serum, serum sickness), and it is believed to be caused by an antigen-antibody reaction.

The allergic reaction in human beings evidently is due to some such antigen-antibody reaction. Most substances that cause allergic reactions are proteins. It is assumed, therefore, that when certain substances enter the organism, either by way of inhalation, ingestion, injection, or contact, they produce antibodies in sensitive individuals. When the offending substance is again absorbed, it sets up an antigen-antibody reaction, which releases histamine and produces allergic reactions. The exact nature of the process that produces allergic symptoms, however, is not yet known.

In order to treat the condition successfully, the doctor must first of all determine the cause of the allergy, for the procedure in treatment of allergy is, first, to eliminate the offending substance from the patient's environment or diet and, second, to administer the substance to the patient in such small doses that it causes little or

[1] Samuel J. Taub, "Clinical Allergy," 2d ed., Paul B. Hoeber, Inc., New York, 1951.

no reaction, so that the organism becomes gradually accustomed to it and learns to tolerate it. This process is called desensitization.

It is generally not easy to determine the substance that has caused the symptoms from which the patient seeks relief. The patient must be questioned about his experiences just previous to the onset of the symptoms. A detailed case history may give a clue; it should include:

1. When attack began
2. Occupation
3. Drugs taken
4. Use of alcohol and tobacco
5. Diet
6. Cosmetics and perfumes used

Identification of a substance which causes allergic reaction is done by means of one of three tests: (1) scratch test, (2) patch test, or (3) intradermal skin test. The assistant will have to prepare the materials for these tests and either assist the doctor in giving them or give them herself. The principle involved is the fact that the skin will react in a characteristic way to the application of a substance to which the patient is allergic, without causing any serious symptoms except the local reaction. A large number of substances, therefore, must be applied in order that the offending one may be discovered. Most physicians use ready-made preparations of such materials as pollen, dust, feathers, animal fur, cosmetics, tobacco, and various drugs and foods. Some doctors prepare their own. This is somewhat cheaper, though time-consuming.

Scratch Test. Materials and equipment needed include:

1. Bottles with all the substances to be tested
2. Alcohol
3. Cotton
4. Needles or dull knife (sterile)
5. Toothpicks (sterile)

The test may be made on the back, arm, or thigh. As many as fifty tests can be made at one time. The skin should be thoroughly cleansed with alcohol. Then small, superficial scratches, no more than ⅛ in. long, are made with the needle or knife, without drawing blood. A drop of the substance to be tested is applied to each scratch and rubbed in with a toothpick. A new toothpick should be used for each scratch (see Fig. 12–1). An exact schedule must be followed in administering the tests, so as to ensure absolutely correct identification of the substance.

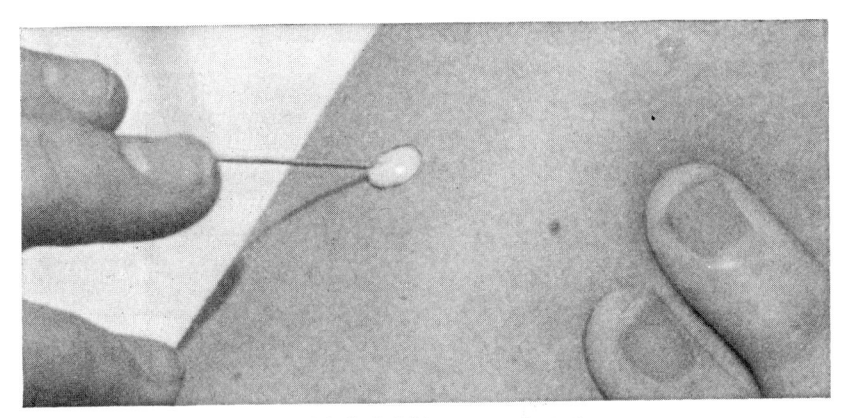

Fig. 12–1. Making scratch test.

After 20 minutes, each scratch is cleaned separately and then the entire area is washed with water. The reaction is then read. A positive reaction is indicated by a small red, swollen area. This usually disappears after about an hour.

Patch Test. In cases where it is undesirable to introduce a substance into the skin, or a contact factor is suspected, or the allergic reaction is a skin manifestation, a patch test is made. The technique for this is as follows:

Clean the skin thoroughly with alcohol or ether. Place a little of the material, which may be dry material, paste, or liquid, on a small piece of gauze, linen, or felt. Cover this with a square of cellophane and attach it to the skin with adhesive tape. The patch may also be sealed with a special liquid adhesive, a form of collodion. The cellophane makes it possible to observe any reaction that may occur during the time the material is in place.

If adhesive tape is used, the name of the test substance may be written on the tape; if not, a strip of adhesive with the name of the test written on it may be attached alongside each patch.

Specially prepared protective covering patches are sold commercially under the trade name Elastopatch. They come in various shapes and sizes, ready to be applied. Attached to each patch is a cellophane disk on which the substance to be tested is placed (see Figs. 12-2 and 12-3). As many as twenty or thirty patches may be applied at one time. The best place to apply them is the back.

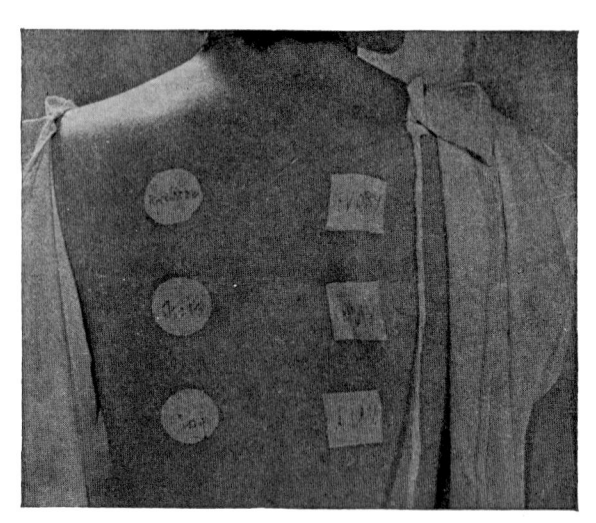

Fig. 12-2. Patch test on back of patient. (*From Warren T. Vaughan and J. Harvey Black, "Practice of Allergy," The C. V. Mosby Company, St. Louis, Fig. 42, p. 203.*)

Patients who have been given a patch test should not leave the office immediately, as a reaction may occur. Itching sometimes develops later, and the patient should be instructed to contact the office if this should happen.

A specific type of patch test is the tuberculin patch test. Prepared patches are available for this test, and these consist of two patches with tuberculin and a center patch for control. The three patches are attached to a square of adhesive. After the skin is cleaned with alcohol or ether, the patch is fastened securely on the skin. The patient should be instructed to leave it in place for 48 hours and to keep it dry. After 48 hours the patient should remove the patch and report to the doctor. If there is any reddening of the skin where the tuberculin was applied, the test is considered positive.

ASSISTING THE SPECIALIST I

Intradermal Skin Test. For the intradermal skin test, a small amount of the substance to be tested is injected between the layers of the skin. The general rules for injections apply to these tests. A 27-gauge, ⅜-in. needle is recommended. Ten to fifteen injections in each arm may be given at one time. A sterile syringe and needle must be available for each injection, so the assistant should ascer-

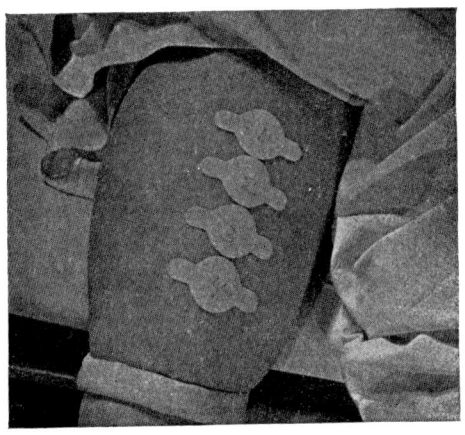

FIG. 12-3. Patch test on arm of patient. (From Warren T. Vaughan and J. Harvey Black, "Practice of Allergy," The C. V. Mosby Company, St. Louis, Fig. 43, p. 203.)

tain beforehand how many substances are to be tested and have that number of syringes and needles sterilized and ready for use. Reaction to intradermal skin tests may not occur for 24 hours.

Gynecology and Obstetrics

In the fields of gynecology and obstetrics the assistant should feel very much at home, as she will be dealing exclusively with women and their special conditions. An assistant with a mature and dignified personality can be of invaluable assistance to the doctor in discussing with his patients many of the details that have brought them to the doctor's office. Many women are embarrassed and hesitate to speak to a male physician about their intimate functions and concerns. If, however, they encounter an understanding office nurse

168   *The Medical Assistant*

who by her professional attitude inspires confidence, they may tell her many things and ask her a variety of questions that will eventually help the doctor in handling the particular case.

Most women have only a vague knowledge of the anatomy of their own reproductive organs. The schematic drawing given in Fig. 12-4 may help the assistant to understand the various gynecological procedures. It may also prove useful when she is talking to the patient and supplementing the doctor's instructions.

Gynecology. Gynecology means the treatment of diseases peculiar to women. The gynecologic patient's first visit usually includes a vaginal examination. The patient should be sure to empty bowels and bladder before the examination. After removing her

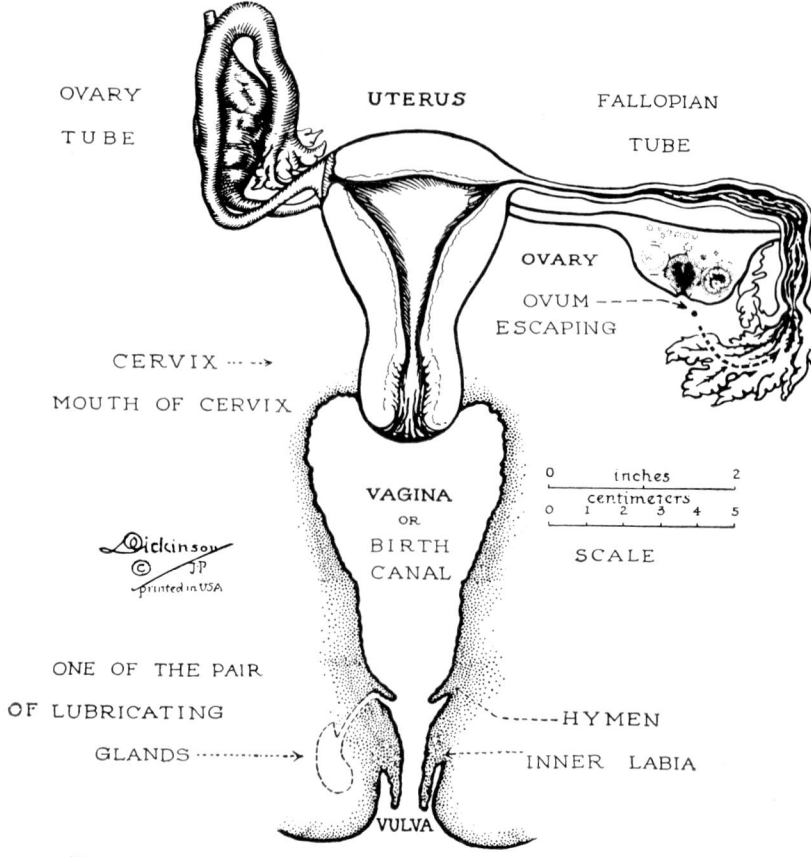

Fig. 12-4. Female reproductive organs. (*Tampax, Incorporated*)

ASSISTING THE SPECIALIST I 169

girdle and lower garments, she is placed on the examination table and properly draped before the doctor enters (see Draping of Patients, in Chapter 4). Although most examination tables have stirrups for the patient's heels, some doctors prefer knee crutches, which are more comfortable for the patient. The office nurse should always be present during the examination. If she is called away, she should leave the door slightly ajar. She should be prepared to hand the doctor the various instruments and materials that he may need.

The setup for a vaginal examination consists of all or most of the following items:

1. Sterile rubber gloves
2. Lubricant
3. Specula in various sizes
4. Dressing forceps
5. Gauze dressings
6. Cotton balls and swabs
7. Basin
8. Towels

A vaginal speculum is illustrated in Fig. 12-5. This comes in a number of different sizes

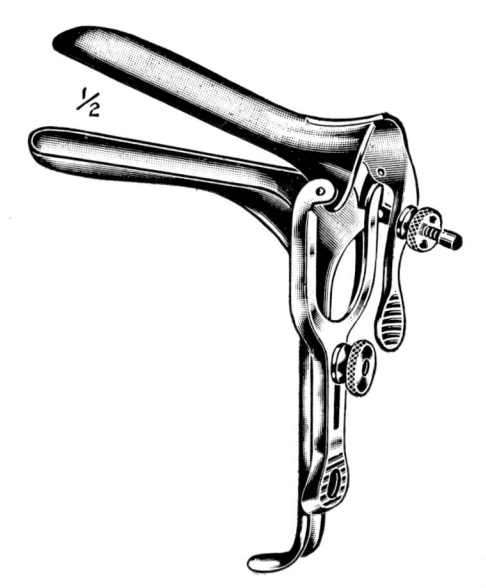

FIG. 12-5. Vaginal speculum. (*Clay-Adams Co., Inc.*)

Smears. A smear may be taken to detect organisms causing unpleasant discharges, such as *Trichomonas*. Smears may be taken with a platinum loop or a cotton applicator. For a dry smear, the specimen is spread on a slide and examined microscopically. For a wet smear, a drop of saline solution is placed on the slide, and the discharge is placed on this and covered with a cover glass. If trichomonads are present they can be clearly seen under the microscope. These examinations are usually the task of the medical office assistant, who is expected to have had some training in routine laboratory techniques.

If a culture is needed, the specimen is taken with a cotton applicator, which is placed immediately into a sterile tube and sent to the laboratory. Another method is to aspirate the material with a pipet attached to an aspirator. For cervical smears, a wooden spatula may be used. If a smear is to be taken, the necessary items must be added to the setup.

Because of the ever-present danger of cancer in the different parts of the reproductive organs, certain examinations are made regularly nowadays—either the Papanicolaou test or a biopsy, both of which have become standard office procedures.

For the Papanicolaou test, aspirations or scrapings are taken from the vaginal canal and from the cervical canal. A kit for the Papanicolaou test is illustrated in Fig. 12–6. If the doctor does not have his own laboratory, slides may be prepared according to the directions given with the kit and then mailed to a diagnostic laboratory. Special slide mailers are available.

Biopsy is the removal of a piece of tissue from a living organism for diagnostic purpose. A biopsy in the gynecologist's office is taken when there is a suspicious lesion. It is usually taken from the cervix. Biopsies may be done in three different ways: (1) with the knife, (2) with a special instrument that literally punches off a piece of tissue, or (3) with an electric loop. Local anesthesia is necessary. The tissue removed should be placed in a fixing fluid (10 per cent Formalin) immediately.

An endometrial biopsy may also be taken. This is a procedure in which portions of the lining of the womb (endometrium) are scraped off with a special instrument (curet) and collected for laboratory diagnosis.

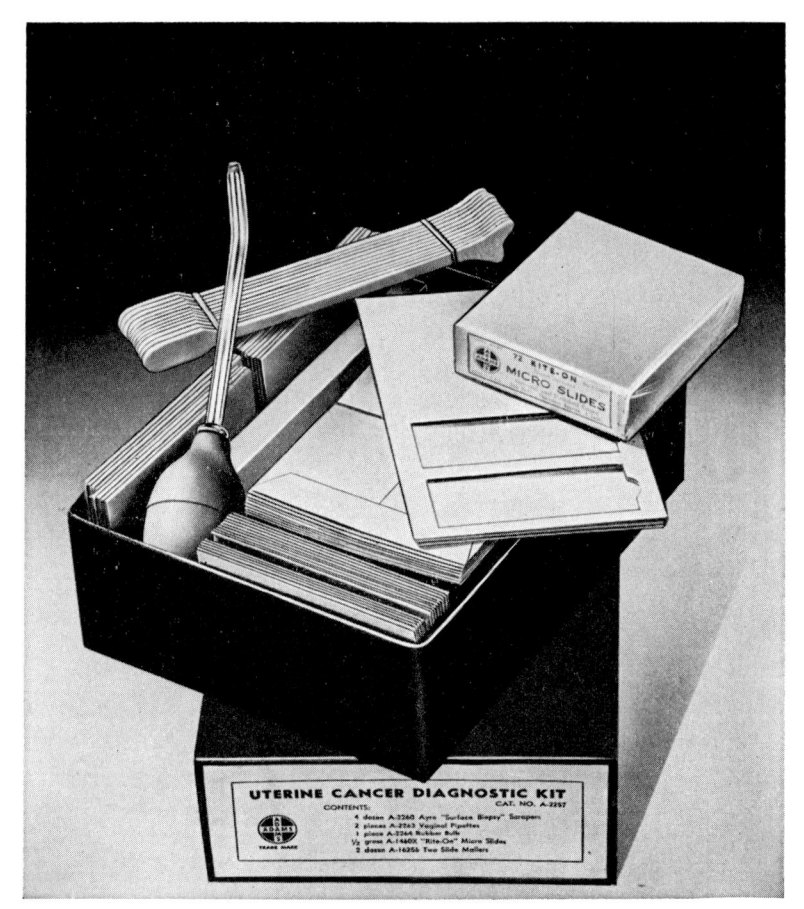

FIG. 12-6. Papanicolaou uterine cancer diagnostic kit. (*Clay-Adams Co., Inc.*)

Examinations for Infertility. The assistant should be cognizant of certain examinations for infertility.

1. Tubal insufflation. This involves blowing carbon dioxide gas through the cavity of the uterus and the fallopian tubes under controlled pressure. There are various machines available for this purpose. The test determines whether or not the tubes are open (patent). If the tubes are patent, the gas of course enters the patient's abdomen, and the patient may have severe pain in one or both shoulders when she sits up. The patient should then be put back on the table for a short period and comforted.

2. Hysterosalpingography (*hystero*, "uterus"; *salpingo*, "tube"; *graphy*, "record"). This is visualization of the lumen (canal) of the tube by x-ray films. For this test a solution that shows on an x-ray film is injected into the uterus, and x-ray pictures are taken at intervals. If the tubes are closed, the radiopaque material will be seen only in the cavity of the uterus. If the tubes are patent, the material will show in the lumen of the tubes and also in the abdomen, in the form of droplets.

Preparation of the patient for these examinations is the same as that for a routine vaginal examination, but a sedative is often given. The setup includes, in addition to those items listed before, the following:

1. Tenaculum (a hooklike instrument)
2. Ring forceps
3. Syringe
4. Special cervical cannula
5. Solution of contrast material
6. Antiseptic solution
7. Sanitary napkin for patient

Needless to say, perfect aseptic technique must be observed.

Cervical Coagulation. Certain lesions of the cervix, such as erosion (benign, reddened areas) and cysts, and suspicious areas may be handled with an electrocoagulating machine. These machines have various attachments, such as wire loops, needles, and ball electrodes. The attachments are self-sterilizing because of the current, but they should be kept clean. (See also Electrosurgery, Chapter 9.)

Obstetrics. Obstetrics deals with the care of pregnant women up to and including the time of delivery and during the period following childbirth, called the post-partum period. At the first visit, the medical history and the physical examination of the patient are the same as those for any other examination; however, as the succeeding visits will require special information, the specially designed medical history forms that are available are most helpful. They include all the questions that should be asked and make it easy to keep the record up to date.

At the beginning of pregnancy, laboratory tests are taken, namely, a complete urinalysis, blood count, blood Wassermann, blood typing, and Rh factor. During the months that follow, the so-called ante-partum or prenatal period, special tests are made regularly, such as measuring the pelvis (pelvimetry), recording the patient's weight, testing the urine for albumin, taking the blood pressure, and determining the growth of the uterus. In the last few months, the doctor listens to the fetal heart. As it is difficult to hear the fetal heart with the ordinary stethoscope, special stethoscopes are used for this purpose. With experience, the assistant can easily learn to distinguish the fetal heartbeat, as might be necessary for her to do during the doctor's absence.

Early pregnancies are usually detectable by laboratory procedures involving the injection of the patient's treated urine into mice, frogs, or rabbits. If such a test is necessary, the patient must bring to the doctor all of her first morning urine. This should be labeled accurately and sent to the laboratory promptly.

Since the patient under prenatal care will be coming regularly to the office during most of the nine months, the assistant should learn what time of day she prefers for her appointments (within office hours, of course) and be sure to remember any particular circumstances pertinent to scheduling the patient's visits. It is most important that the patient be made to feel well known and at home at the office. The assistant should familiarize herself with her doctor-employer's conduct of obstetrical cases. The main issues to be considered relate to the proper diet; avoidance of excessive gaining of weight; dietary supplements, such as vitamins or minerals; suitable exercises; sufficient rest; and proper bowel hygiene, preferably without use of laxatives or enemas.

When the assistant has learned some of the common symptoms that occur during pregnancy, she will be able to discuss them with the patient. Many women, especially during the first pregnancy, are worried and fearful. The assistant can do much to calm these patients by explaining that such symptoms occur in many cases or are, in fact, always present.

The assistant should be familiar with certain obstetric emergencies, as a telephone call reporting such an emergency may come in when the doctor is not in the office. It is of the utmost importance that she have an understanding with the doctor concerning what he wishes to have done when he is not within immediate reach. If the patient reports any bleeding, however slight, this is cause for concern. Certainly if bleeding is profuse, the patient should be advised to go to the hospital. Abdominal pain, constant or intermittent, may also be sufficient reason to hospitalize the patient.

In any event, the assistant should always consult the patient's chart when the patient calls and when the assistant reports to the doctor about the case. It will save considerable time if she has the complete record before her.

Abdominal pain in the later months may, of course, be a sign of labor, and normal labor is often accompanied by a "show" of blood. The symptoms of pain and bleeding, plus the possibility that the fluid surrounding the baby may leak, are usually discussed with the patient early in the prenatal course, so that it should be easy to reassure her when these symptoms occur.

When the time for delivery is drawing near, the assistant may be asked to make a hospital reservation for the patient. At this time she may also engage a nurse and perhaps later a baby nurse. She should have available in accessible form names of such nurses whom the doctor knows and calls on for his cases. Before attending to any of these tasks, she should make quite sure what type of accommodation the patient wishes, as well as how many nurses she wishes and the hours for which she wishes them.

While it is impossible to predict each woman's course of labor, it is well for the assistant to know how normal labor begins. Usually it starts with a low backache, followed by intermittent abdominal cramps. At first the cramps are fleeting, and the interval between them may vary from 10 to 30 minutes. As the interval between the pains lessens, the pains become stronger and last longer. The pains may be accompanied by a show of blood and the leaking of the amniotic fluid (the so-called "breaking of the water"). The patient is usually told to go to the hospital as soon as the pains begin.

Four to eight weeks after leaving the hospital, the patient usually returns to the office for her post-partum checkup. Barring previous complications, the examination at that time attempts to determine if the reproductive system has returned to normal. Excessive post-partum bleeding is one of the more serious complications, which, at times, requires rehospitalization.

Neurology and Psychiatry

The assistant in the neurologist's office will meet situations different from those in all other offices. It must be remembered that though the neurologist deals with diseases of the nervous system that may be caused by infection, poisoning, injury, or aging, or may be of unknown origin, many of these diseases are accompanied by emotional disturbances and abnormal behavior. Most neurologists practice psychiatry in addition to neurology, as it is often necessary to treat a patient from the psychological as well as the physical point of view. Therapy, therefore, may consist of medication, physical therapy, psychotherapy, or a combination of all three, according to the individual patient's requirement.

A psychiatrist who deals with psychiatric disorders and practices psychotherapy exclusively, such as a psychoanalyst, for instance (psychoanalysis being one specific form of psychotherapy), would need a secretary to make his appointments, type case histories, keep his books, and attend to all his secretarial matters, but he would have no special need for a medical office assistant. Some psychiatrists, however, also use certain of the somatic methods of treatment, as does the neurologist. In fact, the line is not sharply drawn between these two specialties, and they are both covered by the same national board of examiners. In the Vocabulary section of the Appendix, the medical terms for these specialties are grouped under the single heading Neurology and Psychiatry.

Psychiatric Disorders. Both the neurologist and the psychiatrist treat patients suffering from behavior disturbances which cannot be traced to any demonstrable physical causes. Disorders without apparent physical cause, such as infection, poisoning, or any other physical change, are divided into two major groups:

1. *Neurosis* is a relatively mild disorder in which the patient has more or less vague complaints—either physical symptoms or states such as irritation, fear, or compulsion. More severe cases are those in

which anxiety occurs without any apparent reason or the patient experiences, temporarily, hysterical states in which he becomes extremely excited and may lose his memory. These conditions are also called psychoneuroses.

2. *Psychosis* is a severe mental disorder affecting the total personality and sometimes causing the patient to lose contact with his environment. Schizophrenia (or dementia precox), paranoia, manic-depressive psychosis, and depression are some of the forms that a psychosis may take.

Senile psychosis and involutional melancholia are caused partially by physical changes during the aging process, though the manifestations may be similar to those occurring in both the neuroses and the psychoses.

The field of psychiatry now disposes of a rich armamentarium in its treatment of mental disorders. In addition to psychotherapy we now have the tranquilizers, insulin shock treatment, electric shock treatment, and psychosurgery (surgery of that part of the brain which affects the disordered behavior, such as lobotomy, meaning removal of a section of the prefrontal lobes; or topectomy, that is, excision of a portion of the cerebral cortex).

The administration of tranquilizing drugs has been found most helpful in quieting nervous as well as excited patients. Tranquilizers are not sedative and do not induce drowsiness or sleepiness; they do, however, seem to make the patient more relaxed, more cooperative, and more ready to understand his own condition and accept psychotherapy, even in fairly severe personality disorders.

According to research by Mortimer Ostow and Nathan S. Kline, the drugs reduce psychic energy and psychomotor activity by their action on a certain part of the brain (the globus pallidus).

Neurological Examination. Patients who consult a neurologist may be suffering from muscle spasms, tics, partial paralysis, and other conditions which prevent muscular coordination, resulting in awkward gait, jerky movements, and peculiar gestures. The assistant must train herself never, under any circumstances, to exhibit distaste or astonishment, for such patients are especially sensitive, knowing full well that they present a sad spectacle. Kindness and sympathy are needed in these cases more than ever, as these unfortunate people are the victims of some of the most devastating and often slowly progressing diseases. Theirs is indeed a long road of sorrow.

The examination in a neurologist's office consists of tests of the sensory and motor mechanisms by touching (percussion hammer) or turning the patient in a specific way, as well as an examination of posture, gait, muscle coordination, and reflexes. The doctor may dictate his findings during the examination to the assistant. Special printed forms are available for neurological medical histories.

When the doctor wishes to test the sensory mechanism, certain materials must be available; therefore, a tray should be prepared with certain items in readiness for testing of the different senses:

1. Taste—sweet, sour, hot, cold substances
2. Touch—pins and needles, cotton, brush
3. Smell—ammonia, camphor, pepper, vinegar, coffee
4. Hearing—tuning fork, clocks, records
5. Sight—eye chart, colors, numbers

Neurological treatments include injections, electrotherapy (faradization, galvanization), massage, and shock treatment.

Shock Therapy. Shock treatment has had an interesting development. It was observed that patients with mental diseases who were suffering from diabetes and were given insulin for this condition sometimes went into deep shock, during which they lost consciousness and had convulsions. When they recovered from the shock, their mental condition was greatly improved. On the basis of these findings, Dr. Manfred Sakel, in 1937, administered insulin to mental patients in sufficient quantities to produce shock. Many of these patients benefited mentally from this form of treatment. The dose of insulin, however, had to be fairly large, and the shock produced was often so severe that patients suffered strong convulsions, and some of them injured themselves. Researchers sought another method, therefore, and eventually shock was produced by electricity. In electric shock treatment a static current is applied to the patient's head; this produces unconsciousness and convulsions that can be regulated as to intensity and duration and that also result in an improvement of the patient's mental condition.

Formerly all shock therapy was given in hospitals only. In the course of the development of this form of treatment, however, machines that were simpler to handle and newer anesthetic methods became available, together with more knowledge about ways of preventing complications. Consequently, it became possible to apply electric shock treatment in the doctor's office. This form of treatment produces prompt results in the case of patients whose frame of mind is disturbed. Depressions especially are benefited by this form of treatment, and patients show up to 90 per cent improvement. Manic states are also benefited, though these have a tendency to recur. Disorders of the whole personality (for instance, states of schizophrenia) are helped through electric shock, but the results are not so good as those obtained in different forms of depression. The mode of action is not yet fully understood.

Technique. As electric shock treatment is now given as a routine procedure in the offices of many neurologists and psychiatrists, the medical assistant in such an office must be familiar with the technique. The doctor must have an assistant for this treatment, and in some cases he may have two. The assistant's duties fall into three categories: (1) before treatment, (2) during treatment, and (3) after treatment.

1. Before treatment, patients who are to undergo shock therapy, especially for the first time, invariably exhibit great fear. Nothing in the entire field of medicine, not even major surgery, seems to frighten patients as much as this form of therapy. A kind, sympathetic attitude on the part of the assistant is therefore of the utmost importance. She should reassure the patient, explaining to him that the treatment is a routine matter and no more difficult than any other kind of diathermy treatment. If there are persons in the waiting room who have had shock treatment in the past, they might help the patient if they can be made to tell of their experiences.

Before shock treatment is started, the doctor must have the written consent either of the patient or, if he is not competent mentally, of a relative. It is the assistant's duty to make sure that the form giving this consent is signed by either the patient or a relative or, best of all, by both. This is of the utmost importance. Standard printed forms can be obtained, but the doctor may devise his own form. A sample is given in Fig. 12–7. An ample supply of such forms should always be on hand. Failure to obtain consent before starting shock treatment may involve the doctor in a lawsuit.

When the patient comes for shock treatment, he should be accompanied by a relative or friend, or it should be arranged that someone come for him before the treatment is completed. The patient should be in the office at least 15 minutes before the time of the treatment.

A chart is prepared for the doctor on which each treatment is entered, showing the date; the medication given before and after treatment; the time of the treatment, which is measured in tenths of a second; the voltage of current used; and any remarks the doctor wants to add.

The following items should be on the dressing table:

1. A sufficient supply of sterile syringes and needles
2. Medication
3. Cotton swabs
4. Towels (cotton or paper)
5. Tissues
6. Mouth gag
7. Electrode jelly
8. Airways
9. Tourniquets

The current for the treatment is applied by an electric unit. A model of such a machine is illustrated in Fig. 12–8. The assistant should check the machine periodically by plugging it in and turning it on to see if the red light functions. If the light does not go on, the fuse may need replacing. Spare fuses should always be kept on hand.

The oxygen tank must be in readiness. This tank also must be checked at regular intervals to ascertain whether it needs refilling. A serious situation might develop if the doctor needed oxygen and found that there was none available because the assistant had forgotten to order it. This actually happened in at least one doctor's office.

Before the treatment the patient is asked to use the bathroom, and then he is taken into the treatment room. He should be asked

RELEASE

for

Electric Shock Therapy

I, _____ hereby consent to a series of Electric Shock Therapy Treatments by Dr. (name of physician).

I have been informed of the nature of the treatment and am fully aware of the risks involved.

I hereby release Dr. (name of physician) and any of his assistants from any and all liability in the case that any complications or unfavorable effects may result from the administration of this treatment.

_____
Signature of Patient

Witness _____

Relationship to Patient _____

Dated _____

Fig. 12-7. Release for electric shock therapy.

ASSISTING THE SPECIALIST I

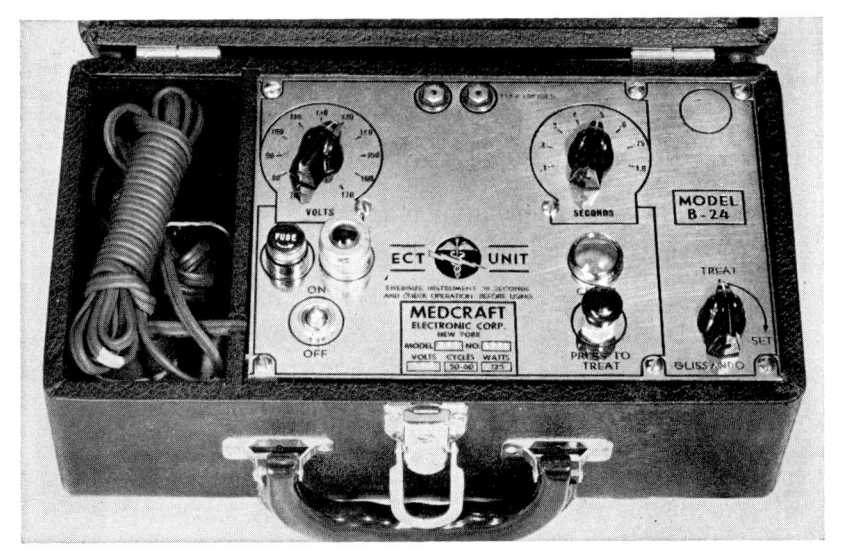

Fig. 12–8. Instrument for electric shock therapy. (*Medcraft Electronic Corp.*)

to remove any tight garments, but it is not necessary that he disrobe entirely. A man should open his vest, belts, and upper two shirt buttons and loosen his tie; a woman may open her brassiere and perhaps take off her girdle. If a patient wears a removable denture, this must be taken out. The assistant should place it in a paper or plastic bag, on which the patient's name is written. All jewelry should be taken off and, for safekeeping, given to the person accompanying the patient. The patient should remove any chewing gum or candy from his mouth.

The patient is then placed on the treatment table and the doctor notified. He will decide whether the patient should have a pillow under his head or lie flat and whether he should be strapped to the table or just wrapped in a blanket. Intravenous medication (anesthesia) might be administered by the doctor. The assistant therefore should have the solution ready and be prepared to hand the doctor the filled syringe, tourniquet, and cotton swab.

The assistant then applies the electrodes to the patient's head. These consist of two small metal disks attached to a rubber strap. The electrodes must be clean. Electrode jelly is applied to both electrodes, and the strap is fastened around the patient's head so that the electrodes are over the temples. Good contact between the electrodes and the skin is essential. One end of the cord is attached to both electrodes, and the other end plugged into the machine.

A mouth gag is placed in the patient's mouth. Such gags may be bought commercially or made in the office. They should consist of some sort of soft elastic material that the patient can hold firmly in his mouth. A plastic sponge or soft rubber, such as rubber tubing or a rubber heel wrapped in gauze, is practical. The texture and size of the mouth gag depends on the individual patient. A patient who has all his teeth needs a harder gag than one who has no teeth at all. After use, the gauze is thrown away, and the gag washed, freshly wrapped, and sterilized in the autoclave; or the gag may be sterilized first and then wrapped in sterile gauze. Such gags may be prepared in spare time.

2. During treatment, the assistant must stand at the middle of the table and with both hands hold the patient's shoulders and upper arms in a fixed position; with her forearms, she should keep the patient's lower arms more or less immobile. With the lower part of her body she should try to keep the patient's lower extremities in place. If there are two assistants, one holds the patient's shoulders and arms, and the other his legs; or one stands on one side, and the other on the other side, each one taking care of one side of the patient.

Holding the mouth gag in place, the doctor turns on the current. The current traverses the patient's head for about 2/10 to 5/10 of a second, and this produces a generalized convulsion during which the patient does not breathe. The cessation of breathing should not be cause for alarm, as patients usually resume breathing 20 or 30 seconds later; the assistant, however, must be prepared to hand the doctor immediately whatever he needs if respiration has to be stimulated. The oxygen tank should be open, the airways sterile, and sterile syringes and needles on hand.

3. After treatment, when the patient starts to breathe, he may be restless for a few minutes. He must be watched then lest he fall down. He will usually drop off into a sound sleep, but he must

be watched constantly in case he again becomes restless. The assistant must not let her attention be distracted even for a moment. The length of this sleep varies with each patient, but he should be encouraged to sleep as long as he can.

When the patient wakes he is usually confused and disoriented. It is advisable to call in the person accompanying him at this point. Seeing a familiar face helps the patient become oriented. When he is fully awake, the assistant should return all his belongings to him, have him dress, and take him into the waiting room to rest another 20 to 30 minutes.

The number of treatments and the intervals at which they are given depend on the individual case. It is advisable to arrange the next appointment with the person accompanying the patient, as the latter's memory will be hazy after the treatment. He should be given a card with the date and time of appointment written on it.

A variation of the so-called "conventional" convulsive therapy is electrical stimulation. For this type of therapy, preparation of the patient is the same, but the current is applied in a different way. It is given in lower intensity, at intervals, and over a longer period of time. The advantage of this type of application is that it does not produce any loss of memory. For these long-period treatments, the electrodes are lined with felt pads to prevent the danger of burns. In other respects the technique is practically the same as for convulsion therapy.

BIBLIOGRAPHY

Decker, Albert: "Practical Office Gynecology," F. A. Davis Company, Philadelphia, 1956.
Hall, Calvin Springer: "A Primer of Freudian Psychology," George Allen & Unwin, Ltd., London, 1956.
Horney, Karen: "Neurosis and Human Growth," W. W. Norton & Company, Inc., New York, 1950.
Speert, Harold, and Alan F. Guttmacher: "Obstetric Practice," Handbook for the General Practitioner Series, McGraw-Hill Book Company, Inc., New York, Blakiston Division, 1956.
Strecker, Edward Adam: "Fundamentals of Psychiatry," 5th ed., J. B. Lippincott Company, Philadelphia, 1952.
Taub, Samuel J.: "Clinical Allergy," 2d ed., Paul B. Hoeber, Inc., New York, 1951.

13

Assisting the Specialist II

The specialties discussed in this chapter are usually included under surgical specialties, to distinguish them from medical specialties such as allergy, psychiatry, and neurology.

Ophthalmology

An assistant to an ophthalmologist needs specialized knowledge if she is to be of real help to her doctor-employer. First of all, she must be familiar with the anatomy of the eye, so that she will understand what the doctor means when he refers to the different parts of the eye. A sketch of the eye is given in Fig. 13-1.

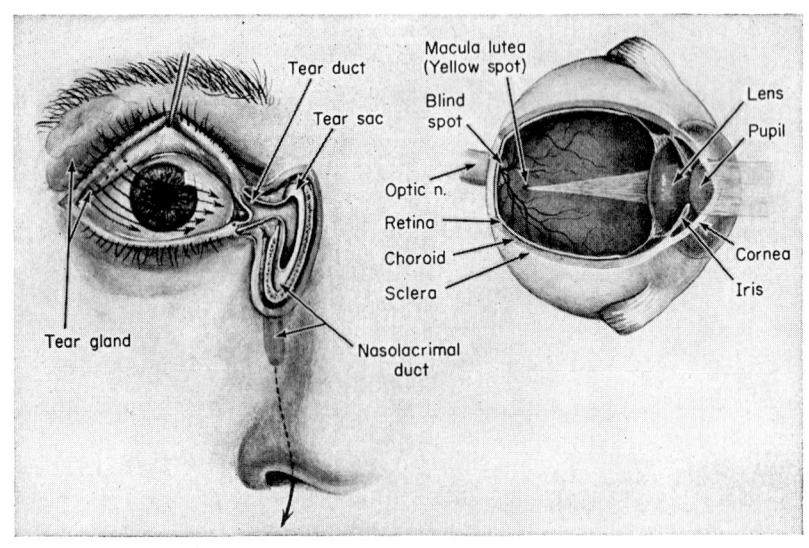

FIG. 13-1. Sketch of the eye. (*From "Blakiston's New Gould Medical Dictionary," 2d ed., McGraw-Hill Book Company, Inc., Blakiston Division, New York, 1956.*)

The principal diagnostic instrument used in this specialty is the ophthalmoscope, which is shown in Fig. 13-2. This instrument is electrically lighted and enables the physician to examine the interior of the eye. Other instruments used are:

1. Tonometer—for measuring the intraocular tension
2. Perimeter—for testing the field of vision
3. Retinoscope—for measuring refraction
4. Ophthalmometer—for detecting any restriction of vision
5. Corneal miscroscope—for inspecting the cornea

Work in the field of ophthalmology falls into two categories: (1) testing of vision and prescription of glasses; and (2) treatment, including surgery, for injuries and diseases of the eye.

Testing and Correcting Vision. It should be realized that an *ophthalmologist* is a physician specializing in the treatment of eyes. He is also referred to as an oculist, but this term is considered out of fashion. An *optometrist* is a technician trained in the measurement of refraction, that is, in the testing of vision. He also prescribes eyeglasses. In most states he must be licensed in order to practice. An *optician* is a person skilled in grinding lenses, making eyeglasses, and fitting them according to a prescription from an ophthalmologist or an optometrist.

Refraction. Visible light can be refracted, reflected, diverted, and absorbed. Light is refracted when it passes through an obstacle that is transparent or translucent. It is reflected when it meets an obstacle that is *not* transparent, such as polished wood, metal, stone, or a mirror. Light is diverted when it strikes an obstacle that directs it to another level (higher or lower) or to the side. As a rule this is the result of light meeting the obstacle in the form of a trans-

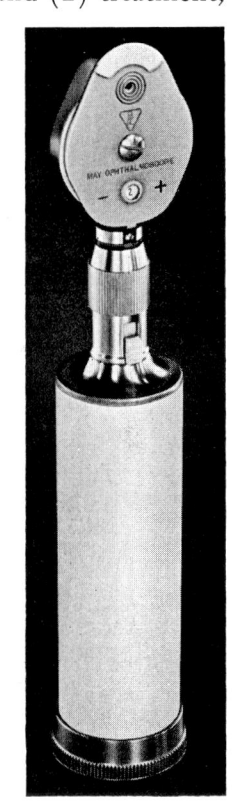

FIG. 13-2. Ophthalmoscope. (*Bausch & Lomb Optical Co.*)

parent prism. Light is absorbed when it enters materials such as are contained in the eyes of living organisms—human beings, animals, insects, and so forth. The process of determining the nature and degree of the refractive errors in the eye and the correction of these errors by glasses is also called refraction. In providing correction for errors of refraction, the curvature and the thickness of the surface of the glasses determine the amount of refraction and the clarity of the picture.

In many offices it is a routine procedure before the examination to put drops into the patient's eyes in order to dilate them. The materials used are called dilators or mydriatics. There are a variety of products on the market, and they differ considerably in the time they require to take effect, which may be anywhere from 15 to 60 minutes. The doctor may use only one type for all his patients (except children, who require a slower dilator), or he may use different types for different patients. In any case, when the patient makes an appointment, ask him whether he is coming for refraction and, if he is, advise him to allow enough time for his appointment. This also affects the doctor's appointment schedule. If a patient has to wait 20 minutes before the dilator takes effect and he is ready to be examined, the doctor can see other patients in the meantime.

It is usually the assistant's duty to put the drops into the patient's eyes when he comes to the office. This can be done in the waiting room. The patient should be comfortably seated, his head tilted back slightly. With a cotton swab, wipe one eye and discard the cotton. Gently draw down the lower lid, ask the patient to look up, release the drops on the center of the inner lower lid, and instruct the patient to close this eye. Repeat the procedure on the other eye and tell the patient to keep both eyes closed for a couple of minutes to allow the medication to spread. At the same time, have him keep his head tilted back for a moment to prevent the liquid from being washed out of his eyes, and hand him a cleansing tissue to use in case it is needed. The dropper must be sterilized before use. It should never touch any part of the eye but must be held just above the lid (see Fig. 13-3).

Vision. Patients consult an ophthalmologist for prescription of

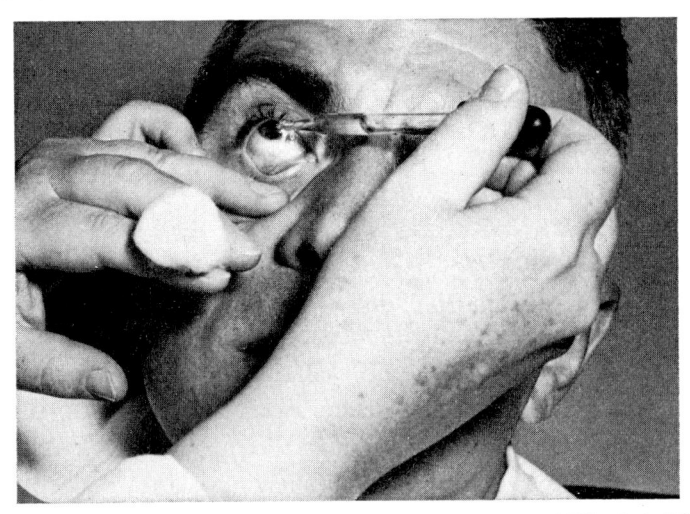

Fig. 13-3. Instilling eye drops. (*From Bertha Harmer and Virginia Henderson, "A Textbook of the Principles and Practice of Nursing," 5th ed., The Macmillan Company, New York, 1956, and Clay-Adams, Co., Inc.*)

glasses when they experience an impairment of sight (or vision). Nearsightedness (myopia) and farsightedness (hyperopia) are the most common conditions for which new glasses are sought. Patients may also be suffering from astigmatism, which is the consequence of irregularities in the curvature of the cornea or the surfaces of the lens. In astigmatism, which is usually a congenital condition, the light rays are not brought into focus at a point in the retina but appear to spread in various directions, depending on the curvature. Myopia, hyperopia, and astigmatism can be corrected by the proper lenses.

Most persons are acquainted with the fact that 20/20 vision means perfect vision, but they rarely know why. These figures refer to the size of letters and the distance at which they can be read. The standard for measuring vision is the Snellen test type, a set of square letters in different sizes. The normal eye can read such letters 20 mm. (approximately 4/5 in.) high at a distance of 20 ft. In the formula 20/20, the first figure 20 refers to the distance (20 ft.), and the second 20 to the size of the letters (20 mm.). In 20–30 vision, for instance, the eye can read letters 30 mm. (approximately 1¼ in.) high at 20 ft., and so forth.

The doctor's aim in prescribing glasses is to find a lens that will give the patient 20/20 vision. When this is not possible, the closest approximation must be accepted.

Lenses. Lenses used for ophthalmics (eyesight purposes) may be of several kinds: spherical, cylindrical, or prismatic. If they are spherical, they represent a segment of a sphere. Spherical lenses refract light equally in all meridians or planes; therefore, when looking through such a lens and turning it, one would find no distortion. Cylindrical lenses represent a segment of a cylinder. These are needed to correct astigmatic areas of the eyes. Such lenses show distortion when rotated before the eye. If spherical and cylindrical values are combined, the lenses are called compound lenses. Prismatic lenses are used to correct muscular imbalances.

Lenses may also be concave, convex, or meniscus. When they are concave (curved inward) they are called minus (−) and are used for nearsighted eyes. Convex lenses (curved outward) are called plus (+) and are used for farsighted eyes. Compound lenses may be plus combined with plus (+ + +); plus combined with minus (+ + −); minus combined with plus (− + +); minus combined with minus (− + −). Spherical lenses may have a plus and minus designation, but one digit will cancel out the other, and such a lens is known as a meniscus.

For example: +7.00 on one side and −6.00 on the other would give a meniscus lens of the value of +1.00. If the signs were reversed to +6.00 on one side and −7.00 on the other, this would produce a meniscus lens of −1.00.

Cylindrical lenses have one line, so to speak, that escapes the effect of grinding. One may picture the lens as a circle with a line drawn through it, either horizontally, vertically, or in any slant of the circle. This line has no power, while on each side of the line there will be either plus or minus power to meet the required prescription of the specialist. This line is known as the axis.

The unit of measurement for lenses is the *diopter* (d.). This represents the adopted standard, namely, a lens which has a focus of 1 m. (40 in.). In other words, a light source or a picture would be seen clearly through this lens at a distance of one meter.

ASSISTING THE SPECIALIST II

In order to ascertain the dioptic power of a lens it is necessary to divide 40 (in.) by the distance at which a clear picture is obtained. For instance, a lens that gives a clear picture (focuses) at 2 in. has a power of 20 d. (40:2 = 20). This would be a magnifying glass.

Prescription. A sample prescription for glasses is shown in Fig. 13–4. The interpretation of this prescription is as follows:

O.D. = oculus dexter, right eye: convex spherical lens of 6 d., concave = cylindrical of 2.5 d., with an axis of 12°, a prism of 2°, with the base of the prism up.

O.S. = oculus sinister, left eye: convex spherical lens of 4 d., concave cylindrical of 1.50 d., with an axis of 10°, a prism of 1°, with the base of the prism up.

One side of the lens would be convex; the other, concave cylindrical. These two lenses would be for distant vision.

For reading, add 2-d. convex spherical power over and above the prescription for distance to both lenses.

A prescription may contain the words "add bifocals" or "trifocals." This would mean that in addition to the correction required

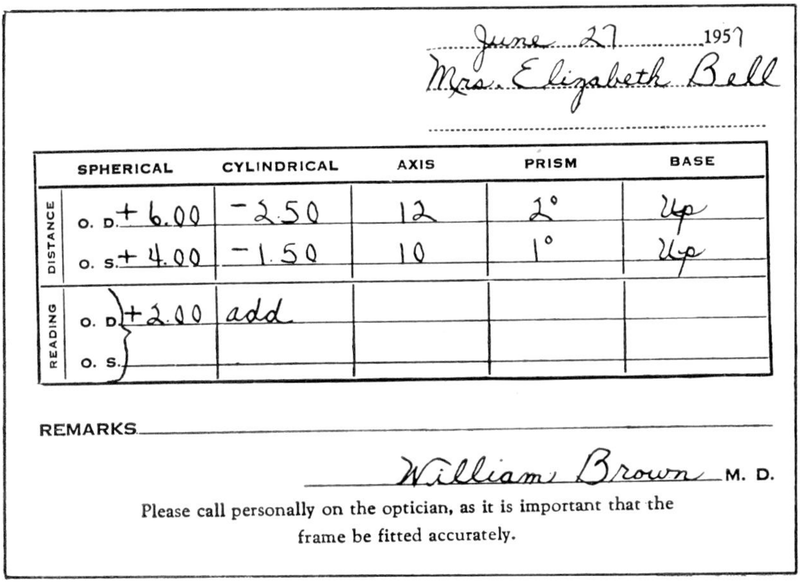

	SPHERICAL	CYLINDRICAL	AXIS	PRISM	BASE
DISTANCE O. D.	+6.00	−2.50	12	2°	Up
DISTANCE O. S.	+4.00	−1.50	10	1°	Up
READING O. D.	+2.00	add			
READING O. S.					

REMARKS

William Brown M. D.

Please call personally on the optician, as it is important that the frame be fitted accurately.

Fig. 13–4. Prescription for glasses.

for distant vision, extra strength is necessary for shorter distances, such as for reading, writing, typing, or playing music. This additional strength is to be incorporated in the lens used for distance. In the bifocal lens, the reading part is in the lower portion of the eyeglass. Trifocals have an additional middle section in the lens to correct eyesight for short distances that are longer than the usual reading distance, such as for typing or reading music while playing the piano or any other instrument.

Checking of Glasses. After the patient has his prescription filled, he is expected to return to the doctor to have the glasses checked. This checking is usually the assistant's task. One method of doing this, called neutralization, is to apply a negative (−) lens to a positive (+) lens of even power—be it spherical, or cylindrical, or compound. The result is zero power; that is, the lens under neutralization loses its power and becomes a plain piece of glass with no power to affect vision. For example, if a lens of −3 d. is placed on the +3 lens to be tested and the assistant rotates both lenses in front of her eyes, all apparent movement stops, and she knows that the prescription has been correctly filled. Neutralization requires much practice with a trial set. A trial set or case consists of standard lenses ranging usually from 0.12 to 20 d. in plus and minus powers.

This checking, however, is rarely done manually nowadays, as very efficient instruments have been developed to do it automatically. Such an instrument is known as a lensometer (see Fig. 13–5). The spectacles to be tested are slipped on the lens holder, and the eyepiece focused; the power of the lens to be tested, that is, its dioptic scale, axis position, and prismatic power, can then be read automatically. Exact instructions are provided with each instrument, and the technique of using the machine is easily learned. The assistant to an ophthalmologist, however, should be acquainted with neutralization, as it is an important part of prescription-lens inspection, and lensometers do get out of order now and then.

Eye Diseases. A large number of the eye diseases seen by the ophthalmologist are infections of various types. Before effective treatment can be instituted, the doctor must discover, through a bacteriological examination, what type of bacteria is responsible for

ASSISTING THE SPECIALIST II

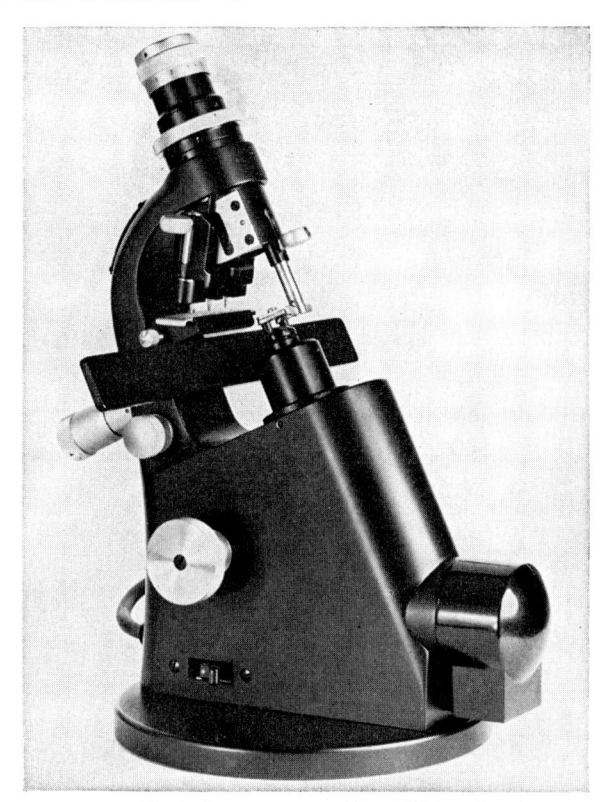

FIG. 13-5. Lensometer. (*Carl Zeiss, Inc.*)

the disease. Some of the exudate from the eye is removed with a stiff platinum loop or a swab. The smear is then spread on a glass slide, covered with another slide, and either examined by the assistant or sent to a laboratory. If the assistant is expected to examine the specimen, she should consult the section on Bacteriological Smears in Chapter 20.

For an eye examination a tray must be set up with instruments, medications, and dressings that the doctor will need. Once the doctor has told the assistant how he wishes the tray to be set up, a check list should be made for future guidance. Aseptic techniques are of the very greatest importance in all eye examinations and treatments.

Smoking is usually not permitted in the waiting room of an eye specialist, because of the irritating effect smoke has on inflamed or sensitive eyes. Lights should be soft and veiled. Patients with bandaged eyes or poor eyesight may have to be assisted to the examination room.

Orthopedics

Orthopedics is a specialty concerned with the proper functioning of the muscular and skeletal systems, as well as with the corrective treatment of deformities. More physical means of treatment are employed in this specialty than in any other branch of medicine except physical medicine and rehabilitation itself. An orthopedist could hardly carry on a practice without an assistant. The assistant, moreover, must be well trained in the many different procedures carried on in his office.

Physical Therapy Exercises. Physical therapy is indispensable in the orthopedist's office. In addition to the various modalities discussed in Chapter 9, certain therapeutic exercises are used. Exercises are essential in restoring the use of muscles that have become weak or atrophied through disuse.

Exercises may be given in the doctor's office, or the patient may be taught certain exercises and instructed to do them at home. In giving such instructions, the assistant must explain the reason for the exercises and actually *teach* the patient how to do them, not just *tell* him about them. She should see that he does each exercise several times in the office until he fully understands the reason for it and the motions involved. Also, she should instruct him carefully as to the length of time that he should exercise and the number of exercises that he should do. Some patients are lazy and fail to benefit from the exercises because they will not do the required amount, while others overdo and harm themselves.

Exercises are usually classified as: (1) active exercises, (2) passive exercises, (3) aided exercises, (4) active-resistance exercises, and (5) progressive-resistance exercises.

1. Active exercises are performed by the patient himself. He may be assisted in these by the operator or by a pulley or weight, or he may perform the exercises entirely unaided. Only active exercises can be prescribed for home treatment without supervision.

2. Passive exercises are those in which the patient remains passive and the operator moves a part of the patient's body. The patient must be completely relaxed. These exercises are usually started very gently and may be gradually increased in strength in the succeeding sessions. It must be understood beforehand whether or not they are to be continued until the patient feels pain. Generally speaking, there should be no pain, or pain should cease immediately when the motion is discontinued.

3. Aided exercises are employed when the patient's muscles are too weak to carry on their functions unaided. In these, the patient attempts to move the affected part and is aided by the operator in doing so. Submarine exercises (swimming) come under the heading of aided exercises, as the extremities lose weight and can be more easily moved in the water. The submarine exercises are used especially in cases of poliomyelitis.

4. In active-resistance exercises, the patient makes an effort to move the affected part, and the operator applies resistance to the motion. The resistance requires the patient to use greater force in making the motion, thereby increasing the strength of the muscles involved.

5. Progressive-resistance exercises have become popular mainly through the work of Thomas DeLorme. As the term implies, increased resistance is provided by the operator at each session; it has been found that no more than four sessions a week should be given.

Plaster Casts. One of the principal forms of treatment in the orthopedist's office is the application of plaster casts. It will be the assistant's duty to prepare the necessary ingredients, to assist with the application, and to dispose of all leftover materials.

Items necessary for applying a cast are:

1. Plaster of paris or acrylic material
2. Pail of *lukewarm* water
3. Bandages
4. Sheet wadding or felt

The materials used for making casts differ in the time they take to set; instructions must therefore be followed carefully. Instead of loose plaster, bandages impregnated with plaster of paris are generally used. As these will set while still in water, they must not be put into the water until just before they are to be used.

Plaster-impregnated bandages are fairly expensive and in an office where many bandages are used would run into a sizable expense. They can be made easily and cheaply by the assistant in her spare time. The procedure for making such bandages is as follows:

1. Place newspaper on the table.
2. Take a roll of gauze bandage.
3. Unwind a strip about 8 in. long.
4. Cover the strip with a thin layer of plaster of paris.
5. Roll it up toward the bandage.
6. Unwind another 8 in.
7. Cover with plaster and proceed as above, until about half the bandage has been covered; then reroll the rest of the bandage.

These bandages can be stored away until needed.

The floor should be covered with newspaper before a cast is put on or removed. Some orthopedists have a special plaster room. The hands may be protected with rubber gloves or with a coating of cream or petrolatum.

The disposal of plaster requires special care. If water in which plaster has been mixed or a plaster bandage has been soaked is poured into the sink, the drains will soon become clogged. There are special paper bags for the disposal of plaster, or, if these are not available, several layers of newspaper may be placed at the bottom of the pail. After the plaster has been allowed to settle for 10 minutes, the water may be poured off, and the paper with the plaster thrown into the trash. It is advisable, even with these precautions, to use a plaster trap in the sink.

Casts are removed with bandage shears, cast cutters, or a cast knife. In working with children or very nervous persons who may be afraid of these instruments, it is better to soak the casts in water until they are soft enough to be torn off. If walking irons, rubber heels, or any other items have been used in the cast, they should not be thrown away. After removal of the cast the patient's skin should be treated with oil or cold cream.

Arch Supports. An important part of the practice of most orthopedists is the prescription of arch supports (inlays) for flat feet or weak arches. For this purpose, a cast is made of the patient's feet and sent to a brace manufacturer, who makes the inlays from the model. Making or assisting in the making of these molds is the duty of the orthopedist's assistant. There are two ways of making a plaster model of the patient's foot:

1. A simple way is to use a plaster-of-paris bandage. The foot is coated with petrolatum, and the bandage is wrapped around the foot, back and forth, in the shape of a ballet slipper. The bandage is wetted and left to harden and can then be slipped off like a slipper. If the bandage has been over the arch, the cast can be cut in the center for ease in removing it. In this case, it is held together with a bandage when the mold is made.

In making the mold, the inside of the cast is coated with petrolatum, and plaster of paris is poured into it. After the plaster has hardened, the cast is broken off, and the mold is ready to be sent off.

2. In the second method, a shoe box or a pan is lined with petrolatum, and some plaster-of-paris cream is poured into the box. The patient places his foot into this plaster. After it has set, a separator (petrolatum, talcum powder) is put on the cast, and more plaster is poured on the front of the foot and allowed to harden. A separator is placed on the back of this cast, and more plaster is poured in the back of the box or pan, so as to cover the foot completely. After this has set, the cast can be taken out in three parts. This cast is the negative. The inside of the negative is then lined with petrolatum and filled with plaster of paris. (The three parts may be held together with a bandage.) After this plaster has hardened completely, the negative may be taken off, and the model is ready for the manufacturer.

It is advisable also to make a paper tracing of each of the patient's feet and to send this along with the plaster mold.

When the cast is removed from the patient, the feet should be cleaned with a paper towel and then washed with water or alcohol.

Splints. In the case of a fracture or dislocation of a joint, or whenever support is needed, a splint may be applied instead of a plaster cast. Lighter than plaster casts (which enclose the extremity completely), splints have the advantage of being easily removable for inspection or massage of the injured part. Splinting materials are aluminum, wood, plastics, plaster of paris, adhesive tape, and stockinet bandages. Hard materials used for splinting are padded with cotton or felt. Before adhesive tape is applied, the skin should be shaved and painted with a compound tincture of benzoin.

Braces. Braces are used for the protection, immobilization, or support of an injured part or for the prevention of deformity. They are usually made to order from measurements supplied by the physician to the manufacturer of orthopedic appliances. A standard method of measuring must be used—the method suggested in the "Orthopedic Appliance Atlas," for instance.

Braces may be made from a great variety of materials—steel, aluminum, plastic, rubber, or leather, to name only a few. The patient should have his brace fitted by the orthopedist, or, if he has been fitted by the manufacturer, he should return to the doctor's office to have the appliance checked.

Most doctors send their patients to one particular brace maker. The assistant should have cards showing the manufacturer's name and address ready to give to the patient together with the prescription.

Crutches. Many patients who come to the office of an orthopedist have had an injury which makes it necessary for them to use crutches. This, at first, is difficult for almost everybody. The patient must therefore be given instructions on how to use the crutches—if possible, in the presence of a relative. This instruction is often the assistant's duty.

With regular crutches, the patient must put his weight on his hands by stretching his elbows, and not "hang" in the crutches. The newer hand crutches, of course, eliminate this necessity. Whichever type is used, it is essential that the crutches be of the proper height.

If one leg is to be kept off the floor, the two crutches are brought forward while the patient stands on the good leg. He then supports himself on the crutches, and the good leg is brought forward. This is the crucial moment, for if the crutches have been brought forward too far, the patient will not have proper control and will feel insecure. If the crutch is serving as a support for a weak foot or leg, the latter is brought forward at the same time as the crutches.

The crutches must always be in front of the patient; otherwise, he may fall backward. He should practice walking with the crutches in the doctor's office until he has completely mastered the skill.

Occupational Therapy. This type of therapy is used a great deal for orthopedic treatments. Patients are usually referred to a trained occupational therapist or an occupational therapy clinic for this, although some simple gadgets, such as a rubber ball for finger exercises, may be kept in the office.

Otolaryngology

The otolaryngologist deals with ear, nose, and throat conditions. This specialty is often divided further. That is, some physicians treat only nose and throat conditions and call themselves laryngologists or rhinolaryngologists, while others specialize in ear diseases and hearing defects only. These are called otologists.

Laryngology and Rhinology. Most patients with diseases of the respiratory tract who come to the physician's office suffer from infections—ranging from that elusive condition the "common cold" to laryngitis, tonsillitis, sinusitis, and bronchitis. The principal diagnostic instruments used are the laryngoscope, the bronchoscope, and the nose speculum.

Treatment usually consists of the administration of medication, especially antibiotic agents, in the form of direct application, inhalation, or irrigation.

Inhalation Therapy. Inhalation therapy is favored by nose and throat specialists because medication can be disseminated throughout the respiratory passages with this method of treatment. There are many different types of inhalators. Some are operated manually; some work electrically. All are operated by the patient himself.

Before leaving the patient, the assistant should observe him for a few minutes to see that he is using the inhalator correctly. As the amount of medication in the inhalator usually lasts for a definite time, it is well to have a time clock as a reminder to return to the patient and relieve him of the apparatus before he becomes impatient. The solution for the inhalator may be bought ready-made or prepared by the assistant.

Irrigations. Irrigations may be given as a means of cleansing extraneous matter from the orifices (nose, sinuses, ears), which is referred to as lavage, or it may be given as a means of introducing medication.

All the materials necessary for each procedure should be ready before the patient enters the treatment room. The solution used may be ready-made, or, again, it may have to be prepared by the assistant. When the assistant prepares the solution herself, accurate measurements are absolutely essential. The amount to be prepared or, if ready-made, to be poured into the irrigator must also be measured exactly, so as to avoid waste. Leftover medication is never returned to the original bottle, but must be discarded. The solution should be of room temperature, unless there is a special reason for using a very hot or cold solution.

The items used may vary from office to office, but as a rule the following materials are needed:

1. Solution
2. Irrigator
3. Nozzle, tube, syringe, catheter (whatever is indicated in the particular case)
4. Receptacle to receive fluid (basin, pail)
5. Rubber or plastic sheet or cape for covering patient's clothing
6. Towels
7. Cotton
8. Tissues

The patient is seated in a chair, with a headrest, if possible. His clothing is covered with a waterproof sheet or cape. This should not touch the patient's skin. A towel must be used. The patient should be given a few tissues.

The nozzle or tube is inserted slowly and gently into the nostrils or the ear, and the solution is allowed to flow evenly. If the patient shows signs of gagging or great discomfort, the irrigation should be stopped for a moment and then resumed.

For nose irrigations, the patient should bend the head forward so that the return flow is facilitated and none of the material flows into other cavities. Before the procedure, the patient must be carefully instructed to breathe through the mouth and not to speak or swallow. The assurance that the irrigation can be stopped instantly at a signal from him if he feels nauseated, gagged, or discomforted frequently relaxes the patient to the extent that he will undergo the treatment without interruption.

Otology. One of the reasons a person consults an ear specialist is the fact that his hearing seems to be impaired. The ear is one of the most complicated mechanisms of the entire body, as can be seen from studying the illustration in Fig. 13–6.

The first step in an examination of the ear is a visual inspection by means of the otoscope. An otoscope is illustrated in Fig. 13–7. As this particular instrument comes with disposable specula, sterilization is unnecessary, for a new speculum is used each time. For the examination, the patient sits on a chair or stool, and a towel is

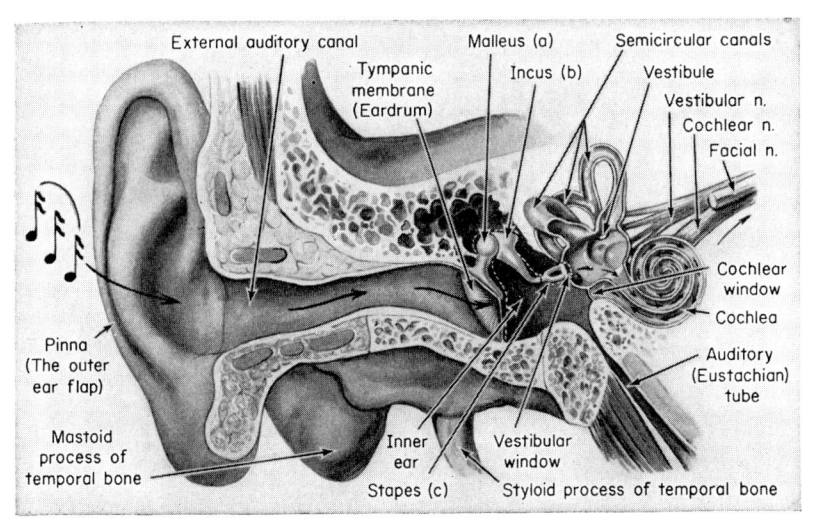

FIG. 13–6. Sketch of the ear. The ossicles, named according to their shape, are: a, hammer; b, anvil; c, stirrup. (From "Blakiston's New Gould Medical Dictionary," 2d ed., McGraw-Hill Book Company, Inc., Blakiston Division, New York, 1956.)

draped over his shoulders. The assistant may support the patient's head.

Often the hearing defect is due to an accumulation of earwax deep in the ear cavity. This can be washed out by irrigating the ear.

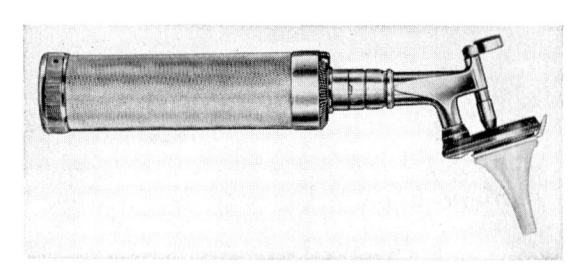

FIG. 13-7. Otoscope. (*Welch, Allyn, Inc.*)

For irrigation purposes, a large metal syringe is used (see Fig. 13-8). These syringes come in various sizes—30 cc., 60 cc., or 90 cc. The ear shield, which is removable, should always be attached when the syringe is being used on the ear. Irrigation with a continuous flow is more pleasant to the patient. He must be told to bend his head to the side which is being irrigated, so that the water may flow out easily. A basin is held under the ear.

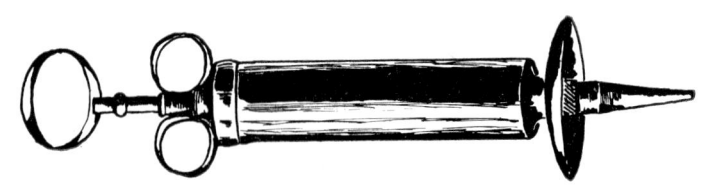

FIG. 13-8. Metal syringe for ear.

The solution used for removal of earwax may be lukewarm water with bicarbonate of soda, a glycerin-and-water mixture, or a soap solution. After the irrigation the ear should be dried thoroughly.

Hearing Tests. If there is no apparent reason for the hearing difficulty, tests are made to determine the degree of loss of hearing for each ear and, further, to establish whether the auditory nerve is affected or loss of hearing is due to otosclerosis (formation of new bone tissue within the ear). One such test is made by means of an audiometer. The assistant who works for an otologist is usually expected to be able to use the audiometer, that is, test the patient's hearing ability, so that the doctor may interpret the results and prescribe a hearing aid.

The audiometer is an apparatus that measures hearing acuity for the different sound levels and frequencies. The standard unit for measuring sound is the *decibel* (db.), which represents the least amount of sound (intensity) at which a note can be heard or the least difference between two sounds that can be recognized. Sounds and noises are thus classified by a scale of decibels; for instance, the noise made by a circular saw is 100 db. (or more).

The frequency of vibrations, or pitch, is measured in cycles per second. A person with normal hearing can perceive a sound of 10 db. in the frequencies between 60 to 8,000 cycles. A person who cannot hear a sound of 20 to 25 db. has what is known as a very slight impairment of hearing; one who cannot hear a sound of 30 to 40 db. has a slight loss; and so forth. Hearing also varies for the different frequencies. As a person grows older, a loss of about 30 db. in the range above 4,000 cycles is usual.

The purpose of testing a person's hearing acuity is to measure the lowest intensity in decibels at each frequency at which he can hear a tone. This point is called the threshold of hearing. From this test the doctor can determine whether or not the loss of hearing is serious enough to warrant prescription of a hearing aid, whether or not one will be effective, and, if so, how much amplification is needed and at which frequency range most amplification is required.

The audiometer is an apparatus which produces sound (pure tone) at the intensity and frequency desired. Various types of audiometer, differing slightly in construction and operation, are on the market. Exact instructions come with each machine, but the general principles of operation are as follows:

One dial regulates the intensity of sound in units of decibels—either 5 or 10. Another dial regulates the frequency or pitch between 125 and 8,000 cycles per second. The machine is equipped with a headband, two air-conduction receivers (earphones), and a bone-conduction receiver. For testing, the cord is plugged in, and the headband is placed over the patient's head with the earphones exactly and snugly over the ears. The patient should be comfortably seated, not facing the controls. The room should be quiet, but need not be soundproof.

If the test is being given for the first time, the purpose and the procedure should be explained to the patient. He should be allowed to listen to a few tones before the test starts and should be told how to signal when the sound becomes audible. Different operators prefer different ways of signaling; the patient may nod his head, or he may keep his hand or finger raised while he hears the sound and drop it as soon as the sound disappears. Most audiometers have a built-in patient signal, so that the patient can press a button which flashes a light on the dial panel. Figure 13–9 shows the testing of a child's hearing.

At the start of the test the audiometer control is adjusted with the frequency selector set at 1,000 cycles and the hearing loss at 50 db. The dial is turned to decrease the sound by 10 db. until the patient does not hear the sound. The dial is equipped with a tone inter-

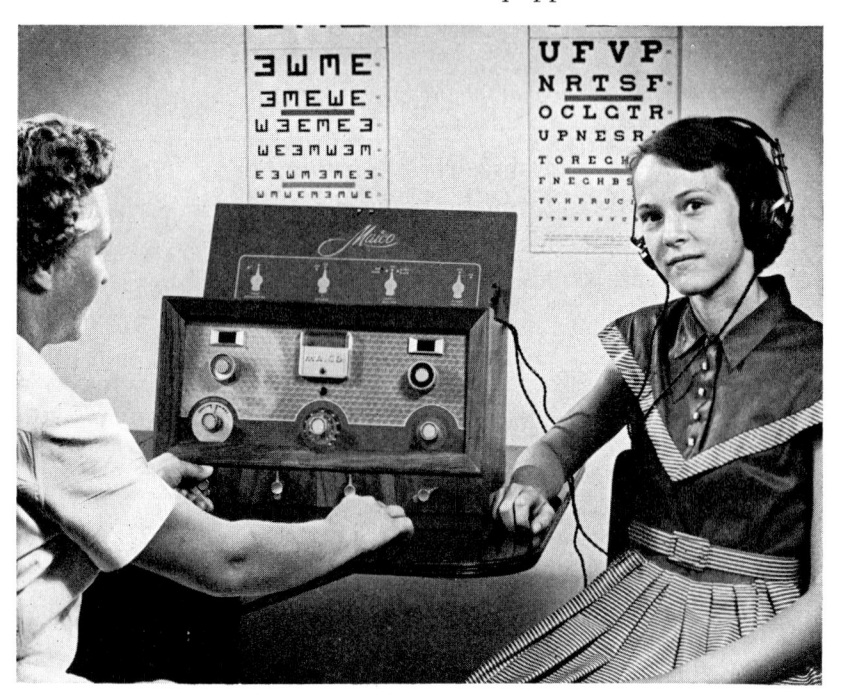

FIG. 13–9. Testing hearing with an audiometer. (*Maico Co., Inc.*)

rupter, which is used to determine the hearing threshold. The operator then switches the dial to the next highest frequency (2,000 cycles) and continues through the higher ranges. After the high ranges have been tested, the dial is switched again to 1,000 cycles, and the lower ranges are tested in the same way. The right ear is usually tested first.

Loss of hearing may be due to a deterioration of the auditory nerve or to other causes. If the auditory nerve is intact, hearing is possible through bone conduction. To determine the cause of the hearing loss, bone conduction must be tested also. For this test, the earphones are taken off, and the bone-conduction receiver is adjusted to the patient's head so that it fits over the mastoid bone in back of the ear to be tested. It may have to be moved back and forth until the spot where the patient hears best is found. The masking tone is turned on, so that hearing in the other ear is blocked out completely, and the procedure described above for air conduction is repeated, first on one ear, then on the other.

The results of the test are recorded on the audiogram. In an air-conduction test, an O mark is used to represent the right ear and an X mark to represent the left ear. During the test, these marks are made on the audiogram at each frequency to show the exact number of decibels at which the patient was able to perceive the tone. After the test is completed, the marks are connected by lines, which are usually drawn in colored pencil—red for the right ear, blue for the left. In a bone-conduction test, the sign < is used for the right ear and the sign > for the left. These marks are then connected by *broken* lines. A complete audiogram is shown in Fig. 13–10.

If the results show that the patient cannot hear by air conduction, but can hear by bone conduction, then the auditory nerve is intact, and the impairment in hearing would be due either to an infection of the middle ear (which may have affected the eardrum so that it cannot vibrate or may have destroyed it entirely) or to otosclerosis, which interferes with air conduction by reduction of the mobility of the three ossicles, which must move against one another in order to transmit sound. This condition may be corrected by an operation called fenestration (from the Latin *fenestra*,

AUDIOGRAM

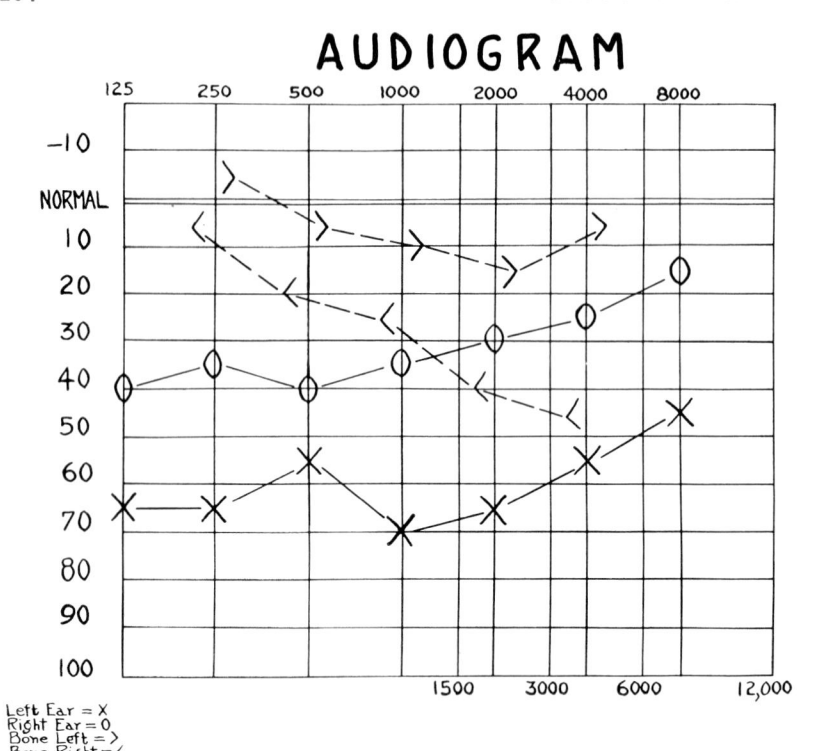

Fig. 13-10. Audiogram.

"window"), in which a small window (opening) is cut into the bone to permit air conduction. Manual loosening of the ossicles is a procedure that has been introduced just recently.

The audiometer measures the hearing ability for pure tone only; it does not give a complete picture of the patient's ability to hear speech. Speech audiometry is therefore given as an additional test in each case of hearing defect. This consists of reading a list of words to the patient and asking him to repeat. Recorded word lists for such testing are available, but many physicians prefer to compile their own list and have this put on a sound recorder. Most audiometers are equipped with a microphone that can be used for speech audiometry. Speech ranges between 1,000 and 3,000 cycles, and a loss of 40 db. in this area of frequency necessitates the use of a hearing aid.

Another test for hearing is the Rinne test. This is performed with a tuning fork. The tuning fork is struck and held to the patient's ear, for air conduction; on the mastoid bone, for bone conduction. If a sound is heard by bone conduction when it cannot be heard by air conduction, the test is called negative. The audiometer test has for the most part taken the place of the Rinne test.

Some abbreviations used in audiometry are:

SRT—Speech-reception threshold
MCL—Most comfortable loudness level
TD—Threshold of discomfort

Another reason for consulting an otologist is, of course, infections of the ear, mastoiditis being one of the most common. Formerly, an operation was almost always necessary to clear up this infection. Today the antibiotic drugs have almost completely eliminated this operation.

BIBLIOGRAPHY

American Academy of Orthopedic Surgeons: "Orthopedic Appliance Atlas," J. W. Edwards, Publisher, Inc., Ann Arbor, Mich., 1952, vol. I.
Davson, Hugh: "The Physiology of the Eye," McGraw-Hill Book Company, Inc., Blakiston Division, New York, 1949.
DeLorme, Thomas L., and Arthur L. Watkins: "Progressive Resistance Exercise," Appleton-Century-Crofts, Inc., New York, 1951.
Howorth, M. Becket: "A Textbook of Orthopedics," W. B. Saunders Company, Philadelphia, 1952.

14

First-aid Rules

In this mechanical age of automobiles, planes, and machines, accidents are a frequent occurrence. A complete course in first aid, such as the one given by the American Red Cross, for instance, might therefore profitably be made compulsory for everyone. Certainly the medical office assistant should be familiar with this important subject. Even if she has had no professional training, she must have at least a rudimentary knowledge of what to do in case first aid must be administered in the office or she is asked for information, possibly over the telephone, when one of the doctor's patients has had an accident.

When the assistant is alone in the office a number of things may happen—someone in the office may faint or suffer an epileptic fit, an accident case may be brought in, or a telephone call may come in from someone who is faced with an emergency and needs advice on what to do. In the absence of the doctor, the medical office assistant must give the necessary help or supply correct information on what to do until the doctor arrives. If the doctor is in the office, she will have to assist him, and there will be no time for him to tell her what to do. She herself must know what to do and do it quickly.

This chapter, therefore, is concerned with accidents or emergencies which may and do occur and for which the assistant should be prepared. The type of emergency for which the office assistant is unlikely to be called on is omitted. There are many good books on first aid, of which the best known is the textbook published by the American National Red Cross.

The assistant should learn from the doctor what information she may give to patients and what aid she may render in case of an emergency in the doctor's absence. She should also know what instructions the doctor wishes her to give to patients or their relatives if they call up about a medical emergency.

It is assumed that the assistant, when confronted with an emergency while alone in the doctor's office, will apply first aid but will immediately get in touch with her employer or, if he is unavailable, with another doctor. The instructions that follow, therefore, deal simply with what to do until the doctor comes.

Emergencies

Abdominal Pain. The causes of abdominal pain vary from a simple gastric upset to a serious infectious condition. Only a physician can interpret the symptoms correctly. The patient should be lying down, and ice compresses may be applied to the painful part. Sips of cold water may be given, but *nothing else*, until the cause has been diagnosed.

Animal Bites. Animal (usually cat or dog) bites always carry the risk of infection. The wound should be treated like any other skin injury. It should be cleaned thoroughly with soap and water, treated with a strong antiseptic applied in liquid, ointment, or powder form, and covered with a sterile dressing and a bandage. If the wound is large, it may require stitches; if the flesh has been torn, some of the mangled tissue may have to be removed. In any case, the assistant should merely wash the wound (rinsing it under running water to remove any saliva) and apply a sterile dressing.

In addition to the possibility of local infection, dog bites carry the danger of rabies. This is a virus disease which is inevitably fatal once it develops. Because the incubation period is longer for rabies than for most virus diseases, it is possible, if a series of vaccinations with rabies serum is started at once, to build up in the patient a resistance to the disease before it develops. This method of treatment was discovered by Pasteur and is usually referred to as the Pasteur treatment. Patients who have been bitten by a dog must therefore make sure that the dog did not have rabies; if this cannot be ascertained, they must be referred to a hospital for treatment.

Apoplexy (Stroke). Apoplexy is the result of a cerebral hemorrhage, which is caused by the rupturing of an artery in the brain. The amount of damage to the brain is determined by the location of the rupture and the extent of the bleeding. Death, unconsciousness, or paralysis results. Some attacks resemble a fainting spell—the patient is pale, with a weak pulse. Other attacks are accompanied by violent pain in the region near the heart and by fear of impending death. The patient may experience shortness of breath, become red in the face, and be gasping for air. The apoplectic patient must not be moved; he should be kept very quiet and covered with a blanket.

Bleeding. Among the most common accident cases treated in the doctor's office are those that involve bleeding from a cut or other injury. It is well to remember that *spurting* blood means a cut artery; *oozing* blood, a cut vein.

To stop bleeding from an artery, pressure must be applied against a firm foundation, that is, where the artery crosses a bone. The pressure points for stopping arterial bleeding should be memorized. Those most important for first aid are shown in Fig. 14–1. They are:

1. Temporal—bleeding of the head, above the eyes
2. Facial—bleeding of the cheek or nose
3. Carotid—bleeding from any part of the neck or throat
4. Subclavian—bleeding of the ear, cheek, neck, or shoulder
5. Brachial—bleeding from the lower arm or the hand
6. Femoral—bleeding from the leg or foot

Pressure may be applied with the thumb until the doctor can tie the artery or apply other methods of controlling the bleeding.

If bleeding occurs from the extremities, apply a tourniquet—above the wound if the blood is spurting, below if it is oozing. If a rubber tourniquet is not available, use a handkerchief, necktie, stocking, or bandage. Fold the handkerchief or piece of material to a width of about 2 in. and wrap it smoothly around the extremity, about 2 in. above the wound. Tie the tourniquet tightly. Remember, however, that a tourniquet is a potential danger. If it is left on too long, the blood will be cut off from that part of the body, and

FIRST-AID RULES 209

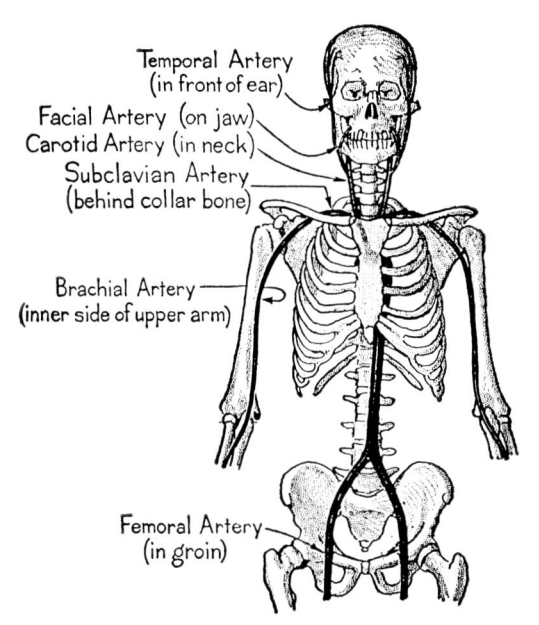

Fig. 14-1. Pressure points. (*From American National Red Cross, "First Aid Textbook," rev. ed., Doubleday & Company, Inc., New York, 1945.*)

the tissue will die. A tourniquet must therefore be loosened every 15 to 20 minutes. Never cover a tourniquet, as it may be forgotten.

If bleeding has stopped, do not tighten the tourniquet again, but leave it in place. Cover the wound with a sterile dressing and apply a bandage firmly (see Chapter 8 under Bandages).

Whenever possible, place the bleeding part higher than the heart, so that less blood will be pumped into it and bleeding will consequently be less severe. Do not disturb a blood clot, which forms a natural barrier to bleeding.

The assistant should also be able to recognize internal bleeding, which is a sign of the gravest danger. The symptoms are:

1. Rapid, weak pulse
2. Excessive thirst
3. Restlessness
4. Anxiety
5. Visible blood (vomiting or discharge)

If these signs are present, the patient should be kept in a horizontal position and as warm and quiet as possible.

Burns. Burns may be caused by fire, heat, electricity, or chemicals, and they are classified as first, second, and third degree. A first-degree burn is simply a reddening of the skin such as is often experienced after too long exposure to the sun (sunburn). In a second-degree burn, the outer layer of the skin is injured, and blisters develop. In a third-degree burn, the skin is completely destroyed, and the underlying tissue is also injured or destroyed, sometimes to the bone.

If the skin is injured as in a second- or third-degree burn and the blister breaks, there will be an open wound in danger of infection. Immediately after a burn, the injured area is completely sterile, as the heat has destroyed any bacteria present on the skin surface. The best possible treatment, therefore, is to protect this clean wound with sterile dressings.

Theories on the treatment of burns have undergone many changes; many remedies have been advocated and later rejected. The most recent thought on the matter condemns the practice of applying unsterile ointments or powders of any kind to a sterile wound.

As petroleum jelly has remarkable healing qualities, a sterile dressing impregnated with petrolatum is currently the method of choice for treatment of burns. Sterile petrolatum gauze dressings, which are available commercially, should therefore be kept on hand in the doctor's office for immediate application. Instructions on how to open sterile dressings must be followed carefully in order to preserve sterility (see Fig. 8-5). If such petrolatum dressings are not available, any sterile dressing is preferable to unsterile ointments. If no sterile dressings are on hand, freshly laundered towels or sheets should be used.

Place the dressing on the burn and bandage the wound firmly, but not tightly, so as to prevent oozing of plasma. Aspirin may be given to relieve pain.

Chemical burns must be washed with large quantities of cold water, so that any traces of the chemical may be rinsed out. Running water is preferable for this, but if it is not available, water may be poured from a glass or pitcher into the burn. When the chemical has been removed, apply a dressing as described above.

Epileptic Fits or Convulsions. A patient who is subject to epileptic fits may suffer an attack in the office or the waiting room as a result of the strain of visiting a doctor. Do not become frightened. If other patients are present, ask them to leave the room. Protect the patient's head and face with pillows or a coat. Remove any objects with which he might hurt himself from his immediate vicinity. Loosen all tight clothing (collar, belt). Using gauze or a handkerchief, grasp his tongue and keep it forward. If his mouth is closed, open it by pressing against the jaw joints and keep it open with a piece of wood (tongue depressor, pencil). Wipe away any foam. When the fit subsides, let the patient lie down on a bed or couch and rest.

Convulsions, while they are distressing to watch, are not in themselves dangerous. They may occur in children for some slight cause, such as a digestive upset, as well as for more serious reasons. The onset is usually sudden, and the convulsion may last from a few minutes to half an hour. The greatest danger during a convulsion is the possibility of injury. The child should be protected as much as possible from striking objects or falling off a chair. It is advisable to wrap him loosely in a blanket. A cold compress applied to the head may be helpful. If the patient is biting his tongue or lips, a gauze pack should be inserted into his mouth. When the attack is over, the child should be kept quiet until he appears completely normal.

Fainting. Some persons faint very easily—at the sight of blood, because of pain, or simply from anxiety about their condition or fear of being hurt during treatment or examination. If a patient seems about to faint, seat him quickly and tell him to bend his head forward between his knees, or bend it down for him, until all pallor disappears. As blood enters his brain, he will feel better.

If the patient has fainted and fallen to the floor, have him lie flat on his back and place a pillow under his shoulders so that his head is slightly lowered. Loosen all tight clothing. Apply cold water to the face, especially to the forehead and temples, but keep the rest of the body warm. Make sure there is plenty of fresh air in the room, and let the patient rest quietly. Smelling salts or spirit of ammonia may help to revive him.

Foreign Bodies. Among the emergency situations with which the medical office assistant is likely to be confronted are cases involving foreign objects that have entered the body through one of its orifices. She should therefore be familiar with the following procedures.

In the Ear. An object that has been pushed into the ear (by a child) or an insect that has flown into the ear should be removed only by a physician. A little lukewarm mineral or olive oil may be dropped into the ear before treatment is administered by the doctor.

In the Eye. The danger of a foreign body, be it only a speck of dust, being blown into the eye is ever present. Patients with "something in the eye" are therefore frequent visitors in the doctor's office.

In attending to a patient's eyes, certain rules must be strictly observed:

1. Wash your hands before touching the eye.
2. Tell the patient not to rub the eye.
3. Do not use any instrument whatsoever.

If the object is embedded in the eyeball, only a physician should remove it. If the object lies on the surface, an attempt may be made to remove it in the following way:

1. Bring the upper eyelid down over the lower lid and hold it there a moment; then move it inward. This often washes out the foreign object.
2. Pull down the lower lid. If the object can be seen on the inside of the lid, remove it with a moistened corner of a clean handkerchief or a moistened cotton-tip applicator. Never use dry material.
3. Using an eye dropper or eyecup, wash out the eye with a solution of boric acid or lukewarm salt water.
4. If the object cannot be removed, instill an anesthetic or a few drops of oil (castor oil, mineral oil, olive oil) into the eye while

the patient waits for the doctor. The anesthetic, of course, must be one that can be safely used in the eye.

Swallowed. Children or irrational persons sometimes swallow objects. If these lodge in the windpipe and cut off the air supply, choking will result. If the air passage is not completely blocked, the patient will nevertheless experience difficulty in breathing and in swallowing. A child may be held upside down and shaken. An adult should be told to bend forward, as far down as possible, and should then be given a sharp slap on the back, which may help to dislodge the object. An object that has passed through the esophagus must be located by x-ray or fluoroscope.

Fractures. Courses in first aid particularly stress the handling of fractures, for they are one of the most common results of accidents. If, however, a patient is able to come to the doctor's office, chances are that first aid will already have been applied. A general rule in dealing with fractures is to keep the injured part immobile and provide support for it.

Heart Attack. Since a heart attack may occur at any time, the medical office assistant must be especially alert to the symptoms of this condition and be able to spot it at once. One indication is shortness of breath and noisy breathing; also, the patient may feel that he is unable to breathe unless he is sitting up. Sometimes the patient has a sensation of pressure in his chest, which may change to a violent pain that often passes down into the left arm. Usually the patient is very much agitated and has a feeling of impending death. This symptom complex is called angina pectoris or stenocardia. In another form of attack, the patient may also feel weak and dizzy, and he may faint and remain unconscious for some time.

Heart attacks may be caused by diseases of the coronary arteries, such as arteriosclerosis (a narrowing of the arteries due to calcium deposits and lack of elasticity); thrombosis (a blood clot in the blood vessels); or an embolus (a bit of matter, a blood clot, fat, or a small piece of tissue) in the blood stream. Angina pectoris may be brought on by heavy exertion or by emotional stress.

If a patient has what appears to be a heart attack, he must lie down and be kept as quiet as possible. The assistant should cover him with a blanket and ask him not to move at all. This is all that can be done until a drug is administered. A victim of a heart attack is usually extremely upset and fearful. It is therefore just as important to calm and reassure him as it is to attend to his physical needs.

Drugs administered in the case of a heart attack ease the pain and dilate the arteries so that more blood flows into the heart. If the medical history of a patient includes past heart involvement, it will probably show the drug to which he is accustomed. Morphine may be lifesaving. The assistant should have whatever medication is to be used ready for the doctor. In the case of a patient who uses nitroglycerin and carries this with him, the assistant may administer the medication.

Insect Bites. A variety of insects can produce painful or itching bites, and some patients have allergies that may cause severe reactions. In treating an insect bite, first determine whether the sting is still in the skin and, if it is, remove it with small tweezers. Then apply a compress to the site of the sting. The compress may be dipped in either a solution of 1 part ammonia and 1 part water or a paste made of baking soda and water. A mixture of 1 part salt water and 1 part vinegar will help to stop the itching.

Nosebleed. Nosebleeds that are not caused by injury are a frequent occurrence and are generally not serious. Some general rules to be observed in case of nosebleed are:

1. Have the patient sit up, with his head tilted slightly backward, and tell him to breathe through his mouth.
2. Loosen his collar.
3. Place cold applications across the bridge of his nose or on the back of his neck. For this, dip a towel in cold water, wring it out, and apply it. If ice is available, place a few small pieces between the layers of the wet towel.
4. Press the nostril on the bleeding side against the central portion of the nose for several minutes. This usually stops the bleeding and gives the blood a chance to clot.

5. If bleeding does not stop, plug the nose with gauze (not cotton, which may stick to the blood).

6. Advise the patient not to blow his nose for an hour or two, so that he will not disturb any blood clot that may have formed.

Poisoning. Poisoning may be accidental or intentional. Immediate action is necessary in either case, for once poison has been absorbed in the stomach, little can be done—though pumping the stomach sometimes helps. As long as the poison is not absorbed, little harm is done, provided that the poison was not an acid or an alkali that caused burns around the mouth and in the esophagus.

Vomiting should be induced as promptly as possible. Make the patient drink large amounts of either soapy water, mustard in water, or baking soda in water. If necessary, force him to swallow. If this does not cause vomiting, make him stick his finger in the back of his throat and tickle.

The exception to this rule would be a case of poisoning by an acid or an alkali, when vomiting should not be induced lest further burning of the alimentary passages result. Acid and alkaline poisons must be neutralized. An acid is neutralized by an alkali, such as sodium bicarbonate; an alkali is neutralized by an acid, such as lemon juice or vinegar.

If the type of poison is known, a specific antidote may be administered; but this would probably have to be done after the patient reaches the hospital, as the doctor is not likely to have all antidotes available. In the meantime, the "universal" antidote mentioned in Chapter 6 under Emergency Drugs should be given. If this is not on hand, it may be made up from substitutes—2 parts scraped burnt toast, 1 part milk of magnesia, and 1 part very strong tea, mixed with a little water.

Intentional poisoning often takes the form of an overdose of sleeping pills. In such cases:

1. Give the patient black coffee if he is able to swallow.

2. Arouse him and keep him awake by talking to him. Make him walk, if this is possible.

3. Take him to the hospital as quickly as possible.

Poison Ivy, Poison Oak, Poison Sumac. The best treatment for poisoning by a plant is to wash the skin immediately with soap (preferably laundry soap) and water. Then sponge the skin with alcohol and rinse it with clear water. To prevent itching, apply a solution of 50 per cent salt water and 50 per cent vinegar or a ready-made lotion purchased at the drugstore.

Shock. The state described by the word *shock*, as a medical term, is not a well-defined condition. Some patients experience a slight case of shock after an injection or a painful treatment. Shock generally accompanies an injury, and as a rule, the more severe the injury, the more profound the state of shock. It varies from a simple feeling of weakness to a state of complete unconsciousness. It may be caused by psychological as well as by physiological trauma.

In shock, all body functions are depressed, especially the nervous system and the blood circulation. Pulse, respiration, blood pressure, and temperature are all affected. The symptoms of shock are paleness, a cold sweat, a weak, rapid pulse, irregular breathing, and perhaps fainting and unconsciousness.

The patient should lie flat on his back with his head slightly lowered. Clothing should be loosened at the neck, waist, and wrist, and the patient should be covered with blankets. If possible, hot water bags should be placed around him.

If the patient is conscious and is not vomiting, fluids should be given—coffee or tea, if available, or a hot-water solution with one level teaspoonful of salt and half a teaspoonful of soda to each quart of water, a proportion which represents almost the same degree of salinity as the blood. In mild cases, smelling salts or spirit of ammonia may prove helpful.

Wounds. Open wounds are classified as abrasions, incisions, lacerations, and punctures.

1. *Abrasion:* a wound in which the skin is scraped off
2. *Incision:* a wound made by a piece of broken glass, a knife, etc.
3. *Laceration:* a wound accompanied by a tearing of the tissue
4. *Puncture:* a wound made by a pointed instrument

FIRST-AID RULES

The first step in treating wounds is to stop the bleeding. This is best done by putting sterile gauze pads on the wound and applying slight pressure, either with the hand or with a bandage. If the wound is on the extremities and the bleeding is severe, use a tourniquet as described earlier, under Bleeding. Do not put cotton, bandages, or adhesive directly on a wound. Do not touch a wound with your hands.

Sterile bandages of gauze with adhesive attached can be bought commercially and are the dressing of choice for small wounds. Wounds with no break in the skin are called bruises. Ice or very cold compresses should be applied to a bruise at once.

Do's and Don'ts

In addition to the specific things that must be done in each of the cases enumerated above, there are some general procedures that should be followed in every emergency by the person called upon to administer first aid. There are also certain things, however, which must *not* be done; for, though meant to help the patient, they might cause further harm. These general rules may be summarized as follows:

Do's

1. Calm and reassure the patient by being calm and cheerful yourself.
2. Work swiftly and systematically.
3. Be sure you know what the emergency is.
4. Move the patient as little as possible.
5. Keep the patient warm.

Don'ts

1. Don't rush through your tasks.
2. Don't let other patients crowd around an emergency case. Ask them to leave the room.
3. Don't give any liquids to a patient who is unconscious or vomiting.

4. Don't disturb a blood clot.
5. Don't cover a tourniquet.

First-aid Supplies

If at all possible, all supplies that may be needed for first aid should be kept separate from other medical supplies. Although it is recommended that other medical supplies be kept under lock and key, a first-aid kit should be quickly accessible and plainly marked. In most doctors' offices, emergencies occur frequently. Not only may patients suffer fainting spells or heart attacks, but persons who live near the doctor's office are likely to call upon him for help when an accident or sudden illness occurs.

The contents of the first-aid cabinet may vary from a few essential items to an elaborate supply of every conceivable material. The following items are suggested for a reasonably complete first-aid kit.

1. Aromatic spirit of ammonia
2. Antiseptic solution
3. Table salt
4. Baking soda
5. Mineral oil
6. Assorted bandages
7. Assorted sterile dressings
8. Petrolatum gauze dressings
9. Cotton
10. Adhesive tape
11. Safety pins
12. Scissors
13. Sterile syringe and needle
14. Tourniquet
15. Flashlight
16. Eye dropper
17. Tongue depressors

Every office should have a first-aid kit, and everyone working in the office should know where it is kept. From time to time, this kit must be examined and old materials replaced.

BIBLIOGRAPHY

American National Red Cross, "First Aid Textbook," 4th ed., Doubleday & Company, Inc., New York, 1957.
"Home Health Emergencies," The Equitable Life Assurance Society of the United States, Medical Department, New York, 1956.

15
Medical Secretarial Duties

Unless the assistant is working for a doctor who also employs a secretary, her duties will include those of receptionist and secretary. The term *receptionist* is used advisedly, for it exactly indicates the assistant's duty—to receive the patients. Usually the assistant is the first person the patient meets upon entering the doctor's office. She should greet him as if she were the hostess in her own home and should act as she would there, making the patient feel at home and welcome. The best way to create good will for the doctor is to greet a patient with a smile and a cheerful welcome. Mention the patient's name. Everybody likes to hear his name spoken. That is the reason hotel personnel cultivate this habit and public relations counsels stress its importance.

If the medical office assistant doubles as a secretary, much of her work will consist in handling correspondence, manuscripts, and many other office routines. Rules governing the appearance and form of letters, as well as rules of grammar and spelling, together with much other helpful information, is available in many secretarial handbooks and is therefore not duplicated here. The author's "Handbook for the Medical Secretary" contains additional material regarding the medical secretarial aspects in a doctor's office.

Receiving the Patient

When the patient enters the office or while he is waiting to see the doctor is a good time to practice some of the suggestions made in Chapter 2 under the heading Public Relations. The assistant must know how to handle people. She must be sincerely interested in people, enjoy helping them, and be by nature a friendly, courteous, and kind person. She will meet many patients whom she will thoroughly enjoy, but she will also meet some who are unreasonable, irritable, and perhaps downright rude. Still, she must keep her composure and her friendly attitude. The patient does not mean to be personal. He is merely "letting off steam" at the nearest vent. Pain, illness, disappointment over lack of improvement, fear of serious and prolonged sickness, anxiety over the doctor's bills—all are factors that contribute to a patient's state of mind. It is surprising, though, how much a little attention and understanding on the part of the assistant, especially while the patient is waiting, mulling over his problems, can cheer him up and calm his fears.

If patients are seen by appointment, the appointment should be checked when the patient comes in to make sure that he is on time and that he is coming at the right hour, or even on the right day. If the doctor has office hours during which patients may come without appointment, it is well to write down each patient's name in the order that he arrives. This serves a twofold purpose: it avoids any question as to who sees the doctor first and provides a record of the patients the doctor has seen on that day.

When a new patient comes to the office, certain information must be obtained: the patient's name, address, telephone number, business address, and business telephone number (in the case of a married woman, her husband's name and his business address and telephone number); occupation, age, and marital status (in the case of a married woman, number and ages of children); who referred the patient, whether he is a member of a health insurance group, and how he wishes to pay his bill. This information forms a permanent record, to which the assistant may frequently need to refer. It is advisable to have the information available on index cards, which may be kept in a file on her desk or in another handy place.

Whether or not the assistant takes down part of the patient's medical history depends entirely on the preference of the individual doctor. Practice in this respect varies widely. Many doctors feel that the assistant's duties should include the taking of the medical history, thereby saving them valuable time that they can spend to better advantage with the patient. Other doctors, however, believe that the assistant should not discuss any medical points with the patient at all. Medical histories are discussed in the next chapter.

Appointment System

One of the most frequent complaints from patients concerns not the doctor's high fees, his inability to bring about the expected cure, or his failure to come to the patient's house as quickly as had been hoped, but rather the time the patient has wasted waiting in the office to see the doctor. In fact, surveys made by various agencies have disclosed that patients complain twice as much about waiting as they do about fees. Patients who come to the doctor's office by appointment at a definite time quite naturally resent being kept waiting from half an hour to an hour, or even more. Yet that is what happens in many offices. This reflects on the doctor's efficiency and, in turn, on his secretary's ability to handle office routine.

The doctor's reputation, and in consequence his practice, must be built on an appointment system that really is a *system* and does not deteriorate into a "catch-the-doctor-as-catch-can." It is well to remember that patients have their own private affairs to attend to. If they are business or professional people, they have their own appointments to keep, or they must return to an office where time off is given reluctantly. They may even have wages deducted for the time they are absent. If a patient has been given an appointment for 12:30, let us say, so that he can visit the doctor on his lunch hour, and he has to wait until 1:10 to see the doctor, he will naturally be disgruntled and exasperated. His feeling toward the doctor will be one of animosity rather than good will. Nothing could be more harmful to a patient's progress toward health—to say nothing of the practical side of such an impression. And on the other hand, a patient who is too ill to work probably suffers every minute that he is sitting in the waiting room—either from fear of the treatment, from the discomfort of being out of bed, or from pain.

The first rule, then, is to make appointments carefully, allowing enough time for each patient. There must also be a margin to allow for an examination or treatment that takes a few minutes longer than expected. This obviously requires familiarity with the doctor's practice and his patients. The receptionist must know—and if she is interested in her work will soon know—for just what type of consultation, examination, or treatment each patient is coming to the office and how much time to schedule for him. If the patient is coming for his first visit and a thorough examination is scheduled, more time must be allowed. If the assistant takes part of the medical history and checks weight, pulse, temperature, etc., the doctor is able to see another patient in the meantime. If a patient takes treatments, such as diathermy or inhalations, during which he can be left alone for 10 to 20 minutes, or if he has to disrobe before seeing the doctor and dress himself afterward, this time need not be reserved for the doctor. Such details depend entirely on the doctor's specialty, but must all be taken into account in planning appointments.

To give an example, let us say patient A, coming to the office for the first time, is given an appointment for 10 A.M. Another patient, B, coming for a checkup, is also given an appointment at 10 o'clock. The doctor sees patient B immediately, while the assistant is busy with patient A, recording the required personal data and taking blood pressure, height, weight, etc. At 10:30 the doctor sees patient A. If the assistant is not needed during the examination, another patient can have an appointment at 10:30 and be prepared for the doctor by the assistant between 10:30 and 11. If, however, she must help the doctor with patient A, no new appointment should be made until 11 o'clock.

Calculating the time that each patient will probably take is therefore an important aspect of the secretary's job. Though it will hardly ever be possible to eliminate all waiting whatsoever, the patient's good will can be earned if waiting is kept to a minimum. There are some doctors' offices in which, because of poor management, patients *always* have to wait from 30 to 45 minutes. These offices are often the place of very unpleasant scenes, as patients become disgruntled and even quite angry. One ear specialist, for instance, has such a poor reputation for punctuality that his patients deliberately come half an hour late for appointments. The chaos in his office is indescribable.

In view of all this, it cannot be stressed too much that long waiting in the doctor's office bespeaks poor medical care and worse public relations. If, in spite of all efforts, the appointments fall behind schedule, it is better to speed up each patient by a few minutes than to let all of them wait a long time. When several patients are scheduled for the same time—one for an x-ray, let us say, one for a diathermy treatment, and one for consultation, delays and backups are bound to occur. If it is found too difficult to run the appointment schedule smoothly, a free period of about 20 minutes, when no appointments are made, should be scheduled in midmorning and again in midafternoon. This allows the schedule to catch up if there has been a delay. To make sure this is not overlooked, the free period should be marked in the appointment book.

Appointment schedules are thrown out of line by various factors: (1) the patient may be late; (2) the patient may take up too much of the doctor's time; or (3) the doctor may have to spend more time with the patient than expected. In each of these eventualities the assistant must step in, in an effort to keep the schedule straight. If a patient is late, he can be told that, because of his tardiness, his time with the doctor will have to be shortened, as other appointments are scheduled. If he is very late, the patient who has the next appointment can be shown in to the doctor before the late patient. The explanation to the patient should be made in the most tactful and courteous way. The lesson will probably sink in just the same. If a patient spends too much time with the doctor, the aide may enter the doctor's room with the reminder that his next appointment is waiting, that the next patient is ready in the examination room, or that one of the patients has to catch a train; or she may call the doctor on the telephone and remind him of the time.

A fourth cause of interrupted appointment schedules is the patient who drops in without an appointment. If the case is not an emergency, an appointment at the next possible hour should be offered. If the patient seems very anxious to see the doctor, the assistant might explain that the doctor will see him for just a few minutes to determine how urgent the situation is; the patient might then see the doctor between two appointments.

Emergencies of course will happen and cannot be avoided. An emergency case takes precedence over any waiting patients. No one resents this, for everyone realizes that he himself may have an emergency someday and he too would want to be treated immediately. It is most important, however, to explain the situation to the waiting patients so that they will understand the reason for the delay.

Making Appointments. A prerequisite for an intelligent and efficient appointment system is obviously an appointment book. This should be one specially designed for a doctor's use, with the time of day indicated in quarter-hours, and, if possible, two columns in which to indicate the service to be rendered. Some appointment books allow one page for each day; others show the six days of the week on two opposite pages, three days to a page. A page from an appointment book is illustrated in Fig. 15–1.

The main points to remember in making appointments are:

1. Be sure you have the name exactly right.
2. Make the appointment for the next hour available.
3. Be sure the date and time are distinctly understood. Repeat them to the patient.
4. Allow enough time for each appointment.
5. Be sure nobody else is scheduled at the same time for the same service.
6. Try to remember the time of day each patient prefers for his appointment.
7. Offer a choice—"Would you like to come today at 5 or tomorrow at 10?"
8. If you have to refuse a request for an appointment at a certain time, explain why this is necessary and try to find another time that is convenient for the patient.
9. Enter the appointment in your appointment book.

MEDICAL SECRETARIAL DUTIES 225

TUESDAY
18
JUNE 1957

MAY
S M T W T F S
1 2 3 4
5 6 7 8 9 10 11
12 13 14 15 16 17 18
19 20 21 22 23 24 25
26 27 28 29 30 31

JULY
S M T W T F S
1 2 3 4 5 6
7 8 9 10 11 12 13
14 15 16 17 18 19 20
21 22 23 24 25 26 27
28 29 30 31

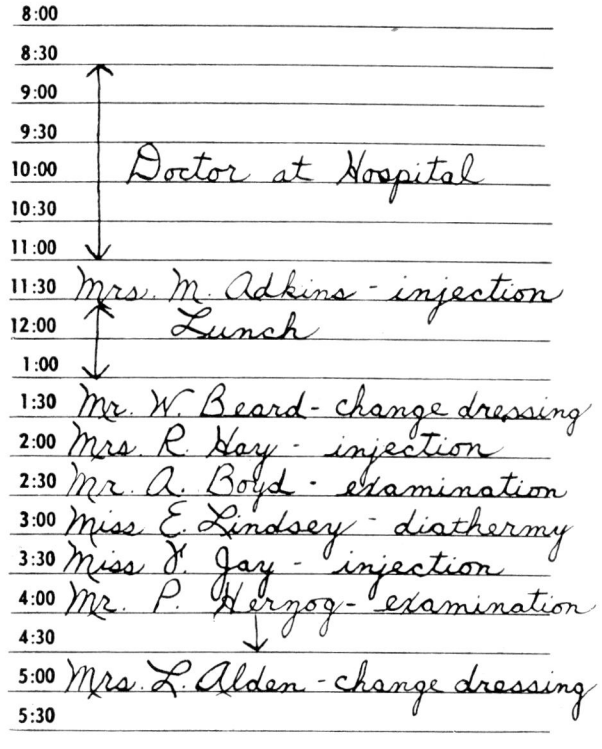

8:00	
8:30	
9:00	
9:30	
10:00	Doctor at Hospital
10:30	
11:00	
11:30	Mrs. M. Adkins - injection
12:00	Lunch
1:00	
1:30	Mr. W. Beard - change dressing
2:00	Mrs. R. Hay - injection
2:30	Mr. A. Boyd - examination
3:00	Miss E. Lindsey - diathermy
3:30	Miss J. Jay - injection
4:00	Mr. P. Herzog - examination
4:30	
5:00	Mrs. L. Alden - change dressing
5:30	

FIG. 15–1. Page from an appointment book.

In a busy doctor's office it is, obviously, rarely possible to give a patient an appointment at exactly the time he would like; however, he should be made to feel that the doctor is available and will see him as soon as possible. A patient who calls for an appointment and is told the doctor cannot see him for two or three days will probably turn to another doctor. If the doctor has a full schedule, therefore, the secretary must ask the patient whether he needs to see the doctor right away, whether he is in pain or has any symptom that requires immediate attention. A patient who calls the office of a nose and throat specialist because he has the first symptoms of a cold and wants to ward it off by prompt treatment would not be helped if he could not come on the same day. On the other hand, a patient who wants to visit an eye specialist to get a prescription for new glasses can just as well come a day or two later if the doctor's schedule is filled up. Excellent judgment is necessary in the matter of making such appointments.

Appointments are made either over the telephone or in the office before the patient leaves. If a patient takes the initiative to call up for an appointment, he is not likely to forget it. It has been found, however, that appointments given to the patient in the office are often forgotten, especially if they are for a date several weeks later. Appointment cards are therefore helpful. If the receptionist reads out the date and time while she is writing the card, the patient hears the information twice (the first time, when the time for the appointment was discussed), and this helps to engrave it on his memory. If appointment cards are used, the secretary should keep a supply on her desk. She must also remember to enter each appointment in the appointment book.

Office Hours. Some doctors, instead of giving each patient an appointment, have fixed office hours, which are made known to the patients. Patients are then seen in the order in which they arrive. The disadvantage of this system is that most patients tend to come during the latter part of the session, which means that the doctor may not be busy at all for the first hour or so and then be forced to stay past the allotted time to see the last patients. This situation can be avoided. If, for example, the office hours are from 4 to 6 o'clock, tell patients who are known to be free to come between 4 and 4:30 or between 4 and 5; or tell about ten patients to come between 4 and 5; another ten, between 5 and 6. Experience in an individual office will soon teach the secretary the best way to handle the particular practice of her doctor-employer.

If patients do not come by appointment, it is most important to keep a record of the order in which each patient arrives, so as to obviate the cardinal offense of ushering in a latecomer ahead of an early arrival. The record may be kept in a book or on special slips of paper that come in pad form. These slips are perforated and have carbon copies. Write one name on each slip and then tear the slip off and hand it to the doctor before, or when, the patient is shown in. This helps the doctor remember the name of the patient he is about to see, and, at the same time, the carbon copy remains on the pad to constitute a permanent record of the patients who visited the doctor on a particular day.

Canceled Appointments. The canceled appointment is the bane of all professional people. To a doctor who has a tight schedule, this can mean real loss of money. There are several points to be remembered in handling canceled appointments:

1. If a patient calls up to cancel an appointment, immediately suggest another time; make sure another appointment is made.

2. Mark your appointment book accordingly; the time is now free for another patient.

3. If another patient had to be given an appointment at a later date than he originally asked for, try to reach him and give him the time that has now been made available.

It is well to keep track of habitual latecomers and people who make a habit of canceling their appointments. Either telephone them shortly before the appointment to remind them of it, or send a reminder by mail. It is also advisable to schedule their appointments at the end of the day, so that the doctor may leave earlier if they do not show up.

If a patient cancels at the last moment or fails to notify the doctor that he is not coming, the doctor may wish to charge for the lost time; but this of course is entirely up to the doctor. Many doctors charge a patient who cancels frequently, but do not like to charge a patient for the first offense.

Doctor's Lateness. Of course, even in the best-run office, the doctor may throw the schedule out of line by being late himself. If he has not arrived on time or if he has called the office to explain that he will be delayed, the secretary should at once explain to the patients why they are being kept waiting. If the doctor will be very late—because of an emergency operation, for instance—new appointments should be offered to those patients who do not wish to wait.

If the doctor's late arrival has thrown the schedule off, try the same remedy as suggested before—hurry just a little with your own preparations; have everything ready for the doctor; mention tactfully to the patient that inasmuch as the doctor was delayed, he would appreciate it if patients did not take any longer than necessary. Some patients like to while away time—theirs and the doctor's —with idle conversation that has no bearing at all on their condition.

Whenever it is necessary for the doctor to cancel an appointment, the patient should be informed immediately—by telephone if feasible; by telegram; or if there is plenty of time, by a note. A new appointment should be offered at the same time.

Telephone Hours

Patients often call the doctor's office to report on their progress or to ask the doctor questions in regard to their treatment or their condition. An occasional telephone call of this sort is a routine matter and needs no special handling; however, many patients abuse the privilege of the telephone call and attempt to obtain advice and prescriptions over the telephone. Such telephone calls are disturbing to the doctor when he is in consultation with, or treating, another patient. Various ways of dealing with this problem have therefore been established.

Some doctors, feeling that such telephone reports or inquiries are to be encouraged, set aside a fixed time each day during which patients can reach the doctor by telephone. A few doctors print this time on their billheads, together with the time of office hours. The telephone time is usually at the beginning of the day, perhaps from 9 to 10 o'clock. If the doctor has a telephone hour, patients should not be connected with the doctor at any other time (except in case of an emergency). But it should be explained to them that a particular hour is reserved for this special purpose. No appointments should be scheduled during the telephone hour.

Other doctors, feeling that patients who telephone the office want a free consultation, make a charge for telephone advice and so inform their patients. As the charge is less than for an office visit, such an arrangement works to the satisfaction of both parties. It saves the patient money and a great deal of time, and the doctor will not have lost the fee to which his services entitle him.

Out-of-office Visits

In addition to their office practice, most physicians visit patients at home or in the hospital. This of course must be taken into account when appointments are being scheduled. If the doctor is on the staff of a hospital, he will no doubt be at the hospital at fixed times, either every morning or on certain days of the week. These times must be noted in the appointment book. If these hours are crossed out in the book, appointments will not be made in error. But some patients do not have to see the doctor himself. If a patient is coming for injections, certain treatments, changing of dressings, exercises, checking of glasses, or one of the many services that may be rendered by the office nurse, this should be remembered when the appointment is made. The time when the doctor is not in the office is the best time for such visits, for the assistant will then be free to help the doctor when he sees other patients.

A record of the doctor's house or hospital visits must also be kept at the office, and this often presents a real problem. If the doctor makes a regular round of visits each day, the secretary should work out a list of calls according to the location of each patient's home and the urgency of each case. She should give the doctor a copy of this list and when he returns check it with him to ascertain the services rendered at each visit, the fee involved, and whether the fee has been paid or is to be charged. This information is then transferred to the patient's record. Or the doctor may carry with him a pad of house-call slips, which he completes at each patient's home and hands to his secretary when he returns to the office. Such a slip is illustrated in Fig. 15–2.

An excellent method was suggested in an article that appeared in *Medical Economics* in November, 1954. The doctor keeps a sim-

OFFICE VISIT		DATE	19	BAL.	
HOUSE "				FRD.	
NIGHT "	CHARGE TO				
HOSPITAL "				CHG.	
EXAMINATION	ADDRESS				
CONSULTATION					
CONFINEMENT				TOT.	
ANESTHETIC					
OPERATION	PATIENT			PAID	
SURG. DRESSING					
MEDICINE	ADDRESS			BAL.	

AP.   SLEEP   BOWELS   T.   P.   R.   B. P.

DIAGNOSIS

SYMPTOMS

TREATMENT

FORM NO. 105 PROFESSIONAL PRINTING COMPANY, INC., NEW HYDE PARK, NEW YORK

FIG. 15-2. House-call slip. (*Professional Printing Company, Inc.*)

ple pocket notebook, using two facing pages per day for all entries. On the left-hand page the assistant enters the names and addresses of the patients and possibly the time when the doctor expects to arrive. On the opposite page the doctor enters remarks about the service rendered, the patient's condition, and the amount to be charged or payments received. The assistant can rule the pages according to the number of columns needed and insert headings.

The larger the notebook is, the more columns it can hold; but if the book does not fit comfortably into the doctor's pocket, its value is lost. This book serves a manifold purpose. It gives the doctor a record of his out-of-the-office appointments, which the assistant usually lists for the doctor anyhow. As he visits each patient, he checks off the name. This book is a permanent record of all visits, progress reports, charges, and payments. When the doctor returns to the office from such a visit he hands the book to his aide, and she transfers the entries to the patient's record and writes out the list of appointments for the next day.

Handling the Telephone

The telephone is one of the most important instruments in everybody's life today. It keeps us in touch with the world around us, even though we ourselves may be completely alone within our four walls. Many people have a telephone installed expressly for the purpose of being able to call a doctor when necessary. The doctor's telephone, therefore, must be handled with the utmost skill and care.

The doctor's individual preference will determine the manner in which the telephone is to be answered and how calls are to be handled. Whether to say, "Good morning. Dr. Clark's office," or simply, "Doctor's office," also depends on whether the doctor occupies his office alone or whether he shares it with one or more colleagues.

The first requisite for good telephone technique is a good telephone voice. The voice should be pitched low. The secretary must speak more slowly than usual and show no hurry, excitement, or irritation at any time. A high squaky voice or one that is listless or monotonous is to be avoided by all means, lest it send the caller to another doctor, where he may expect to find more interest in his affairs.

It is surprising how much can be conveyed merely by a person's tone of voice. The same words can create an entirely different impression according to whether they are uttered in a listless, monotonous, indifferent tone with a certain edge to it, as if the secretary were just a bit annoyed at having to answer at all, or in a firm, cheerful voice with an inflection that indicates interest and willingness to help the caller. The task of handling calls can be made easier by a pleasant telephone manner; for it is sometimes quite difficult to obtain from the caller the reason for his call, or even his name, or to understand him clearly, and he will be far more cooperative if the secretary's voice communicates a desire to be helpful.

It is unlikely that the doctor will want to speak to everybody who telephones regardless of who it is or the reason for the call. Most doctors expect their secretaries to screen the telephone calls for them and to take care of as many as they can. In order to handle a call intelligently, the first information that must be obtained is the caller's name. While almost every person knows that he will be asked for this information, very few give it right away. If the caller does not identify himself, it is therefore necessary to ask, "Who is calling, please?" or, "May I have your name, please?"

Needless to say, it is of paramount importance to have the name right. Unpleasant or embarrassing mix-ups might occur if a name is mistaken for one that is similar. It is much easier for the secretary to grasp what the other person wants if she knows with whom she is speaking. If the name is difficult to understand, she should ask to have it spelled out, as this is less annoying to the caller than having to repeat it several times. Perhaps she could say, "I want to be sure I have understood your name exactly, so won't you please spell it for me?" In the case of a common name like Brown, Jones, or Smith, it is advisable to ask for the initials or the first name also, as the doctor may know several people by that name.

The next piece of information that must be elicited is the reason for the call. The majority of people do not give the reason for their call, but simply ask "to speak to the doctor." If there are several doctors using the same office, the secretary must find out tactfully which one is meant. Most patients assume that only "their" doctor occupies the office. Much time could be saved if every patient would make a simple statement such as "This is Mrs. Bennett. I want to make an appointment." But this is rarely the case. After finding out the name, the secretary must usually ask, "May I help you?" or "Do you wish to make an appointment?" Or she may say, "The doctor is busy with a patient right now. Perhaps I can give him a message."

The next step is to attend to the request at once. If an appointment is desired, it should be given at the next hour available; if that hour is not convenient, another hour should be suggested.

If a patient wants to know something concerning the treatment he or someone in his family is receiving, you must know exactly how much information you can give over the telephone. Probably the doctor will have given you instructions regarding certain routine procedures. Some doctors prefer to be called to the telephone as little as possible and want to know who is calling and for what reason before they answer the telephone themselves. They expect their secretaries to handle calls independently.

Be sure to get instructions from the doctor on how to deal with cranky patients—for instance, those who call up several times a day just to ask foolish questions. You must know whether the doctor will back you up if you tell such a patient that the doctor is busy and that you will be able to answer the question.

If the doctor does not wish to speak to anyone without knowing his name—and the majority of doctors don't—it is best to ascertain the name at once. If the secretary makes a statement of any kind to the effect that the doctor is out or is busy, the caller may just hang up with the remark "I'll call back later," and the call will have been wasted. If the caller turns out to be someone to whom the doctor wishes to talk, the secretary will be in an embarrassing position.

The situation becomes a little more complicated when the caller refuses to give even his name and demands to speak to the doctor on a "personal matter." A friend of the doctor will not hesitate to give his name and mention that he is a friend. When a person hedges about giving his name or his reason for calling and insists "it's personal," the chances are that his reason is something that will be of advantage to himself only. This is especially true when a caller assumes a tone of authority and implies that if he is not connected with the doctor at once, without further questioning, he will make a complaint. Many a secretary, new in her job, has become frightened and called the doctor to the telephone, only to be told later that he was interrupted unnecessarily and was put in the position of having to refuse to buy tickets for a ball game.

The best way to deal with such a caller is to tell him that the doctor cannot be disturbed unless the caller states his name or the reason for his call. The secretary may suggest that he write to the doctor and explain his business; or, if he asks to see the doctor, she may inquire whether he wishes to make a professional appointment. Usually when the caller realizes that he cannot speak to the doctor unless he identifies himself, he will state the reason for his call. Not wishing to be charged for his visit, he will usually be quick to say that he does not want a professional appointment. If his errand is legitimate, there is no reason for him to be secretive about it.

You need not fear that your employer will miss an important call if you refuse to connect a reticent caller. Any professional man who has something important or confidential to discuss with the doctor will say so quite clearly. If a caller identifies himself as a doctor, you must of course connect him without further questioning. Medical etiquette requires this act of courtesy.

Sometimes the secretary of another physician will call up to find out whether the doctor is in, as her employer wishes to speak to him. In this case, connect your doctor's telephone after the other doctor is on his line. Telephone etiquette prescribes that the person who originated the call do the waiting.

All telephone conversations should be kept as brief as possible. "Visiting" over the telephone with patients, as well as with personal friends, is to be discouraged.

Making a Memorandum. A memorandum should be made of every telephone call *immediately*. This memorandum should contain the following information:

1. Date
2. Time
3. Name of person who called
4. His telephone number in case he is to be called back
5. The main points of the conversation
6. What the secretary did about the call
7. Some comments on the conversation if they seem necessary

Pertinent comments might be "The patient seemed very much excited," or "The caller was very impatient." Some doctors like to have a memorandum made of all telephone calls from patients, even if the secretary has attended to the call herself, and they like to have these memoranda filed in the patients' folders.

Whenever a patient calls, the secretary should take his record from the file and either consult it herself, if she is handling the call, or give it to the doctor so that he can refresh his memory while talking to the patient.

Emergency Calls. When there is an emergency call, the secretary must above all remain calm herself, even though the person who is calling may be very excited and upset. The questions to be asked, in addition to the name and address, concern the nature of the emergency and any relevant details. If the doctor is not in the office, tell the caller you will try and reach him as quickly as possible. Be sure you have the caller's telephone number, so that you or the doctor can call back to let him know when the doctor will arrive. Waiting is one of the worst ordeals for a patient who is in severe pain or who has had an accident.

If you know that the doctor will not be able to be reached by telephone for any length of time, remind him before he leaves the office to call you at intervals. Then, when he calls, have all messages for him by your telephone in the order of their importance.

Summary. The rules for handling the doctor's telephone can be summarized as follows:

1. Answer the telephone as promptly as possible.
2. Keep a pad and pencil next to the telephone at all times.
3. Find out the caller's name.
4. Ascertain the reason for the call.
5. Handle as many telephone calls as you possibly can without disturbing the doctor.
6. If the doctor prefers to speak to patients, call him to the telephone after telling him who is calling. Take out the patient's medical history and give it to the doctor.
7. Whenever possible, if you cannot handle the matter alone, take a message for the doctor, so he can read it at his leisure and tell you what to do or call the person back when he has time.
8. Make a memorandum for the doctor of every telephone call. Use printed telephone memorandum pads that show date, time of call, name of caller, telephone number, and message.
9. Always know where to reach the doctor. If the message is urgent and the doctor is not in the office, telephone him at once and give him the message.
10. If the doctor cannot be reached, have the message by your phone so you can read it to him when he calls you.
11. Learn how much medical information the doctor wishes you

to give over the telephone. Patients frequently call the office because they have forgotten the doctor's instructions about treatments or medications. If these instructions are clearly stated in the medical history, it may be possible for the assistant to repeat them to the patient.

12. End all telephone conversations on a friendly note. In general, let the caller be the first one to hang up or say good-by.

Outgoing Calls. A piece of advice about outgoing calls might assist in keeping the office running efficiently. If you have to make a number of telephone calls, allow an interval of about 5 minutes between such calls. This will give a person who is trying to reach the doctor's office a chance to make the connection. A constant "busy" signal may discourage a patient and cause him to call another doctor.

Have a list of the numbers you call often on your desk and keep this up to date. It will save valuable time.

Be careful about making calls to patients when other patients are in the waiting room (if that is where your desk is) or near your desk.

BIBLIOGRAPHY

Bredow, Miriam: "Handbook for the Medical Secretary," 3d ed., Gregg Publishing Division, McGraw-Hill Book Company, Inc., New York, 1954.

Hutchinson, Lois: "Standard Handbook for Secretaries," 7th ed., Gregg Publishing Division, McGraw-Hill Book Company, Inc., New York, 1956.

16
Patients' Records

The appointment book, discussed in the preceding chapter, provides a record of each patient who has visited the office; however, a great deal more information regarding each patient is needed. It has been mentioned that at the patient's first visit it is necessary to obtain so-called "statistical" data, that is, the patient's name, address, and so forth. Additional points that may be included are the parents' names, in the case of a minor; the person to be billed; the patient's mailing address; his business telephone number, if it is all right to call him at his place of business. This information should be typed on a card and kept in the most accessible place for quick reference.

The Medical History

After a new patient has given the secretary his name and address and such general data, the doctor must learn something about the patient's medical condition. He must learn why the patient is consulting him, the symptoms of which he complains, how long he has had the condition, what he has done about it, and many other facts. This information, together with the doctor's diagnosis, the treatment prescribed, the progress of the disease, and the patient's improvement and cure, forms the patient's medical history. Without such a record, the doctor could not remember from one visit to another just exactly what he had found and just what he had prescribed in each case; nor would he be able to form an opinion on the progress of the patient. The medical history is a permanent record that may be referred to over a period of many years, every time the patient comes to the doctor's office—sometimes at intervals of several years.

Medical histories are "privileged communications"; that is, they are confidential records. They belong to the doctor and must not be given out; nor must any information from them be disclosed without the express authorization of the patient, except to another doctor whom the patient has subsequently consulted. All medical histories should be locked up except when they are on the doctor's desk.

The information that is obtained from the patient on his first visit and entered on the medical history should include the following points:

1. Description of the present major complaint and minor complaints
2. Date when the condition first began
3. Treatments for the condition prior to coming to this doctor
4. Past medical history (operations, illnesses, accidents, or congenital conditions)
5. Family history (the state of health of parents, brothers and sisters, and any important medical facts regarding other blood relatives)
6. Diagnosis (results of examination)
7. Treatment prescribed
8. Prognosis (outlook for the development and cure of the patient's illness)

Points 6, 7, and 8 are, of course, added by the doctor after he has seen and examined the patient.

Each time the patient returns to the office or the doctor visits him at his house or at the hospital, his condition is recorded, together with any new treatment prescribed or any change in the instructions previously given, such as change in the dosage of medication, change in diet, etc. This record is called the progress report. It is important that each entry be dated.

To facilitate the taking and keeping of medical histories, many different types of printed forms are available. Some are cards of different sizes, either 3 by 5 or 4 by 6, for specialists who do not need much medical data—an ophthalmologist, for instance. Some are double cards that provide ample space for medical information and may be filed either folded, in conventional card-filing cases, or flat, in manila folders. Further, some forms are standard letter size, 8 by 11.

Medical history forms are available for use in general medical practice as well as in the different specialties. For each of the different specialties the headings necessary are provided so that the specific data may be easily recorded. A number of printers of professional stationery manufacture their own copyrighted forms, each of which is preferred by doctors in the different specialties. One such form for internal medicine is illustrated in Fig. 16–1.

Many doctors, however, do not like to be restricted to a standard outline and prefer to write up case histories in their own way. Some of the firms specializing in professional printing or in filing equipment will print cards or forms according to the doctor's specifications, with his name and address, if he so wishes. Or the doctor may dictate his case histories and have them typed on plain white paper. In the latter case care must be taken to use proper headings, so that the history may be read easily. If laboratory examinations have been made or x-rays taken, the findings should be entered on the medical history.

In many doctors' offices, the medical office assistant takes part of the medical history, that is, points 1 to 5 of the above list, herself, before the patient sees the doctor. This saves a great deal of the doctor's time. There are, however, varying opinions about this practice. Some doctors wish their secretaries to take all medical histories; others are very much opposed to this and do not allow their assistants to ask any medical questions at all. The doctor's wishes are the deciding factor, and the assistant is advised not to ask the patient any medical questions unless she has been specifically instructed to do so.

If the assistant does take the medical history, she should make sure, first of all, that no other patients are listening. No one likes to reveal personal data in front of strangers. In fact, the medical his-

NAME Edith M. Carlson (Mrs. Joseph A.) Final Diagnosis Gastric Ulcer File or Hosp. No.
Address 70 Metropolitan Avenue Referred by Dr. Max Johnson Date May 3, 1957

Age	Sex	Color	S (M) W D	Occupation	'Phones	Nearest Relative and Address
36	F	White		Housewife	EL 7-3478	Joseph A Carlson, husband

COMPLAINTS Upper abdominal pain. "Heartburn"

PRESENT ILLNESS Had much heartburn while at college but this disappeared when she took medicine. (does not remember name). Later, whenever she had recurrence of heartburn she took bicarbonate of soda which gave relief until recently. Pain now very frequent and at times severe. No nausea or vomiting.

RESPIRATORY	Rhinitis	0	Sinusitis	0	Sore Throat	0	Epistaxis	0	Post-Nasal Discharge	0		
	Cough	0	Sputum	0	Hemoptysis	0	Chest Pain	0	Night Sweats	0	Chill	0
CARDIO-VASCULAR	Vertigo	0	Headache	0	Cardiac – Pain	0	Radiation	0	Rhythm	0	Rate	0
	Palpitation	0	Cyanosis	0	Pallor	0	Petechiae	0	Claudication	0	Mental Symptoms	0
GASTRO-INTESTINAL	Dysphagia	0	Nausea	0	Anorexia		Flatulence		Indigestion	✓	Vomiting	
	Hematemesis	0	Pain	✓	Location	Upper Abd.	Radiation	yes	Relieved by	—		
	Constipation	0	Diarrhea	0	Hemorrhoids	0	Melena	0				
UROLOGIC	Polyuria	0	Oliguria	0	Anuria	0	Hematuria	0	Dysuria	0	Colic	0
GENERAL	Fever	0	Dyspnea	0	Edema	0	Loss of Weight	no	Asthenia	0	Allergy	0

NEURO-MUSCULAR SKELETAL average

MENSTRUAL HISTORY Began at 14, 28 days cycle, 4 days Children 3 Ages 13, 10, 8 Abortions 0

USE OF Alcohol Mod. Tobacco Mod. Narcotics 0 Food Habits poor, irregular meals

FIG. 16–1A. Medical history form for internal medicine. (*Physicians' Record Co.*)

PAST HISTORY					
Diphtheria	Measles ✓	Chicken Pox	Mumps	Scarlet Fever	Poliomyelitis
Small Pox	Typhoid Fever	Malaria	Pneumonia	Dysentery	Gonorrhea
Syphilis	Tonsillitis	Nephritis	Influenza	Rheumatic Fever	Chorea
Cancer	Injuries		Operations *appendix removed at 16*		

FAMILY HISTORY Father 68, l. & w. Mother 60, "nervous" Grandparents ✓
Siblings *An older sister also has "stomach trouble" and is nervous* Other ✓

PHYSICAL EXAM. Height 5'3" Weight 118 Temp. *normal* Physique *stocky* Nutrition ✓ Color *fair* Development ✓

Skin *fair*
Head and Neck Scalp
Eyes — Right / Left
Nose
Tongue / Oral Hygiene / Teeth / Mastoids
Buccal Mucosa *not examined*
Pharynx / Tonsils / Larynx
Parotid Gland / Submaxillary Gland
Thyroid / Cervical Nodes

Chest Circumference / Expansion *not examined* / Shape / Symmetry / Respiration Rate
Lungs

Heart Rate—At Rest 72 / After Exercise / Return to Normal / Thrill / Radial Pulse 72
Rhythm / Blood Pressure 125/75
Apex / Right Border
Heart Sounds

FIG. 16-1B. Medical history form for internal medicine (*continued*). (*Physicians' Record Co.*)

Abdomen Scaphoid	Obese	Distended		
Musculature	Good	Poor	Tenderness *in epigastric region*	Peristalsis
Fluid	Liver		Spleen	Kidneys
Masses				Herniae
Rectal Examination				
External Genitalia				
Pelvic Examination				
Spine	*not examined*			
Extremities				
Reflexes Triceps	Ulnar	Patellar	Abd.–Right	Left	Cremasteric	Babinski	Oppenheim	Gordon

LABORATORY EXAMINATION Urine – Amount 800 cc S.G. 1.015 Albumin 0 Sugar 0 Blood 0 Pus Casts

Blood – Hgb. 11 grams R.b.c. 3,500,000 W.b.c. 6,500 C.I. Platelets 0

Differential Count *normal* Morphology *normal*

Gastric Analysis – T.A. 50 cc obtained F.A. 80 Blood *Positive* Mucus 0 Lactic Acid 0

Feces *Occult blood in stool*

Blood – N.P.N. 0 Urea 0 Creatinin 0 Ca. 0 Phos. 0 Chlorides 0

B.M.R. *not taken*

RADIOGRAPHIC EXAMINATION *Xrays show an irregular erosion of the gastric mucosa 5 cm from the pylorus on the greater curvature*

Electrocardiograph *not taken*

TENTATIVE DIAGNOSIS *Gastric Ulcer*

TREATMENT *Special bland diet. No alcohol. Anti-acid medication. Patient to return in one week.*

FIG. 16–1C. Medical history form for internal medicine *(continued)*. (*Physicians' Record Co.*)

FOLLOW-UP RECORD

VISITS (Dates)	COMPLAINTS	EXAMINATION	TREATMENT
May 10	Had two attacks, pain less severe		Continue previous treatment

Fig. 16-1D. Medical history form for internal medicine (continued). (Physicians' Record Co.)

tory should not be taken even in the presence of friends or relatives who may be accompanying the patient. The patient may be embarrassed to tell the secretary all he would like the doctor to know about himself, and yet, at the same time, he may hesitate to ask to speak to the secretary alone. She should therefore make it easy for him by suggesting that they go into another room. If that is not possible, she should invite the patient to sit next to her desk, while she finds a chair farther away for the friend or relative and gives him something to read, thus implying that he is not expected to listen. Some friends are extremely curious, and it may be necessary for the secretary to be quite firm in telling such a person that the doctor's instructions are that she question the patient alone, without anyone else listening. Modern interiors of doctors' offices provide a certain amount of privacy for the secretary by partitions or plants that set off her desk from the waiting room, without obstructing her view.

While asking the patient medical questions, the secretary should make note of relevant things the patient may mention that may be of help to the doctor in dealing with the case. A doctor may find that patients talk more freely and at greater length to his secretary than to him, sometimes providing hints that prove profitable in the management of the case. For instance, a woman who complains of a skin rash may mention casually to the secretary that she has changed to a new brand of face powder—a fact which she might consider too trivial to mention to the doctor but which would give him an important clue.

It must be remembered that case histories are legal documents and may have to be produced in court. For instance, if the patient had an accident and were suing for damages, the doctor's testimony would be of the greatest importance. Or, if the doctor were suing the patient for nonpayment of his bill, the case history would be the proof of the services the doctor has rendered and for which he asks payment. All the information contained in the medical history, therefore, should be accurate, legibly written (if it is not typed), and as complete as possible. Dates of the patient's visits are especially important. A well-kept history may have important bearing on the outcome of a legal case, as it will help to substantiate the doctor's testimony, while a sketchy, badly written-up form may prejudice the doctor's case.

Personal Health Record

In addition to the medical history, which is kept by the doctor, there have recently been introduced personal-health-record booklets, which are to be kept by the patient himself, regardless of whether he is currently under the doctor's care or not. This booklet provides space for his family medical history, listing in systematic form various types of disease that a close relative might have had. It includes a check list of many medical conditions or symptoms that a person might easily forget to mention when in the doctor's office. It also contains space in which to enter any circumstances related to employment that may have a bearing on the person's health.

The purpose of this record is manifold. It helps the doctor who may be treating the patient to check on the patient's daily reaction to the treatment. If the patient consults a new doctor, the doctor can read this record and form an opinion about the patient's condition by studying his medical background. The record will serve as a reminder of some medications and treatments prescribed for the patient that he might wish to have repeated.

An excellent personal-health record is the one designed by Dr. Carl A. Dragstedt and published by the Military Service Publishing Company of Harrisburg, Pennsylvania. In addition to headings for keeping the personal-health record, this booklet contains much valuable information on first aid, medical abbreviations, weights and measures, etc. Such a personal-health record may well be recommended to a patient.

Filing of Medical Histories

Medical histories should be filed separately from all other material, preferably in a special filing cabinet, but certainly in a separate drawer. A manila folder should be made for each patient. This folder should contain all material pertaining to the patient—his medical history (unless this is kept on cards and filed in special filing boxes), all laboratory reports, and all correspondence with and about the patient.

Folders are filed in alphabetic order according to the last name of the patient. Rules regarding alphabetizing and filing in general can be found in every secretarial handbook. If the assistant has had no special training in the art of filing, she is strongly advised to study it in one of the many secretarial manuals.

In offices where it is desirable to preserve the anonymity of the patient, folders may be kept by numbers. For this system, a book is kept with a list of consecutive numbers, and each time a folder is made for a new patient, his name is entered opposite the next free number. This number is entered on the folder, and the folder is filed numerically, that is, the last number last. A key must be established for this system. The name of each patient and the number of his file folder are entered on cards, and these are kept in alphabetic order. It is necessary to consult this key to find any patient's folder. Doctors who treat venereal diseases sometimes use such a system.

In an alphabetic file the manila folders are placed behind alphabetic guides. If many folders accumulate, the sections are divided according to second or third letters (Aa–Al, Am–Az, etc.). Guides may be purchased in any desired number of divisions. About ten folders should follow each guide. For efficient filing, ten to twenty papers are kept in one folder.

In order to prevent a filing cabinet from becoming so crowded as to cause delay in finding a folder, all the folders of patients actually under the care of the doctor should be kept together in an *Active* file. When a patient is discharged, the folder can be removed to an *Inactive* file in another filing cabinet, from which it can always be transferred to the active file if the patient returns to the doctor. If a patient dies, moves to another city, or definitely ceases coming to the office, the folders can be stored in a *Closed* file. The Inactive and the Closed files can be placed in storage rooms. They certainly need not take up valuable space in the front office.

The question of how long to keep records often arises. Many

doctors never throw away a medical history, and this is often good practice. A patient may return after many years, or his children may be benefited by their doctor's having access to their parents' history; however, storage space is also a decisive factor. If the doctor does not like to discard any medical histories, microfilming is one way of solving the dilemma; but there is really no need to save histories of patients with routine conditions who are no longer under the doctor's care and will not return to his care.

Filing Practices

Cross References. For efficient filing, a cross-reference system is important. This works in the following way: If a letter from Dr. Arthur Hill, let us say, dated July 15, 19—, deals with several patients—Mrs. Anthony Bates, Miss Roberta Jones, and Mr. William Barker—the original letter is filed in the folder of the patient first named in the letter (in this case Mrs. Anthony Bates) or in the folder of the patient with whom the greater part of the letter deals. A cross-reference sheet is placed in each of the folders of the other two patients mentioned, with the notation "For the letter from Dr. Arthur Hill, dated July 15, 19—, *see* folder of Mrs. Anthony Bates." The rule governing cross references may be stated thus: Whenever a paper may be looked up under two or more names or subjects, a cross reference must be made. Printed cross-reference sheets are available. In any case, it is helpful to use colored paper, as this is quickly spotted in a folder.

Out Cards. Whenever a paper is taken out of the file, a notation to that effect is made. A description of the paper, the date, and the person to whom it was given is entered on such a record. This is placed in the folder in place of the paper that was taken out, and it remains there until the original paper is refiled. Making such a record has saved many a secretary from being accused of losing or misfiling a paper. A paper taken out is easily forgotten. When a paper is not in its proper place, only an "out" card will help to locate it promptly.

Filing by Subject. Whenever the subject is of more importance than the writer, the material should be filed *by subject*. For example, if a doctor is corresponding with a number of physicians regarding their experience with treatment by ultrasonic therapy, it would be better to have all this correspondence filed in one folder labeled Ultrasonic Therapy, than to have the letters scattered alphabetically according to the names of the writers.

A cross-reference system is important whenever the filing is done according to subject. For instance, in the example just mentioned, the doctor may also correspond with other doctors or collect articles on different types of treatments for arthritis of the shoulder—of which ultrasonic therapy is one. The doctor may have a folder in his scientific file labeled Arthritis of the Shoulder. A cross reference is made, showing that the material on ultrasonic therapy is filed in the folder of that name, and this note is placed in the folder on arthritis of the shoulder.

Patients' Ledger Cards

In addition to the medical history of the patient, a record of his financial transactions must be kept. The book in which the record is kept is called the patients' ledger, and the individual card or sheet, the ledger card or ledger page. Many of the printed medical history forms include ledger information. Doctors who use these forms believe that it is simpler to keep both together and that it is quicker to enter all information on the patient's record at the same time. Other doctors, however, object to keeping medical and financial information together and therefore have separate forms for each. Certainly, there is some objection to disclosing medical data to accountants or income tax agents who may need to have access to the financial records; moreover, it may not be advisable to disclose financial transactions when submitting medical records to another doctor. Also, considerable time is saved when the billing period comes around if all the ledger cards are kept separate and together, rather than filed in the folders with patients' medical histories. Most medical bureaus, therefore, advise that medical and financial records be kept separate.

Although ledger books with individual pages for each patient are used by a few doctors, cards are the usual method of choice. A card is made out for each patient. It must contain the patient's name, address, telephone number, and any information relevant to the procedure of billing. For instance, if the patient does not want to have his bill sent to his home address, or if he wishes to be billed on a certain date, or if the bill is to be sent to another person instead of to the patient, this is entered on the ledger card.

The entries should show the date on which the doctor rendered any service to the patient, the type of service rendered (office visit, house visit, laboratory tests, office surgery), the amount charged the patient, the amount paid, and the balance due, if any.

The ledger card must be brought up to date every day. The information may be taken from the appointment book and from the receipt book, and great care must be taken that correct entries are made. Otherwise, either the patient may be charged for treatments for which he has already paid, the doctor may not receive payment for his services, or the bills may be made for incorrect amounts.

When patients do not pay at each visit, the doctor's charges are entered each time on the ledger card. Each time a patient makes a payment, whether in person or by mail, this is also entered. If the payment does not cover the total amount or if the patient has incurred additional charges since the last bill was sent and paid, this balance appears on the ledger card and represents the amount to be billed. For example:

1. A patient was billed on the 1st of the month for $120. He sends a check on account for $70. The ledger card will show a balance due of $50, for which a new bill is sent the following month.

2. The patient is billed for $120 and sends a check for $120, but visits the doctor's office during the following month. A new bill is sent for the new charges.

3. A bill is sent for $120. The patient does not pay anything in the ensuing month, but incurs an additional $100 charge. The bill at the end of the second month will be for $220.

The ledger card gives an up-to-date picture of the patient's account at all times—showing the doctor what his earnings have been, how much of this has been collected, and how much money is still outstanding from each individual patient. As ledger cards show

how much money each patient owes, the bills are made out from these cards.

The ledger card shown in Fig. 16–2 is punched for rotary filing. Rotary-filing cards are kept on a circular or a curved rod (see Fig. 16–3). Both sides of the card are accessible for writing without the

FIG. 16–2. Patient's ledger card (*Wheeldex & Simpla Products, Inc.*)

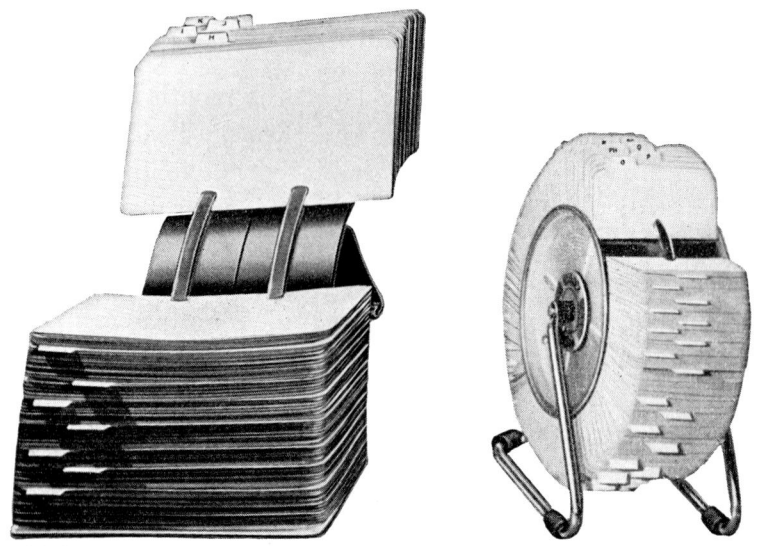

FIG. 16–3. Two types of rotary card file. (*Wheeldex & Simpla Products, Inc*).

card having to be removed. As such a file takes up less space and weighs less than a box, it can be kept on the secretary's desk when needed and locked up in a cupboard at night. Cards for vertical filing are of course also available and may be obtained in various sizes. Some general practitioners, who see the same patients over a period of years, may need the larger cards.

17

Financial Matters

In addition to the medical care rendered patients in a doctor's office, there are also economic matters to be taken into consideration. There is a business side even to the practice of medicine, and the doctor's secretary is very much involved in it. She may be the one who discusses the doctor's fee with the patient. She sends out his bills and collects his fees. She keeps a record of the doctor's earnings, his collections, and his expenses. She must be a combination secretary–credit manager–bookkeeper.

The Doctor's Fee

In the preceding chapter, under Receiving the Patient, it was stated that a number of questions must be asked of a new patient. One of these was "How do you wish to pay?" Obviously the answer to this question is of great importance to the doctor, who makes his living from his practice, and to the assistant, who acts in the capacity of the doctor's collection agent.

Doctors traditionally dislike discussing financial matters with patients. An efficient secretary should be able to take this task off the doctor's shoulders almost entirely. Once she is familiar with her employer's way of handling matters, she should be able to answer patients' questions about the various aspects of bills and fees. The less the doctor's name enters into it, the better pleased he will be. The most important thing is to keep accurate accounts, so as to avoid mistakes in billing. Patients become irate if they are charged for something they did not receive or for something for which they have already paid.

If it is the assistant's duty to discuss fees with the patients, she

FINANCIAL MATTERS 253

will have to develop good judgment, so that she may learn to evaluate a patient's ability to pay. Many persons, unfortunately, plead poverty so that they will be charged smaller fees, because many doctors do adjust their charges according to the patient's financial status. It is extremely difficult to prevent abuse of this generosity. Ideally, a doctor should have a fixed fee schedule. This would ease the problem of quoting fees considerably. But before making a revision downward, the doctor should investigate the patient's financial status in order to learn whether he is a needy case. Instead of paying a lower fee, the patient may prefer to pay the regular fee but be given a longer time in which to pay it; or, if the patient belongs to a low-income group, he may be referred to a clinic or a welfare agency.

Doctors' fees have been subject to a great deal of criticism—the size of them, from the patient's point of view; the unwillingness of the patient to pay them, from the doctor's. Many professional people, such as accountants, public relations counsels, and administrators of medical credit bureaus, have put in much thought and effort in order to improve this thorny side of medical practice and of doctor-patient relationship.

According to the conclusions that have been reached, the first point to remember in handling doctors' fees is that whenever possible the fee should be discussed in advance. Some doctors still feel embarrassed to quote a price for their services, which to them represent an act of humanity rather than a purchasable commodity. Yet experience has shown that failure to inform the patient, at the beginning of what may turn out to be a lengthy treatment or before an operation, what the fee will amount to, at least approximately, is the cause of more disagreements regarding payment of the bill than any other. Once the patient knows about what his medical bill will be, he can accept it, or he can make the necessary arrangements to meet it. He may even wish to discuss with the doctor his inability to pay the sum mentioned. When the amount of the fee has been agreed upon, one point that could lead to later misunderstandings has been removed.

Fees are more easily collected if as many patients as are able pay cash. Whether this is feasible or not depends on many factors—custom in the particular vicinity, the doctor's type of practice, whether the patient is expected to see the doctor only once or twice or over a long period. Some patients expect to pay cash at each visit, and this should be encouraged. It saves bookkeeping and later efforts at collecting. Many patients hesitate to offer to pay cash unless it is suggested to them first. If there are a number of persons paying by cash, it is important to keep a supply of small bills on hand in order to make change. A receipt book with a carbon slip for duplicates should be on the secretary's desk, and a receipt should be given the patient for each payment made. It is well to remind the patient to keep this receipt (which must be dated) for income tax purposes, as medical expenses are deductible but must be proved. The carbon copies that remain in the receipt book provide a permanent record of payments, and no individual financial record card would be needed for those patients who always pay cash. It is good practice, nevertheless, to have a ledger card for each patient, showing all financial transactions.

Bills

Some patients prefer to be billed. Bills should be sent out promptly on the first of each month. If they are received together with all other bills, they are likely to be paid at the same time. Many persons habitually pay their bills between the 5th and 10th of the month, and if a bill is received after that day, it is left on their desk until the following month. Prompt billing is a sign of an efficiently run office.

Before bills are sent out, accounts should be carefully checked. All charges still outstanding from previous months must be included. If the doctor has a laboratory and an x-ray department, the technician in charge must be consulted about charges for services rendered by these departments. On the other hand, billing a patient for an item already paid for will surely annoy the patient.

The question of whether or not to itemize bills has been under discussion in medical circles for quite some time. One thing is certain: it saves a lot of questioning later, and patients certainly prefer to receive itemized bills—there is no question about that. Some doctors, however, simply do not like to send itemized bills. For these doctors, therefore, the old formula, "For services rendered, April—$120.00," may be the best way, if only office visits are involved. Whenever services include house visits and office visits or any extra services such as a laboratory test, x-rays, or medications dispensed, the bill should be itemized.

Patients are apt to forget the details of their visits to the doctor, and a bill for a large sum that does not specify what charges the bill represents elicits an angry reaction at what is considered an exorbitant fee. On the other hand, if all the services are listed, the patient may realize that the doctor's bill is a reasonable one.

The trend is definitely toward itemized bills. It has been predicted that by 1965, itemized bills will be the rule, and not the exception as they are today. A sample bill is shown in Fig. 17–1.

If a patient requests a bill as soon as his treatment has been terminated, it should be sent at once. There is no need in this case to wait until the end of the month to send the bill.

In addition to the methods of payment already mentioned, there is the practice among some patients of paying a fixed amount each week. Persons who receive a weekly pay check find this method of payment the easiest. Whenever a large fee is involved, the secretary may ask the patient whether he would prefer to pay a fixed amount every week. Most patients are very grateful if this cooperation is shown them.

Collections

Unfortunately, sending the bill does not necessarily complete the transaction. Many patients are negligent in paying their bills, some are unable to do so, and a few simply do not like to pay bills. It is therefore necessary to watch all patients' accounts so that no unpaid bill is overlooked and allowed to remain open in the books without an attempt being made at collecting it. This requires first of all that accounts be examined regularly. Bills that are more than three months old should be actively followed up. Usually a simple reminder that the account is still open is sent first; some doctors do

```
                    PHONE 133 J


                              FREDERICKSBURG, TEXAS    May 31         1957



            Mrs. Joseph A. Carlson
                       70 Metropolitan Avenue
                   TO  DR. ROY CLARK
                       353 EAST 12TH AVENUE

            FOR PROFESSIONAL SERVICES:

               Examination              $25.00
               X-rays                     10.00
               Laboratory tests           15.00
               Office visits
                 5/10, 17, 24 @ 5.00      15.00
                                         ──────
                                          65.00
               Paid on account
                 5/17                     25.00
                                         ──────

               Balance due              $40.00



                                                         $ 40.00
```

Fig. 17–1. Sample bill.

not wait three months but insert such a reminder with the third or even the second bill. Suggestions for such reminders are:

1. Please remit.
2. Payment of this bill is now due.
3. Payment of this bill is overdue (or past due).
4. May I remind you that this bill is overdue. Your prompt attention to this bill will be appreciated.

These notations may be typed directly on the bill or on a separate slip to be attached to the bill.

If such a reminder brings no results, a letter should be sent to the patient. This may be written either by the doctor or by the secretary. Here are a few examples:

1. In looking over my records I find that your account is still open. If you will send your check now, I shall not need to trouble you further.

2. You have not replied to my letter of April 10, in reference to your unpaid bill. I am wondering whether this is because you find it difficult at this time to pay the entire amount. If you would like to pay one-third now and the balance in two monthly installments, this will be agreeable to Dr. Clark.

3. Not having received your check for the enclosed bill, I am wondering whether it may have gone astray, as you have always paid your bills so promptly in the past. If you have sent us your remittance, would you be good enough to ascertain whether the check was returned to you and, if so, let me know the date of the bank's endorsement. I could then correct what may have been an error here in the office.

4. Time passes quickly, and you may not realize that you have not yet settled the enclosed bill. Won't you please send us your check today.

5. Dr. Clark has been much surprised that you have allowed your bill to remain unpaid for three months. He feels that he has shown you considerable leniency and requests that you send him your remittance without further delay.

Collection letters should be friendly and sympathetic, assuming that the patient has failed to pay only from forgetfulness or inability to do so. Only when such a letter is not given the courtesy of a reply should letters become somewhat more urgent and forceful in tone. Eventually the doctor may turn over the account to a collection agency or bring suit against the patient. He will probably want to warn the patient beforehand that he will do so unless he receives payment by a certain date.

In addition to collection letters, there is of course the possibility of following up unpaid accounts by telephone. If handled by a competent, tactful person, who has been specially trained in soliciting by telephone, this method is highly desirable. The assistant, however, will probably be too busy, and the office too crowded, during the day to undertake such calls. Also, if the patient is not home during the day, the telephoning must be done in the evening. At any rate, the assistant may wish to give it a try.

If a patient dies, the doctor's bill is rendered to the estate of the deceased. It is expeditious to obtain the name of the executor and send the bill to him. If a relative of the patient is not accessible, this information may be obtained from the county surrogate court.

It is often a question of how long financial records should be kept. Assuming that the doctor is not interested in having his financial records microfilmed, it has been suggested that financial records be kept until the period specified by the statute of limitations has expired and no possibility of any legal action exists. The period determined by the statute of limitations, during which the doctor can bring suit for collection of his bill, varies in the different states. Once it has expired the doctor can no longer sue a patient. The Bureau of Internal Revenue requires records as far back as three years.

Bookkeeping

In order that the doctor may have a correct picture of his financial situation, detailed records of his financial transactions must be kept. He must be able to judge whether his income is sufficient to cover his expenses and provide a profit, whether the expenditure for a particular item is excessive, and whether his method of collection is satisfactory. But most important of all, he must have these details for his income tax declaration. Complete financial records are therefore indispensable. Keeping the doctor's books is the duty of the doctor's secretary.

The requirements for keeping doctors' accounts are relatively simple. In addition to the patients' ledger, which shows what each patient was charged, has paid, and may still owe, the doctor must keep a record of the following items:

1. His daily income (money actually collected) and expenses
2. The amount of money earned each day, but not necessarily collected
3. His total annual income
4. His total annual expenses (itemized)

Income tax is paid on an individual's net income available for personal use. The salary a person earns represents his net income. Before the doctor can earn any money for his personal use, he must pay the expenses of his office, such as rent, salaries, light, telephone, supplies, and many others. These expenses, which are necessary for maintenance of his office and continuance of his medical practice, are deductible from his income for tax purposes. That is, income tax is paid only on the amount that remains after all necessary expenses have been deducted—in other words, on the doctor's profit from his practice. All expenses, however, must be shown on the income tax declaration. It is for this reason that an accurate and permanent record must be kept, as it may have to be produced for an income tax inspector. If the records are unsatisfactory the doctor may be assessed for additional income tax.

A classic double-entry bookkeeping system can be adopted to any doctor's office and would give the doctor all the information he needs. With its built-in safeguards of checks and balances, mistakes in addition, subtraction, and copying, which occur only too frequently, are easily caught. A double-entry bookkeeping system also provides an exact and complete record of the doctor's assets and liabilities, profit and loss at all times.

Such a system, however, with its many ledger books and entries is too complicated and time-consuming for the average doctor, and most doctors do not feel that the check against errors and irregularities is as necessary for their offices as it is for a business concern. In most doctors' offices, therefore, a single-entry system is used, which provides a simple record of the doctor's income and expenses.

Special Bookkeeping Systems. To assist the doctor in keeping his financial transactions in accurate form, a number of bookkeeping systems have been designed especially for physicians. What they all have in common is that they are simple and concise, easily learned, and that all entries can be made quickly and with little chance for mistakes, as many printed headings are provided.

The principal advantage of all these systems is that all records are combined in one volume, with pages for daily entries as well as monthly and annual summaries. Pages for payroll records are also included. Each of these systems has its advantages and its disadvantages, and each doctor will probably have a preference for one or the other. The best known of these systems and their publishers are:

"The Daily Log for Physicians," Colwell Publishing Company

"The Fagell Simplified Record-system for Physicians," William Fagell and Warren-David Publishing Company

"Histaccount Bookkeeping System," Professional Printing Company

"Penn-way Professional Business System," Physicians' Record Company

As the Fagell system is the most recently published, in fact the first new system to have come out in over twenty years, this is used here as an illustration of how such a bookkeeping system is handled.

The volume, which is a handy, 8 by 10 loose-leaf or ring binder, is divided into five sections. The first section, entitled Daily Record of Cash Receipts and Charges, serves for entering each day:

1. The names of patients seen
2. The type of service rendered
3. Charges made
4. Fees collected from patients seen on that day
5. Bills collected from patients seen on previous occasions
6. Any receipts from other sources, such as any salary, royalties, or dividends the doctor may receive.

Columns are provided, with headings for each of these classifications (see Fig. 17-2).

A new page should be started on the first of each month, but

FINANCIAL MATTERS

MONTH OF *May 1957*

DAY	PATIENT'S NAME	SERVICE RENDERED	CHARGES	CASH REC'D CASH-PAY PATIENTS	CASH COLL. CHARGE PATIENTS	SUNDRY RECEIPTS
	BROUGHT FORWARD					
2	Mr. Greto Hugo	Consultation		25 00		
	Mr. S. Henderson	Office Visit		5 00		
	Mr. Daniel Field	Home Visit	10 00			
	Mr. D. Burton	Pd. in full			60 00	
	Miss Linda Rice	Pd. on account			15 00	
	Mr. Frances Worth	Office Visit	10 00			
	Mr. Wm. Roberts	Xrays	15 00			
31	Amer. Tel. and Tel.	Dividends				225 00
	TOTALS FOR MONTH TO DATE		565 00	485 00	970 00	225 00

FIG. 17-2. Sample page: record of cash receipts and charges. (*William Fagell and Warren-David Publishing Company.*)

the author suggests leaving only three blank lines between the days of the month, so as not to waste pages on which, for example, there may be only two or three entries. All columns are totaled at the bottom of each page, and the totals are transferred to the top of the next page.

The second section is entitled Disbursements, Daily Record. A double page is used for this record. There are two columns for entering all payments made by check. These are entered in numerical order with the name of the person or firm to whom it was made out and the amount of the check. For classification purposes, additional columns are included for a second entry of the amount of the check under the appropriate heading. That is, the headings show whether the check was for office expenses, automobile expenses, salaries, equipment, supplies, or for the doctor's personal use. Each column is labeled, and the appropriate entry is made on the same line as the first entry of the check (see Fig. 17-3).

A special column is provided for payments made by cash. Cash payments may be entered once daily or even once a week in one amount, but must be broken down according to the various types of expenditure the sum covers, exactly like payments made by check.

In both sections, all columns are added up at the foot of the page, and the totals are transferred to the following page. At the end of the month the monthly totals of all columns are transferred to the third section, entitled Annual Summaries. In this section, one

MONTH OF May 1957

DAY	PAID TO	BY CHECK NO.	AMOUNT	BY CASH	DEDUCTIONS S.S.	I. TAX	EMPLOYEES SALARIES (GROSS AMT.)	MEDICAL SUPPLIES & DRUGS	LAB. FEES & ASSIST. DRS. AND NURSES
	BROUGHT FORWARD								
2	Eastern Pharmacy	252	23 75					23 75	
	Wheeler & Company	253	275 00						
	Westside Garage			12 00					
	Bell Tel. Co.	254	23 60						
	Jane Bailey	255	61 50		1.50	12.00	75 00		
31	State Tax Commission	285	175 00						
	TOTALS FOR MONTH TO DATE		1753 85	12 00	6 00	48 00	300 00	87 70	

FIG. 17–3A. Sample page: record of disbursement by check and cash. (William Fagell and Warren-David Publishing Company.)

page provides columns for each month of the year, corresponding to the daily pages of the first section. This is illustrated in Fig. 17–4. A double page corresponds to the daily-disbursement page in the second section, with lines for each month of the year, so that the monthly totals can be transferred (see Fig. 17–5).

In addition to the annual summary of the daily cash receipts and disbursements, the third section contains a page for a Detailed Analysis of Other Office Expenses by month. On this page the items included in the column headed Office Expenses are entered by month, according to the type of expense they represent, such as rent, light, telephone, etc. At the end of the year, the columns are totaled and represent the yearly totals for each type of expenditure.

This section also contains a Schedule of Depreciation, on which the doctor enters all his equipment on which depreciation is still being charged, the date when he acquired it, the price he paid for

FINANCIAL MATTERS

it, the amount of depreciation already charged, the estimated life of the equipment, and the depreciation for the current year.

Some equipment may wear out in five years, and therefore a charge of 20 per cent depreciation annually for five years would

MONTH OF May 1957

OTHER OFFICE EXPENSES		ALL AUTO EXPENSES	(SPARE)	DOCTOR'S PERSONAL DRAWINGS	TAX PAYMENTS TO		SUNDRY PAYMENTS	
DESCRIPTION	AMOUNT				FEDERAL	STATE-LOCAL	DESCRIPTION	AMOUNT
Rent	275 00							
		12 00						
Telephone	23 60							
							Equipment	200 00
					175 00			
	413 65				175 00			350 00

FIG. 17–3B. Sample page: record of disbursement by check and cash (continued). (*William Fagell and Warren-David Publishing Company.*)

be correct. A piece of furniture, however, may last twenty years and would then be depreciated at a rate of 5 per cent annually for twenty years. The amount of depreciation is an allowable expense for income tax purposes, while the purchase price is not. Equipment is considered an investment, not an expense.

	CHARGES	CASH REC'D CASH-PAY PATIENTS	CASH COLL. CHARGE PATIENTS	SUNDRY RECEIPTS
January	565 00	485 00	970 00	225 00
February	345 00	255 00	750 00	—
March	680 00	440 00	875 00	175 00
December	530 00	410 00	835 00	75 00
TOTALS FOR YEAR	3,750 00	6,500 00	11,500 00	545 00

FIG. 17–4. Sample page: summary of cash receipts and charges. (*William Fagell and Warren-David Publishing Company.*)

	BY CHECK	BY CASH	DEDUCTIONS		EMPLOYEES SALARIES (GROSS AMT.)	MEDICAL SUPPLIES & DRUGS	LAB. FEES & ASSIST. DRS. AND NURSES
			S.S.	I. TAX			
January	1750 00	135 00			300 00	87 45	
February	1277 00	45 00			300 00	57 80	
March	1345 00	60 00			375 00	67 35	
December							
TOTALS	11,340 75	1,865 90			3,900	876 40	

FIG. 17-5A. Sample page: summary of disbursements by check and cash. (*William Fagell and Warren-David Publishing Company.*)

This section finally contains an Annual Statement of Income and Expenses. The yearly totals from the summaries of Receipts and Charges, Disbursements, Office Expense Analysis, and the Schedule of Depreciation are transferred to this page at the end of the year.

The fourth section is entitled Employees' Earnings Records. As the law requires that every employer withhold social security and income taxes from his employees and keep specific records of the salaries paid and the deductions made, this section contains pages for several employees, set up in the manner prescribed by law. Each week the employee's gross salary, social security and income tax withheld, and net salary paid are entered. A separate page must be used for each employee. The regulations concerning payroll deductions are discussed later.

The fifth section entitled Nonprofessional Receipts—Disbursements, provides a record of any income the doctor may have outside of his practice, such as dividends and interests from stocks and bonds. It also supplies pages for recording expenses the doctor has incurred for purely personal purposes.

Precise and exceptionally clear instructions precede each section in this volume, so that a person without any knowledge of bookkeeping can learn to keep this record system efficiently and in a minimum of time. The doctor can see at a glance how much he has earned, what he has collected, and what his expenses have been. The columns are comfortably wide, and the lines are not crowded.

FINANCIAL MATTERS

OTHER OFFICE EXPENSES	ALL AUTO EXPENSES	(SPARE)	DOCTOR'S PERSONAL DRAWINGS	TAX PAYMENTS TO		SUNDRY PAYMENTS
AMOUNT				FEDERAL	STATE-LOCAL	AMOUNT
410 00						
40 00	89 35		1250 00	540 00		75 00
124 00	95 00		800 00			65 00
237 00	101 40		975 00			83 00
3,226 90	963 45		11,752 00	2,875 00	175 00	788 65

Fig. 17–5B. Sample page: summary of disbursements by check and cash. (*William Fagell and Warren-David Publishing Company.*)

A bookkeeping system such as this would be easy for the secretary to keep and would assure the doctor of accurate records. (An appointment book, of course, is also necessary, as well as the patients' ledger, which is a separate record altogether.)

At the end of the year all the pages in the volume may be taken out of the cover and filed away intact, thereby taking up very little space and being readily accessible for later reference. The annual summaries greatly facilitate the preparation of the income tax declaration.

Cash and Checks. To keep the financial aspects of the doctor's practice straight, a few basic rules should be observed. When checks arrive in the mail or are handed to the assistant by a patient, they should be endorsed immediately with a rubber stamp reading "Deposit to the account of (doctor's name), M.D." Cash should be placed in a cash box, which is best kept in the assistant's desk and, if possible, fastened to the drawer in such a way that it cannot be quickly lifted out. It should be kept locked. Sufficient bills of small denominations should be kept on hand to make change for a $20 bill. If the doctor collects money on his out-of-office visits, he should, in order to have his accounts kept correctly, give this to his assistant, together with a charge slip showing the patient's name, service rendered, amount, and date.

All money received in the office should be deposited in the bank —whether checks or cash. In an office where much cash is taken in, bank deposits should be made every day. If the doctor needs cash for himself, he should draw a check on his personal account and cash it, that is, replace the cash he takes from receipts with his check. In this way the daily bank deposits always equal the day's income. If for some reason a bill is to be paid in cash, the same procedure should be followed; that is, a check should be drawn to cash on the doctor's professional account and placed in the receipts to replace the cash paid out. However, because so many doctors do not follow this accepted bookkeeping procedure, but use cash on hand without bothering to draw a check to replace it, the bookkeeping systems for doctors provide separate columns for expenditures by check and by cash.

Payroll Records. Every person in the United States who has an income of over $600 annually, regardless of the source, must pay a Federal income tax. The amount to be paid depends on three factors: (1) the amount of the income (as the income increases, so does the proportion of the tax); (2) the number of dependents (called exemptions); and (3) the rate set by Congress. If a person earns a weekly or monthly salary, the employer must withhold an amount for income tax from the employee's pay. A booklet published by the United States government and sent to every employer sets forth the amount to be deducted, according to income bracket and the number of exemptions claimed.

In addition to withholding income tax, the employer must deduct the social security tax of 2½ per cent of the employee's salary, up to an annual salary of $4,800. That is, if a person earns $100 weekly, $2.50 would be deducted from his salary for forty-eight weeks of the year.

The payroll record that is included in the bookkeeping system mentioned above shows the name of the employee, address, date on which employment began, gross salary, income tax deducted, social security tax deducted, and net salary paid (see Fig. 17–6). This record must be kept. If the doctor does not use a special doctors' bookkeeping system, which provides pages for the payroll, a payroll book can be bought at most stationery stores.

The doctor must of course turn over to the Federal government the money that he has deducted from his employee, plus 2½ per

FINANCIAL MATTERS

S.S. NO. 083-45-776

NAME Jane Bailey   ADDRESS 54 Northern Blvd   EXEMPT CLAIMED 1

WEEK ENDING	GROSS SALARY	DEDUCTIONS FOR S.S.	I. TAX	OTHER	NET PAID	WEEK ENDING	GROSS SALARY	DEDUCTIONS FOR S.S.	I. TAX	OTHER	NET PAID
5/2	75.00	1.50	12.00		61.50						
5/9	75.00	1.50	12.00		61.50						
5/16	75.00	1.50	12.00		61.50						
1ST QUARTER	975.00	19.50	156.00		799.50	3RD QUARTER	975.00	19.50	156.00		799.50
2ND QUARTER	975.00	19.50	156.00		799.50	4TH QUARTER	975.00	19.50	156.00		799.50
						ENTIRE YEAR	3900.00	78.00	624.00		3198.00

FIG. 17-6. Sample page: employee earnings record (based on a 2 per cent social security deduction). (*William Fagell and Warren-David Publishing Company.*)

cent of the salary as his contribution to the social security fund. For instance, if he has deducted from an employee who earns $100 a week, $21 for income tax and $2.50 for social security tax each week, he must turn over to the government this $23.50 plus $2.50 as his own contribution, that is, $26.00 in all for one week. This money can be paid to any bank, and a special form is provided on which the details of the payments are entered. Payments to the bank are usually made once a month.

Every three months, that is, during January, April, July, and October, a report must be sent to the government setting forth the names of all the persons employed during the preceding quarter, their social security numbers, the total salaries paid, the total amount of income tax deducted, the total amount of social security tax deducted, and the amount of social security contribution paid by the employer for the preceding quarter. Forms for this are sent out by the government, and failure to file these reports on time involves a fine.

Petty Cash. In every office there are occasions for very small expenditures, such as tips to delivery men, postage, purchase of a notebook, and many others. In order to avoid entering such small sums in the bookkeeping record, a petty-cash fund is set up. This may vary from $5 to $50, depending on the needs of the individual office. For the average doctor, a $10 or $20 petty-cash account is adequate.

If the account is to be started with $20, let us say, a check for this amount is drawn. This check is entered like all others in the regular daily and monthly records. The check is cashed, and the currency placed in a special petty-cash box. As this money is to be used for small expenditures, it is necessary to obtain enough pennies, nickels, dimes, quarters, and dollar bills to serve its purpose; therefore, it is necessary to tell the bank teller when cashing the check just what denominations are wanted. It is best to figure this out beforehand and attach a slip with the breakdown to the check.

All moneys spent from this petty-cash account are entered in a special expense book. Whenever possible vouchers, receipts, or bills should be obtained, and these may be kept in a special folder marked Petty-cash Vouchers. At the end of the month the entries are totaled and checked against the currency in the box. That is, if the entries amount to $18.50 and the amount in the box is $1.50, the account balances. In other words, the amount of the expenses plus the amount of currency in the box should always equal the original amount.

To replenish the account, a check is drawn for the amount spent—in the above example, this would be for $18.50. The check is cashed, and the currency is added to the money in the box, which would again equal the original amount of $20. The check for $18.50 (or whatever the amount) is entered on the daily record.

BIBLIOGRAPHY

Freeman, M. Herbert, J. Marshall Hanna, and Gilbert Kahn: "Bookkeeping and Accounting Simplified," Gregg Publishing Division, McGraw-Hill Book Company, Inc., New York, 1953.

Mayne, F. Blair, and Gerald Crowningshield: "Accounting for Secretaries," 2d ed., Gregg Publishing Division, McGraw-Hill Book Company, Inc., New York, 1957.

18

Insurance in Medical Practice

Not all patients who visit the doctor's office actually pay for the services they receive. Many are covered by some type of insurance. This may be a commercial health insurance policy, a voluntary health insurance (prepaid medical care) plan, or Workmen's Compensation insurance. Whenever the patient is covered by such insurance, the billing procedure is different. Also, certain forms may have to be filled out. The medical office assistant must therefore know just who will pay the patient's bill and the procedure necessary to collect payment. A question about any insurance carried by the patient should therefore be included in the information that is obtained at his first visit.

Health Insurance

If a person wants to insure himself for payment of his medical bills and his family's, he must join some sort of medical care plan or take out a health insurance policy. In the latter case the patient collects from the insurance company directly when he is ill. The amount he collects depends on the amount of the premium that he pays and the type of policy he has selected. The doctor does not enter into the transaction at all, except perhaps to certify that the patient was ill and state the amount of his bill. Some insurance companies have special forms to be filled out, which they send to the doctor. When the doctor has completed this form and returned it to the company, the company pays the patient the amount to which he is entitled according to the terms of the policy. But the doctor's bill is sent to the patient, and he is responsible for payment of it.

Such insurance policies are too expensive for the majority of people. Yet, the threat of "catastrophic" illness hangs over everyone. In many countries the government has stepped in, in order to ease the financial burden caused by prolonged illnesses, and compulsory health insurance has been introduced. That is, each person must pay a specific tax for health insurance, in return for which medical treatment is rendered free of charge to the patient. The doctor is paid by the government. The mechanics of the plan vary in the different countries. In England, for instance, all medicines and even surgical appliances are included. Private practice is still carried on, but has dwindled to a very small percentage of doctors and patients. According to the doctors in these various countries, under compulsory health insurance the number of patients each doctor has to see is too great, and adequate care cannot be given.

In the United States the answers to the problem of meeting medical expenses have been the voluntary health insurance policies offered by commercial insurance companies, and nonprofit, prepaid medical care plans. The principle on which the medical care plans are based is that a person who wants to join such a plan pays a definite sum annually—the sum is the same for all members of any one plan—for himself alone and, if he wishes to include his family, additional amounts for the different members. When the subscriber becomes ill, his doctor's bills are paid partly or in full by the plan, according to the type of contract he carries or the type of organization he has joined.

There are many such prepaid medical care plans, with a variety of methods of reimbursing the patient for his medical expenses. In some cases, the doctor signs a statement, and the patient pays the doctor in the regular way, but collects from the insurance plan. In others, the insurance plan pays the doctor directly. Certain funds pay the doctor a fixed sum per patient per month, regardless of the service rendered. This is called "capitation," in contrast to the "fee-for-service" plans, which pay for each service that the doctor renders to the patient. Some organizations pay all the patient's medical expenses; others pay only part of them.

Whenever a patient states that he belongs to some insurance plan, it is important for the assistant to know the regulations governing that particular plan. The report to the insurance association must be made out in accordance with their requirements. If the insurance plan pays only part of the doctor's charges, the patient is billed for the difference. These records and accounts must be kept accurately and carefully if the doctor is not to lose money because of faulty billing.

The best known health insurance plan is the Blue Shield medical care plan, which operates under different names and in slightly different ways in the various states. This plan is associated with Blue Cross hospital insurance. Many persons carry Blue Cross insurance only, which provides for payment of hospital expenses—room, board, operating room, routine examinations, and hospital services—but not for doctors' or surgeons' fees. Much confusion exists in regard to this plan, and patients often are under the impression that their Blue Cross insurance includes the payment of doctors' fees.

The fact that a patient belongs to an insurance plan should be noted on his record when his medical history is first taken. If a patient states that he belongs to Blue Cross, it is well to make sure that he is correctly informed regarding his insurance coverage. The assistant should ask for the patient's membership card and make careful note of the type of insurance and the type of contract and whether it is still in effect. Patients frequently are not aware of the kind of coverage provided by their contract. The assistant should discuss this aspect fully, in order to avoid confusion when the doctor sends his bill for services the patient thought were covered by his insurance contract. The assistant should also be thoroughly familiar with the provisions of Blue Cross insurance in her vicinity, as patients will often ask her for this information. The benefits provided by Blue Cross, as well as the requirements for membership, vary from time to time. The nearest Blue Cross office will supply informative literature, and copies of these pamphlets may be kept in the waiting room for patients to read and perhaps take home.

If the majority of the doctor's patients belong to one particular insurance plan, the assistant should acquaint herself with the rules and regulations of that particular plan. If the doctor is a member of any of the Blue Shield plans, she might well attend one of the lectures given periodically by this organization to instruct medical office assistants in the workings of the plan and the procedures that must be followed by subscribers. If no such lectures are being given, she might ask to speak to a representative, who will be glad to explain the routine to her.

The provisions of the Blue Shield plans differ somewhat in the different states and vary from time to time. In the following paragraphs the plan is described as it operates currently in New York State.

Three different types of contract are offered: (1) one that pays all surgeons' fees; (2) one that pays all doctors' fees while the patient is in the hospital; (3) one that pays general medical expenses.

An individual or a family whose income is below a specified amount (an amount established from time to time) is entitled to service benefits. That is, the doctor is paid the fees fixed by the Blue Shield organization for each service. The doctor must agree to accept this fee in full payment for his services. If the patient's income is above the specified amount, he is not entitled to service benefits. The doctor is paid the same fixed fees, but the patient must pay the difference between the amount received by the doctor from Blue Shield and his regular fee. It is important, therefore, to know whether the patient is entitled to service benefits and the doctor is to be paid by Blue Shield only or whether a bill must be sent to the patient for the difference between the fixed fee the doctor will receive from Blue Shield and his regular fee.

When the assistant has ascertained the type of contract the patient has, she must complete a special form issued by Blue Shield and send it to the head office. This form may be sent either monthly or once the patient has been discharged. An ample supply of these forms should always be on hand. A sample is illustrated in Fig. 18–1. The upper part of the form should be completed and signed

INSURANCE IN MEDICAL PRACTICE 273

FIG. 18-1. Medical report form. (*United Medical Service, Inc.*)

by the patient. The assistant must be sure to ask the patient to fill this out before he leaves the office on his final visit. He may request her to fill it out for him and then sign it himself.

The lower part of the form is filled out by the doctor's office from the patient's record. Dates must be given, together with the services that the doctor has rendered. Full details should be given, and the data must be precise and clearly stated, as payment is made on the basis of each service rendered. The doctor signs this form and it is then sent to the head office. Care must be taken that the form be filled out correctly and completely, signed, and dated. No questions should be left unanswered. If a question does not apply, a dash or a zero mark will indicate that it has not been overlooked.

Payment to the doctor is made on the basis of this form. The amount received should be entered on the patient's ledger card, with a notation that it was received from the insurance plan. If the patient is not entitled to service benefits, he is sent a bill for the difference. A rate book of the amounts paid by the Blue Shield for various services is sent to the doctor when he agrees to accept patients under Blue Shield coverage. This is used to compute the amount of the bill sent to the patient. Certain diseases, as well as operations for cosmetic surgery, are not covered.

Workmen's Compensation Insurance

If a person is injured or becomes ill as a result of his employment, his doctor's bills are paid by an insurance company with which his employer is insured for this very purpose. It is the law in practically all forty-eight states that every employer with more than four employees must carry such insurance. An employer with fewer than four employees has the option of taking his chances that no accidents will befall his employees or, if an accident does happen, of paying the expenses himself. Doctors as a rule do not carry Workmen's Compensation insurance for their employees, but they usually carry a personal liability insurance policy, which offers protection to anyone injured while in the office, but not as a result of the doctor's medical services. Almost every doctor, however, treats patients whose bills are paid by an insurance company under the Workmen's Compensation law. The details of this law vary in minor aspects in the different states. In the following remarks, the law as it applies in New York State is described.

When a patient visits the doctor under the Workmen's Compensation law, he has usually been sent by his employer. The law provides that each person have free choice of a physician, but most persons either do not have a physician of their own or, in the case of an accident, must consult a doctor close to their place of work. The doctor, in order to be able to treat patients under this law, must register with the local bureau under which the law is administered for the specialty in which he practices. A registration number and a code number designating his specialty are then assigned to him. This registration must be renewed annually.

At the patient's first visit, information in addition to the routine data must be obtained: (1) the name of the patient's employer; (2) the name of the insurance company; (3) the date of the accident; and (4) a statement in the patient's own words regarding the accident or onset of illness. (Illness is also covered, provided that it occurred as a result of the person's work, or was aggravated by it.)

After the doctor has examined or treated a patient, prescribed forms must be sent to the government bureau under whose jurisdiction the law is administered. In most states this is the Department of Labor. A copy of the form is usually also sent to the insurance carrier, and another one to the patient's employer. As one copy must be kept in the doctor's office, an original and three carbon copies of this form must be made.

The forms vary somewhat in the different states, but the principle is always the same; that is, all the questions must be answered. When a question does not apply, a mark should be made to show that it has not been overlooked. The doctor's registration and code numbers must be included, and the form must be dated and signed by the doctor.

These forms must usually be sent soon after the doctor has first seen the patient, from time to time while the patient is under treatment, and after he has been discharged. (This last form is marked Final Report.) The regulations regarding these matters vary in the different states. Some states have a fixed time limit for each form. There are also various forms to cover different contingencies. The assistant should familiarize herself with the law as it operates in the state in which she is employed. As Workmen's Compensation insurance is a very important part of the practice of most physicians, the regulations covering the insurance must be carefully observed.

The office should always have a supply of the blank forms. Copies may be obtained, by a letter over the doctor's signature, from the nearest bureau or government office under whose jurisdiction the law operates. Return postage should be included.

One reason why it is very important that a carbon copy of each form be kept in the doctor's office is the fact that certain disputes may arise. Occasionally there may be a question as to whether the patient's illness is the result of his employment, whether his work has aggravated or brought on an existing or latent condition, or whether the illness is unrelated to his employment. At other times, the insurance company may question the amount of the bill, either because of the number of visits or because of the type of treatment given. In all such instances, the case is brought before an arbitration board for review before a decision is made. It is essential for the doctor to present accurate, well-kept records, dating from the time of the patient's first visit, in order to substantiate his claim.

Bills for patients provided for under the Workmen's Compensation law are sent to the insurance carrier—not to the patient. They must be fully itemized and must also show the patient's name and address and the employer's name and address. The charges must conform to those set by the official agency that regulates the Workmen's Compensation law. A list of these fees is available on request and is given to the doctor when he registers for this type of practice. Some doctors have exclusively a Workmen's Compensation practice.

Medicare

In accordance with Public Law 569, 84th Congress, 2d Session, which went into effect on December 8, 1956, all dependents of members of the armed services on active duty will be hospitalized in civilian hospitals and receive medical care while in the hospital from civilian physicians when there is no government medical care available in the community. Under this law, the government will turn over funds to a so-called "fiscal agent," who will administer the law in each state. At present the Blue Cross organization is handling the hospital aspect of this law, and Blue Shield or the state medical society is handling the doctor's side of it.

The fees to be paid the doctor are determined by each state. Once these fees have been set, the doctor who wishes to treat dependents under this law must accept these amounts as full payment for his services. In addition to the medical care rendered while the patient is in the hospital, the government will pay up to $75 for diagnostic procedures at the doctor's office prior to hospitalization and up to $50 for aftercare following hospitalization.

Before the doctor accepts a patient under this law, the latter should present a medical authorization, DD Form 1173, identifying him as a dependent of a member of the armed services who is on active duty. The form must be signed by the person on active duty. The doctor should not undertake any form of treatment before this form is presented. Upon termination of treatment the doctor must submit the proper form, in duplicate, to the fiscal agent. Another copy should always be made for the office. One section of this form contains the patient's name and address; the name, address, branch of service, rank, and service number of the patient's sponsor; and the patient's signature. The doctor fills out another section of the form, certifying to the length of the hospital stay, the diagnosis, services rendered, and the charges. The doctor is then paid by the fiscal agent. Copies of this form may be obtained from Blue Shield or the state medical society—whoever acts as the fiscal agent. It is advisable to keep a supply in the office.

Malpractice Insurance

In addition to the various types of insurance the patient may carry for his protection, there is at least one type of insurance the doctor must carry to protect himself. This is malpractice insurance. If, in connection with the doctor's practice, a patient is injured, either by accident or by negligence on the part of the doctor, the patient can sue the doctor for damages. Various kinds of accidents can and do happen in a doctor's office. Burns from diathermy or ultraviolet lamps are the most common accidents and causes for damage suits. Other causes of infections resulting from injections with broken needles or improperly sterilized equipment, cuts from broken glassware, and injuries from a surgical knife. In order to make a claim for damages, a patient must prove negligence on the part of the doctor or one of his assistants. The fact that the patient was not cured or perhaps even grew worse under treatment is not a cause for a damage suit. If the doctor prescribed the wrong treatment, this is legally considered "error of judgment" and not negligence, unless it can be proved that the doctor did not exercise reasonable care in examining and treating the patient.

In the case of a lawsuit instituted by a patient who is suing the doctor for malpractice and for damages, the doctor must present his side of the case. The assistant may be called on to testify. If the assistant was responsible for the accident, both she and the doctor may be held liable. If the patient wins the suit, the damages are paid by the doctor's malpractice insurance, up to the amount for which the doctor was insured. For instance, if the doctor carries $5,000 worth of malpractice insurance, a claim up to that amount would be paid by the insurance company, but if the damages awarded were more than $5,000, the doctor would be liable for the difference. Specialists in physical therapy and x-ray treatments and surgeons therefore carry higher insurance than, for example, general practitioners.

The premiums for this insurance are usually paid annually or semiannually, and the policy must not be allowed to lapse. Policies should be kept indefinitely, as claims may be presented many years after the accident happened or is supposed to have happened.

19
Housekeeping Hints

The training of a technical person includes instruction in the care of all tools and equipment used in his work. The medical office assistant's duties include responsibility for the supervision of the entire office. The doctor's practice would be severely handicapped by haphazard care of his equipment. A patient coming to a doctor's office expects to find every room neat, attractive, and spotlessly clean. The assistant's efficiency will be judged by the appearance of the office of which she is in charge.

Care of Office

The assistant's first duty in this regard is to see that the cleaning is done properly by whoever is responsible for this work. The assistant must attend to all other details herself. Many things are necessary for a well-kept doctor's office, just as they are for a well-kept home.

The doctor may occupy rooms in a building that provides cleaning service without extra charge, the charge being included in the rent; or he may engage a cleaning contractor for daily cleaning and special weekly and monthly jobs; or he may hire one person to clean every day. In any case, the assistant must exercise constant supervision to make sure that everything is done and done well. The following check list may be useful:

1. Wash ashtrays.
2. Empty trashbaskets.
3. Wash enamel table tops.
4. Wash sinks, basins, toilets.
5. Dust and polish furniture.
6. Vacuum and dust open bookshelves.
7. Vacuum rugs.
8. Vacuum upholstered furniture.

9. Scrub and wax floors.
10. Clean windows.
11. Clean mirrors and picture frames.
12. Polish metal fixtures and parts on apparatus.
13. Brush silk lamp shades, wipe parchment shades.
14. Wash venetian blinds.
15. Wash window curtains and clean drapes.
16. Clean upholstered furniture.
17. Wash or dry-clean slip covers.

Some of these things must be done daily; others, once a week. Some can be done once a month, and still others, only at the change of the seasons. Once a schedule has been decided upon, the assistant should make sure everything is done properly and on time.

In addition, small details must be attended to almost constantly —light bulbs must be changed, old magazines thrown away, and paper towels, toilet paper, and soap supplied. Trivial things in themselves, each one of these details is important in that together they convey the impression of a carefully supervised office.

A public relations counsel once asked a group of doctors, "Have you looked at your waiting room lately?" It is revealing to look at this room from the point of view of a stranger walking in for the first time. Too frequently the waiting room, once it has been furnished, remains the same for years and soon looks old-fashioned, shabby, unfriendly. The waiting room is the "display case" of the doctor; it provides the patient's first impression. If the waiting room is not attractive, the patient will be unfavorably influenced right from the beginning.

What makes a pleasant waiting room? Light, good-looking furniture helps. Comfortable sofas and chairs, as patients may have to sit on them for quite some time. Cheerful wallpaper or light paint. Sufficient small tables to hold ashtrays and magazines. Good lighting facilities for reading, and pictures that are pleasant to contemplate. Patients seem to dislike and object to extreme modern paintings, they do not take kindly to striking color combinations. A doctor's waiting room should have a restful look.

Flowers and plants help to create a pleasant atmosphere, but only if they are fresh. Unless the assistant has the time to care for growing things, it is better not to have them in the office. Also, it should be kept in mind that some patients are allergic to flowers.

Patients are usually nervous or ill at ease when they come to the doctor. A friendly atmosphere in the doctor's office, especially in his waiting room, is therefore of the greatest help in making the patient feel relaxed. The appearance of the waiting room may mean the difference between the patient's liking and disliking the doctor, even before actually meeting him.

Examination and treatment rooms must be spotless, or the patient will depart with indignation—and rightly so. A few minutes' attention, after each patient leaves and before the next one is called in, is really all that is needed. Remove all soiled linen and used instruments and any medication that was administered. Pick up any hairpins that may have dropped on the floor. Wipe away liquids that may have splattered on a chair or table. Iodine stains on a dressing table, for instance, spoil the entire professional appearance of the treatment room.

Care of Equipment

The doctor's equipment represents a considerable investment of money and deserves the best of care. All machines, such as an electrocardiograph, a basal metabolism apparatus, diathermy machines, and ultraviolet lamps, will quickly deteriorate if left unprotected. Dust that settles in the machinery can ruin it far more quickly than actual use. Any piece of equipment that is not used frequently should be protected with a plastic cover and wiped clean from time to time. Uncovered machines must be dusted daily.

Wooden cabinets are much improved by an occasional polishing with furniture oil; metal parts, with metal polish. Clean, gleaming equipment is the efficient assistant's pride. A soft dustcloth kept in a handy place and run over the machine just before and after use produces the well-groomed look every medical office strives for.

Electric equipment must be checked from time to time for mechanical defects. Especially, cords must not be allowed to become frayed. As a rule, only a skilled electrician should attempt to fix equipment in need of repair, but the assistant is responsible for either telling the doctor of the need or sending for the repairman herself.

Instruments, too, are expensive. Unless kept in perfect condition, they are useless to the doctor. One of the first rules in caring for instruments is to see that none are thrown out by mistake, either with soiled dressings or with the water from the sterilizer. Used instruments must be washed and dried; otherwise they will rust. Hinged instruments should be taken apart. A drop of oil may be put on the joints before they are stored. More details regarding the care of instruments, rubber goods, and glassware are given in Chapter 3 under Methods of Sterilization.

Supplies

Supplies are divided into two types, medical and administrative. The supplies in a doctor's office are usually the assistant's responsibility. She ought to keep in mind that they are expensive and that it is her duty to look after them carefully. New supplies should be ordered in ample time, as it is most embarrassing to run out of something like absorbent cotton, for instance. A good rule is to order a new supply whenever the first half of a box or bottle is used.

Medical Supplies. Medical supplies consist of medications, bandages, dressings, cotton, adhesive, thermometers, syringes, needles, applicators and the many items that have been mentioned throughout this book. Obviously, the materials and the amount to be kept on hand depend on the doctor's specialty. As there is a considerable saving in ordering supplies in large quantities, this should be taken into consideration.

Medications need special attention. If the doctor keeps vaccines, the expiration dates must be checked, and unused material exchanged in time. The same is true of certain types of injection material. The assistant must know which medicines can be exchanged when they expire and which cannot. Of the latter, no more than absolutely necessary should be kept on hand. If the doctor uses some materials in the assistant's absence, he should be asked to leave the empty container on her desk.

HOUSEKEEPING HINTS

Some medicines must be stored in a cool, dark place. A special cabinet may have to be reserved for these, unless a refrigerator is available. A refrigerator must be defrosted regularly, and the person defrosting it must make sure that nothing in it will deteriorate if the temperature is raised.

Regarding narcotic drugs, notwithstanding the fact that the doctor himself is the only one legally responsible for them, he will appreciate it if the assistant keeps an eye on them too. When she files the patient's medical record she might read at a glance what has been administered to the patient. This does not take much time and may be of great help to her in her work. If she notices that a patient has been given codeine, morphine, or another narcotic drug, she should check the narcotic record book to see whether the doctor has entered it. It is easy to forget such matters, and once forgotten, they are hard to track down. He has an assistant to help him remember.

Medical supplies that come in different sizes, such as syringes, needles, bandages, etc., are preferably stored in order of their size. Everything should have its place and should always be kept in that particular spot. This saves time when something is needed in a hurry. In some offices it is possible to paste labels on the shelves as a guide.

Closets, cabinets, and cupboards should be cleaned regularly, and the shelves lined with fresh paper. Plastic-coated paper that can be wiped with a damp cloth will last a long time. As this cleaning cannot be done when there are patients around, it is a good idea to plan to clean one or two shelves at a time before or after office hours.

Administrative Supplies. These consist of all types of stationery —letterheads, envelopes, prescription blanks, billheads, calling cards, charge slips, appointment cards, copy paper, carbon paper, medical history forms, insurance blanks, memorandum pads, pencils, erasers, clips, staples, blotters, index cards, rubber bands, file folders, and perhaps other items that a particular office may need. Much time is saved if a sufficient supply of each item is kept on hand and stored in a definite place. It would be rather annoying for the doctor and embarrassing to the assistant if she had to hunt for any item in the middle of a busy morning. An efficient assistant is always one step ahead of the doctor, and it should not be necessary for him to ask her for any of these common articles that he may need. These things should always be in or on his desk.

When ordering supplies, remember that it takes time to fill an order. Printing or engraving often takes from three to four weeks. Also, engraved stationery is expensive. Do not waste it for drafts or to jot down a memorandum!

This word of warning applies to all supplies, whether medical or administrative. Do not waste them. A little care at all times will in the long run mean a great deal of saving, which the doctor will be sure to appreciate. Careless use of every type of supply can soon add up to a considerable amount of money.

When an assistant starts a new job she will do well to tour the office and inspect closets and cupboards, in order to become familiar with the supplies that the doctor uses. This will save her from not being able to find something that is needed and appearing foolish, as well as from ordering unnecessary supplies.

Ideally, a list is kept of all supplies in the office, and an inventory is taken once a year, but this involves a lot of work and is seldom done in private offices. If, however, the office is shared by several doctors, this practice will repay the amount of time consumed. The medical supplies, especially, should always be listed on a running inventory.

Bills for supplies must be checked carefully and compared with former bills. When the assistant notices that the price of a certain item has increased over a period of a few weeks, for instance, she should ask for an explanation. Bills should be initialed by the assistant before being submitted to the doctor, so that he may know she has checked them. This is particularly important when several doctors share an office and when there is more than one assistant.

Laundry

Laundry is used extensively in any doctor's office. Items needed are:

1. Towels
2. Sheets
3. Pillowcases
4. Doctor's gowns or coats
5. Assistant's uniforms
6. Patients' examination gowns

Just what items and how many are needed in any particular office depends, like so many other matters, on the doctor's specialty and his individual preference.

The majority of physicians rent their laundry from a linen-supply firm that makes weekly deliveries. These companies, as a rule, rent a certain number of each item—towels, sheets, etc.—at a flat rate. Let us say, the doctor rents fifty sheets a month at a given rate. Each week the laundryman will leave as many clean sheets as he takes away soiled. If the total number of sheets used during the month exceeds fifty, an additional charge per sheet is made. For this reason it is advisable to estimate as closely as possible the number of each item needed and to arrange for rental of this amount. If it is found that fewer or more of any particular item is used, the arrangement can be changed accordingly.

When the laundry is delivered, it should be carefully checked. Articles with stains, buttons missing, rips, or too many mended places should be not be accepted. Doctors' gowns and uniforms should be the right size. Too often the garments that are delivered are too small or too large. Patients' gowns, of course, are wide and large and are not expected to fit. Dealers soon discover whether the assistant is alert and watches deliveries.

If the doctor uses his own linen, this is sent to a regular laundry. A list must accompany the soiled laundry, and a copy should be kept at the office to check the clean linen when it is delivered. If pieces are stained or torn, the doctor must decide what he wishes to do with them. They can be sent out to be mended, but this is usually more costly than replacing them.

Laundry bills must be carefully checked; mistakes do happen.

Like all other supplies, sufficient laundry must always be kept on hand. The assistant must learn to judge how many of each item the office is likely to need within a given time and order a sufficient supply. Waste, however, must be avoided. There are a number of ways of saving on laundry, such as placing a towel over the pillow instead of putting on a fresh pillowcase. In a clinic it would be impossible to supply a clean sheet for every examination. If the patient does not have to undress, a towel on the pillow and a rubber sheet at the bottom of the table for the feet will be sufficient. Sometimes a bath towel is enough covering for the patient during an examination when he is only partially disrobed.

A patient who comes daily for a series of treatments, a gastric series, or something similar can be given a gown on his first visit, with his name on a tag pinned to the gown. No patient will object to using one gown throughout the treatment.

A little thought will reduce the number of towels used to a surprising extent. Towels are not intended to be used for dusting furniture, cleaning shoes, or wiping tables. Nor is it necessary for the assistant to use a fresh towel every time she washes her hands. She might keep a towel for her own use in her desk and change it every few days.

Fresh linen should always be put on the examination table in the presence of the patient. He is apt to reject linen that is already on the table when he enters the room.

Removal of Stains

No matter how orderly and clean the office may be kept, the appearance is spoiled if there are stains anywhere. Stains are unavoidable in a doctor's office, with medicine being used freely and blood being drawn. Quick removal with the right substance is the only solution to the problem.

In deciding on a stain remover, not only the type of stain but also the surface from which it is to be removed must be considered. A remover might be successfully used on metal, enamel, glass, or any other hard surface and not be suitable for any fabric. Among fabrics, it is important to know what the cloth is made of. Cotton and linen can be cleaned with solutions that completely ruin silk

HOUSEKEEPING HINTS

or wool, and nylon, as well as the other synthetic fibers, must be treated entirely differently.

A few suggestions for removing stains such as are most likely to occur in a medical office are given below. As was mentioned, *prompt action is necessary*. A stain that has set is often impossible to remove. A stain may also set if the wrong material is used for removing it. Hot water and soap will set some stains; cleaning fluid, others. Before attempting to remove a stain, be certain of the type of stain and the surface from which you are trying to remove it.

1. Adhesive plaster—use benzin or any cleaning fluid that is commercially available.
2. Blood—use cold water (never hot) until the blood is dissolved. If this does not remove the stain completely, sponge with hydrogen peroxide; wash with soapsuds afterwards and rinse.
3. Gentian violet—wash with pure alcohol.
4. Grease, fats and oils—use benzin, ether, or any cleaning fluid. If the material is washable, hot water and soap or detergent will remove the stain. On delicate materials use cornstarch, chalk, or talcum powder, or place the spot between white blotting paper and press with a warm iron.
5. Ink—use a blotter; then soak in milk. (Milk stains are easily removed with soap and water from washable materials, with cleaning fluid from nonwashable ones.) If milk is not available, use glycerin and water or soap and water. For old spots that have dried use oxalic acid (*poison*), 3 tablespoons to a pint of water; this is a bleach and may take out color.
6. Iodine—soap and water will remove a fresh stain. Alcohol (diluted for synthetics or colored materials) will remove stubborn stains.
7. Iron rust—on hard surfaces, use commercial rust removers; on materials, use lemon juice and salt and, if possible, place the article in sunlight to bleach. When the stain disappears, rinse well. Or, use a few drops of the oxalic acid mixture mentioned under ink stains and rinse in hot water.
8. Mercurochrome—use equal parts of alcohol and water to

loosen the stain. Follow with glycerin, which should be worked into the stain until color disappears. On white materials, if the stain does not disappear, use a bleach.

9. Silver nitrate—soak the article in salt water; then apply iodine. Remove the iodine in the way suggested above.

10. X-ray developer—cover the stain with iodine and proceed as above.

Because stains are so much more easily removed if they are treated at once, some of the cleaning materials mentioned should be kept on hand. A bottle of commercial cleaning fluid will also be especially appreciated by patients who not only may get a spot on their clothes in the office, but may come to the office with stains on them. They will be grateful if the assistant helps them to remove a stain.

A sponge, a supply of clean rags, a soft cloth, and a small handbrush or nailbrush should also be kept in the office.

Many more useful hints are contained in a booklet that may be obtained free of charge from the Government Printing Office. Write to the Superintendent of Documents, U. S. Government Printing Office, Washington 25, D.C. for "Stain Removal from Fabrics," Farmers' Bulletin 1474, U. S. Department of Agriculture.

The Doctor's Bag

Whenever the doctor makes house visits, he must take along certain medications, instruments, and supplies. This necessitates certain duties on the part of the assistant.

1. Make sure that everything the doctor needs is in his bag.
2. After his return, check the bag for specimens that must be refrigerated, tested, or sent out to a laboratory.
3. Sterilize syringes, needles, and rubber gloves.
4. Replace items that have been used up.
5. Refill containers that have been emptied.
6. Check to see that each instrument is in proper working condition (batteries in flashlight; scissors sharp).

The contents of the bag depend upon the specialty of the doctor and on his personal preferences. Everything must be kept in perfect condition, as the doctor depends entirely on this limited supply during the time that he is visiting patients in their homes. The assistant should test needles, see that rubber gloves are not torn, and supply an ample amount of anything that the doctor may dispense.

If your doctor's practice necessitates many emergency calls, the bag must be ready at all times. Never leave the office without checking on its contents. Only one person should be responsible for the contents of the bag.

While doctors' preferences vary considerably regarding the contents of the bag, a check list should be made and might include the following:

Instruments

1. Hypodermic syringes and needles
2. Scalpel
3. Probes
4. Otoscope
5. Ophthalmoscope
6. Thermometers (oral and rectal)
7. Blood pressure apparatus
8. Stethoscope
9. Tourniquet
10. Pencil flashlight
11. Percussion hammer
12. Head mirror

Medications

Ampules, vials, capsules, or tablets of:

1. Adrenalin
2. Amytal
3. Codeine
4. Morphine
5. Antibiotics
6. Ear drops
7. Eye drops
8. Skin sterilizer

Accessories

1. Scissors
2. Tongue blades
3. Wooden applicators
4. Cotton
5. Sterile dressings
6. Bandages of assorted sizes
7. Adhesive tape
8. Gauze
9. Safety pins
10. Fountain pen
11. Prescription pad
12. Sterile gloves and lubricant

13. Containers for specimens
14. Fixer solution
15. Staining solution
16. Slides (6)
17. Aspiration equipment

Before making up such a check list, the assistant should discuss it with her employer to make sure that she has included everything he wishes to have in his bag and omitted those things he does not need. Once this check list has been made, it should be consulted every time the bag is prepared, until the assistant is so thoroughly familiar with her doctor's habits that there is no chance of her forgetting to include anything.

20

Laboratory Techniques[1]

It has been said that the human organism is a chemical factory. The foods we eat and the fluids we drink are broken down in the body into their constituents. They are utilized for growth of new tissue, for repair of injured parts, for the production of heat and energy, and for the many other functions performed by the organism. Waste products are isolated and eliminated.

If any one of these chemical processes breaks down at any point, or is inadequately performed, traces of substances that have not been properly utilized may be found in the urine, indicating to the physician what may be wrong and helping him in the diagnosis. The blood too may show indications of faulty chemical processes. Blood and urine, therefore, are examined when the doctor tries to determine the state of a patient's health.

Many doctors have a laboratory in order to have some of these relatively simple examinations made at their office while the patient is there, and they expect the medical office assistant to be able to perform them. The techniques are therefore described in this chapter.

The procedures for urinalysis in a hospital laboratory are fairly complicated and time-consuming. More streamlined tests have been devised, which use prepared ingredients and are quickly performed. While the tests made with prepared tablets or solutions may not be quite so accurate as the more detailed ones, they are sufficient to indicate to the doctor whether or not a certain patho-

---

[1] Based on a manual of medical laboratory techniques by Peter A. Moschetta and Frank O. Waters, Jr.

logical condition exists. These tests are used almost exclusively in doctors' offices and are the only ones described here.

The section on Hematology includes only those tests that are made routinely in a doctor's office. For more elaborate examinations a fully equipped hospital laboratory would be necessary, and the operator would have to be a trained medical technologist.

URINALYSIS

Collection of the Specimen. All specimens of urine should be collected in clean containers of a suitable size. The technician is warned against accepting specimens in containers that may have contained drugs that will result in possible false-positive reactions. Greater control is possible in the hospital laboratory, where suitable containers are supplied to the patients. This, however, is not always the case in a physician's office, where specimens are sometimes delivered by the patient.

Preservation. If the urine cannot be examined immediately, refrigeration is the best method of preservation. The examination should not be delayed too long, however. Specimens should be examined as soon as possible after being voided.

Physical Examination

Quantity. When it is desirable to know the volume of the urine, pour the specimen into a volumetric cylinder and record the quantity. This procedure is usually necessary only in the case of either day, night, or 24-hour specimens.

Color. Observe the color of the specimen and report as "colorless," "straw," "amber," "red," "greenish," "brown," etc. Normally the color of the specimen is straw to amber.

Appearance. Examine the specimen and record as "clear," "cloudy," "cloudy with sediment," "shreds," etc.

Odor. Record as "normal," "medicated," "ammoniacal," "strong," "putrid."

Reaction. Dip a strip of blue litmus paper into the specimen. If it turns red, the urine is acid. If it does not change, dip a strip of

LABORATORY TECHNIQUES

red litmus paper into the urine. If it turns blue, the specimen is alkaline. If neither paper turns color, the urine is neutral. If both change color, then the reaction is amphoteric due to the presence of both alkaline and acid phosphates.

Specific Gravity. A specific gravity has been established for every substance, that is, its weight in relation to the weight of the same volume of a substance that has been established as a standard. For solids and liquids, distilled water is the standard, the maximum weight of which is 1 Gm. per cc. at 4°C., and its specific gravity is expressed as 1.000. The specific gravity of a solid or liquid, therefore, is its weight compared with the weight of an equal volume of water, or the number of times a certain volume of that substance is as heavy as an equal volume of water. The normal specific gravity of urine varies between 1.015 and 1.025. If it is below or above this figure, disease may be present, and further tests are indicated. For this reason the doctor may request a reading of the specific gravity of a patient's urine. Figures 20-1 and 20-2 illustrate the technique for this test.

Total Solids. Under normal conditions the total amount of solids passing through the kidney in a 24-hour period is approximately 60 to 70 Gm. Factors influencing this amount are weight, age, exercise, diet, metabolism, and kidney function. An estimation of the total solids, therefore, may be of value to the physician as an indication of the functional efficiency of the kidneys.

The total solids in 1,000 ml. of urine may be roughly calculated

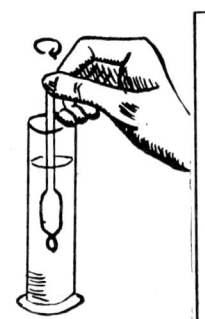

The cylinder is filled 3/4 of the way with urine sample (well mixed). The float is then placed in the urine and given a gentle spin with the thumb and forefinger, causing the float to spin. This prevents the float from adhering to the sides of the cylinder. If there is insufficient urine to float the urinometer, report q.n.s. (quantity not sufficient.)

FIG. 20-1. Determining specific gravity of urine.

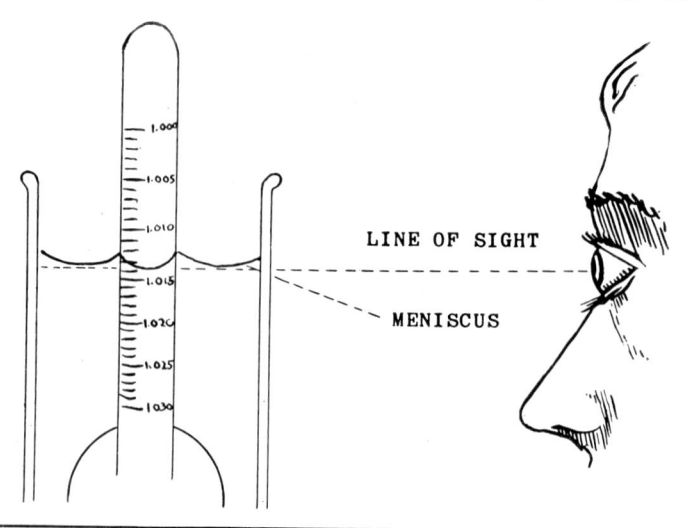

The cylinder is placed so that the lower line of the meniscus is at eye level. Reading of the specific gravity is then made by imagining a line drawn at the point where the lower line of the meniscus crosses the scale on the urinometer.

In the above diagram, the specific gravity would be read as 1.014.

FIG. 20-2. Method for reading and reporting specific gravity.

by means of Long's coefficient, which is 2.6. The last two digits of the specific gravity at 25°C. are multiplied by 2.6.

Example:
$$\text{Specific gravity at } 25°C. = 1.015$$
$$15 \times 2.6 = 39 \text{ Gm. in 1,000 ml. of urine}$$

To determine the solids excreted in a 24-hour period, multiply the value obtained in 1,000 ml. of urine by the volume (in milliliters) of the 24-hour specimen and divide by 1,000.

Example:
$$\text{Volume of 24-hour specimen} = 1,200 \text{ ml.}$$
$$\text{Solids in 1,000 ml. of the 24-hour specimen} = 39 \text{ Gm.}$$
$$\frac{1,200 \times 39}{1,000} = 46.8 \text{ Gm. of solid matter in 1,200 ml. of urine}$$

Microscopic Examination

Obtaining Sediment. Mix specimen to stir up any sediment that may have settled at the bottom. Place 10 cc. of urine in a centrifuge tube and centrifuge 4 to 5 minutes at 1,500 r.p.m. Pour all the urine from the tube into the original container. The urine in the container may be used for chemical analysis. Several drops of urine will remain along the wall of the tube and flow back down into the sediment. Mix by tapping the tube with the finger and transfer a drop to a slide with the aid of a capillary pipet or several applicator sticks held together. Cover the drop with a cover glass and examine with the low- and high-power objectives. *Avoid use of too much light.* The field of the microscope must be darkened by almost completely closing the diaphragm. This is absolutely necessary if hyaline casts are to be found, because of their low refractivity. Identify and report the approximate number of crystals, cells, casts, etc.

Casts are usually reported in approximate (average) number per low-power field. Red and white blood cells are usually reported in approximate (average) number per high-power field. Other elements, e.g., crystals and epithelial cells, are usually reported as "occasional," "few," "moderate number," "many," depending on the number seen per average field.

Figure 20-3 shows urinary sediments.

CRYSTALS OBSERVED IN URINE
Acid urine: uric acid; calcium sulfate; sodium urate
Acid, neutral, or feebly alkaline urine: calcium oxalate; hippuric acid
Alkaline urine: calcium phosphate; ammonium biurate; calcium carbonate
Alkaline, neutral, or feebly acid urine: triple phosphate; calcium phosphate

Figure 20-4 illustrates amorphous material usually observed in urine.

Chemical Examination

Tests for the determination of acetone, albumin, blood, or sugar in the urine can be made by the use of special tablets. These tests

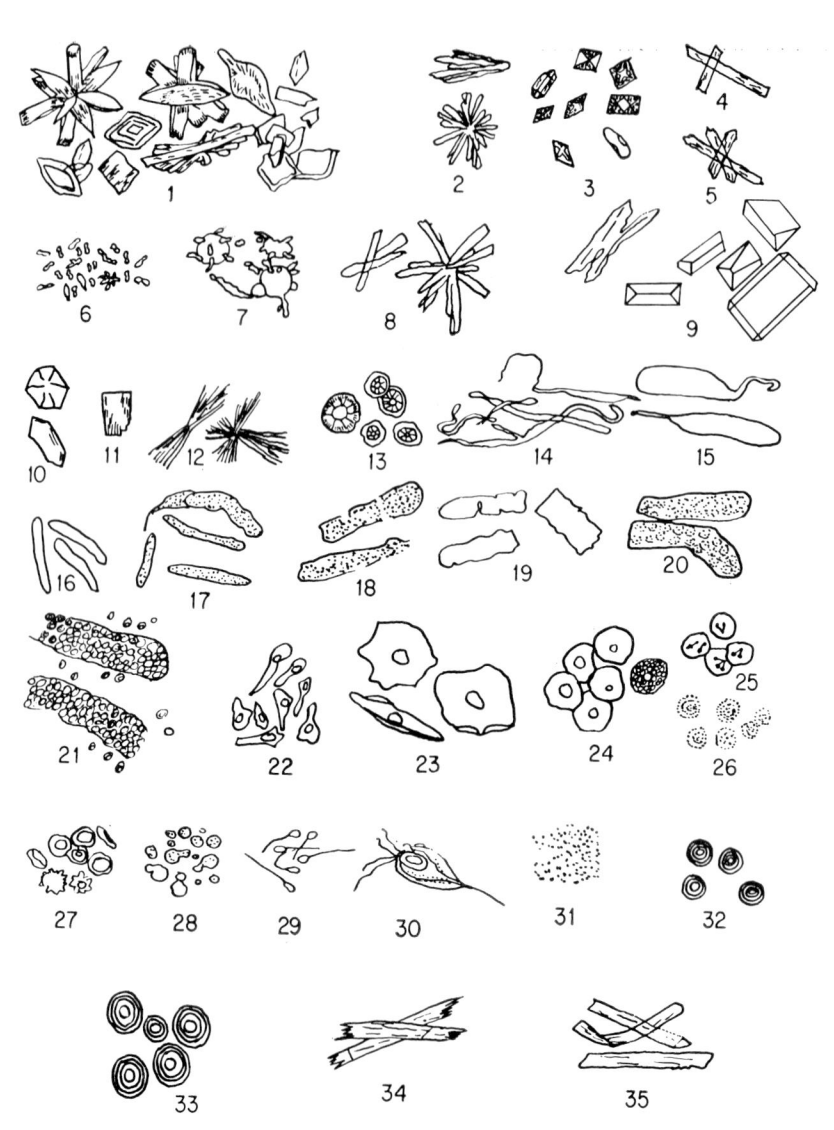

Fig. 20-3. Urinary sediments. *1*, Uric acid crystals; *2*, sodium urate crystals; *3*, calcium oxalate crystals; *4*, calcium sulfate crystals; *5*, hippuric acid crystals; *6*, calcium carbonate crystals; *7*, ammonium biurate crystals; *8*, calcium phosphate crystals; *9*, triple phosphate crystals; *10*, cystine crystals; *11*, cholesterol crystals; *12*, tyrosine crystals; *13*, leucine spheres; *14*, mucous threads; *15*, cylindroids; *16*, hyaline casts; *17*, finely granular casts; *18*, coarsely granular casts; *19*, waxy casts; *20*, pus casts; *21*, RBC casts; *22*, caudate epithelial cells; *23*, squamous epithelial cells; *24*, round (renal) cells, one showing fatty degeneration; *25*, leukocytes; *26*, pus cells; *27*, erythrocytes; *28*, yeasts; *29*, spermatozoa; *30*, *Trichomonas vaginalis*; *31*, bacteria; *32*, oil globules; *33*, air bubbles; *34*, flax fibers; *35*, cotton fibers.

LABORATORY TECHNIQUES 297

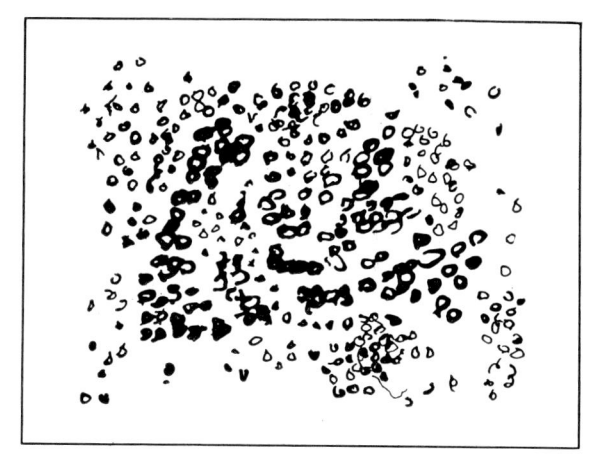

FIG. 20-4. Amorphous material usually observed in urine.

are simple to perform and take a minimum of time. They are therefore especially practical for a doctor's office.

The tests described below are made with the various reagent tablets put out by Ames Company, Inc., and the directions given are taken from the instruction leaflets supplied by the company.

Test for Acetonuria. Using Acetest reagent tablets:

1. Place the reagent tablet on a clean white sheet of paper.
2. Put a drop of urine on the tablet.
3. After 30 seconds, compare the resulting color with the color chart enclosed with the tablets.

Test for Albuminuria. When albumin is found in the urine, the patient should have a thorough examination; for the finding of albumin must be correlated with other laboratory and clinical data in arriving at a diagnosis. Using the Bumintest reagent tablets:

1. Place equal parts of the Bumintest reagent solution and urine in a test tube. (Reagent solution [5%] is prepared by dissolving four Bumintest reagent tablets in 1 oz. [30 cc.] of water.)
2. Shake the tube gently.
3. The amount of albumin is estimated by the degree of turbidity.

A newer test is the Albutest, which employs a new and different principle from other tests, the presence of protein being indicated by a color change on the tablet surface instead of a precipitate in a solution. Albutest consists of a tablet containing an indicator, a buffer, an agent which adsorbs protein, and an inert carrier.

When a drop of urine containing protein is placed on the tablet, the protein is adsorbed on the tablet surface. Following the addition of 2 drops of water, a considerable quantity of the urine is washed away, but the protein, indicator, and buffer remain at the surface of the tablet, and the indicator maintains a blue color. The intensity of the blue color is proportional to the amount of protein present in the urine.

1. Place the tablet on a clean surface and put 1 *drop* of urine on the tablet.

2. After the urine drop has been absorbed, add 2 *drops* of water and allow penetration before reading.

3. Compare the color on top of the tablet with the color photograph supplied with each package of tablets (see Fig. 20–5).

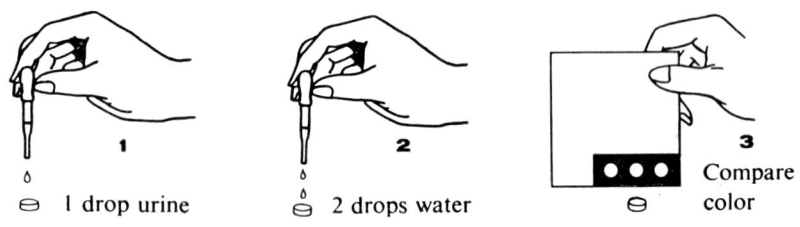

FIG. 20–5. Directions for Albutest. (*Ames Company, Inc.*)

Important: It would appear that reporting weak positive reactions in this test is too indefinite. Insignificant negative reactions, on the other hand, could be interpreted as positive by this method.

Test for Occult Blood. Using Hematest reagent tablets:

1. Place 1 drop (or smear) of urine on filter paper that rests on a clean, dry surface.

2. Place the tablet in the center of the specimen.

3. Add 2 drops of water. Blue color on the filter paper indicates a positive finding.

A more recent test is the Occultest, which the manufacturers maintain is more sensitive. Occultest reagent tablets are used. Dropper and working area must be clean and free from traces of blood.

1. Place 1 drop of well-mixed, uncentrifuged urine in the center of a square of filter paper.
2. Put the Occultest tablet in the center of the moist area.
3. Place 2 drops of water on the tablet.
4. Diffuse blue color appearing on the filter paper around the tablet within 2 minutes indicates a positive finding. The amount of blood present is proportionate to the intensity of blue color, its area on the filter paper, and the rapidity of color development. If no blue color appears on the filter paper at the end of 2 minutes, the finding is negative.

Test for Glycosuria. Determination of excess sugar in the urine is a classic criterion for the detection and control of diabetes mellitus. Recent clinical experience with ACTH and cortisone indicates the need of frequent checking for glycosuria. Using Clinitest tablets:

1. Place 5 drops of urine and 10 drops of water in a test tube.
2. Add the Clinitest reagent tablet. Watch the reaction.
3. Shake and compare the solution with the color scale enclosed with the tablets.

This test may also be performed with the newer Clinistix reagent strips. These are strips of enzyme-impregnated paper. The technique is as follows:

1. Dip the test end of Clinistix in the urine and remove. (Alternatively, the test end may be placed in the urine stream momentarily or moistened with a drop of urine.)
2. If the moistened end turns blue, the finding is positive. If no blue color develops, the finding is negative. When sugar is present, blue color normally appears in less than a minute but may occasionally be delayed a minute or so, depending on the nature of the urine.

Important: The test end of the strip should not be allowed to come into contact with fingers or other objects that may be contaminated with glucose or other chemicals, since misleading reactions may result. Similarly, the wetted strip should either be held in the air or laid on a thoroughly clean surface before the reaction is read.

HEMATOLOGY

The methods used in hematology are simple. It is suggested, however, that if the medical office assistant does not have any previous training, she try them out on herself or some of her friends, rather than on a patient. This will give her confidence as well as proficiency. Also, most patients are quick to spot the novice.

Obtaining Blood

For most routine hematologic procedures, very small quantities of blood are needed. A skin puncture made with a suitable sterile instrument is therefore satisfactory.

SITES FOR SKIN PUNCTURE
1. Palmar surface of the finger tip
2. Ear lobe
3. Plantar surface of the heel ⎫
4. Plantar surface of the great toe ⎭ Infants

SITES TO BE AVOIDED
1. Edematous areas
2. Cyanotic areas
3. Scarred areas
4. Traumatized areas
5. Heavily calloused areas

INSTRUMENTS USED FOR SKIN PUNCTURE
1. Disposable, individually packaged, sterile lancet. (See Figs. 20–6 and 20–7.)
2. Automatic lancet.

LABORATORY TECHNIQUES

3. Hagedorn needle.
4. Bard-Parker No. 12 scalpel blade. (The blade should be embedded in a cork in such a manner that only 3 to 4 mm. of the blade is visible. The cork acts as a safeguard against puncturing too deeply.)

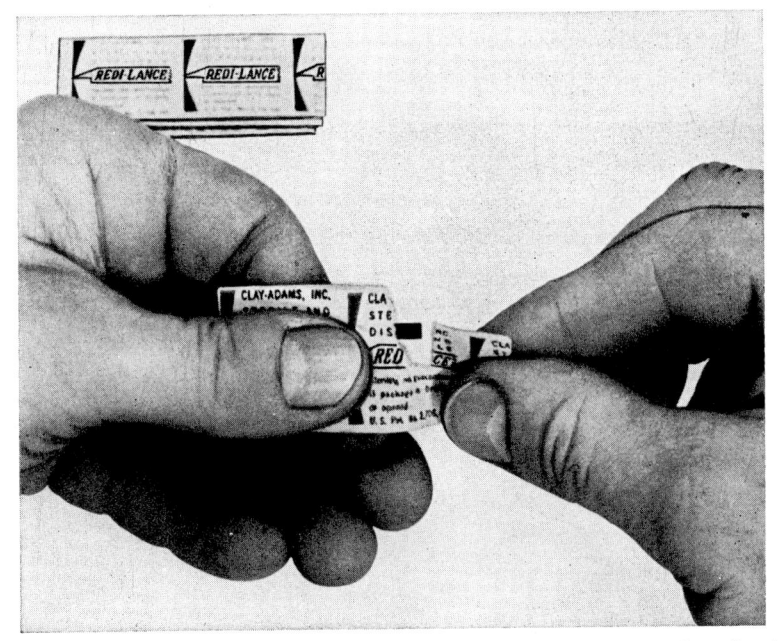

FIG. 20-6. Removal of lancet from its wrapper. (*Clay-Adams Co., Inc.*)

INSTRUMENTS TO BE AVOIDED
1. Rusty instruments. Discard these at once.
2. Instruments that are dull or have burrs.
3. Round pins and needles. The wound produced by them will seal before the required amount of blood is obtained, thereby necessitating two or more punctures.

Important: It has been established that viral hepatitis can be transmitted by means of a common hematologic puncture instrument; therefore, only an instrument sterilized by autoclaving should be used. Individually packaged, sterile, disposable lancets, which are commercially available, are the method of choice. The

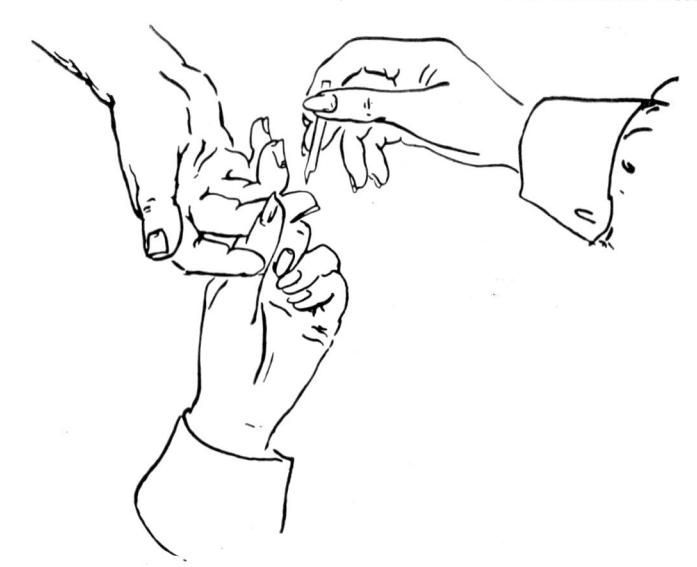

FIG. 20–7. Technique of using a lancet. (*Clay-Adams Co., Inc.*)

other instruments that have in the past been in common use cannot be adequately sterilized by a brief exposure to alcohol or other antiseptic solution. When it is necessary to use the automatic lancet (as for bleeding-time estimation), it should be wrapped or tubed and autoclaved in advance.

MATERIALS AND EQUIPMENT
1. 70% isopropyl alcohol
2. Absorbent cotton sponges
3. Sterile puncture instrument
4. Appropriate instruments for the procedures to be done (pipets, diluting fluids, slides, etc.)

PROCEDURE
1. Select a finger. The thumb and index finger should be avoided, since they are more heavily calloused than the other fingers. It is difficult to obtain good results from a cold finger. A warm pack may be used to promote circulation.
2. "Milk" the finger gently to promote circulation to the tip.
3. Cleanse the puncture area thoroughly with an alcohol-saturated absorbent cotton sponge. Allow the area to dry. Do not

LABORATORY TECHNIQUES

blow on it and do not touch it or allow anything to come into contact with it.
4. Using your thumb and forefinger, grip the patient's cleansed finger at the middle joint. Using a sterile lancet, firmly gripped in your other hand, puncture the palmar surface of the distal phalanx to a depth of 3 to 4 mm., using a quick, clean, stabbing stroke. Remember that a puncture of 3 to 4 mm. causes no more pain than a puncture of 1 mm. There should be an immediate flow of blood. The blade should be held at a right angle to the "fingerprint" striations of the patient's finger. This will result in a cutting wound that will produce drops of blood that will not flow down the finger. Gentle pressure exerted at a distance from the wound should cause the blood to flow freely. Squeezing will liberate tissue juices, which in turn will dilute the blood and cause inaccurate results.
5. Wipe away the first drops of blood with a dry cotton sponge, as these are greatly diluted with the tissue fluid that was liberated when the cells were punctured.
6. Use gentle pressure to cause a drop of blood to form that is large enough for the particular procedure you are performing (e.g., a comparatively large drop for a white cell count and for hemoglobin; a small drop for a red cell count).
7. Wipe the finger dry and work from a freshly expressed drop of blood for each procedure. This will prevent using blood that has begun to coagulate.
8. If the pipets must be laid down for a period of time or must be moved, care should be taken that no fluids are lost. There are various closure devices available that may be used to prevent loss.
9. Carefully identify each sample to prevent confusion of reports.
10. The proficient technician is able, routinely, to obtain a complete blood count from a single puncture. The complete blood count (CBC) consists of:
    a. A red blood cell (RBC) count
    b. A white blood cell (WBC) count

c. A hemoglobin (hb) estimation
d. A differential count

Blood Counts

Counting Chamber. The counting chamber with improved Neubauer ruling consists of 9 sq. mm. The four corner squares are each divided into sixteen squares. The central ruled square millimeter is divided into twenty-five double-ruled squares, each of which is divided into sixteen squares, each small square being the equivalent of 1/400 sq. mm. (see Fig. 20-8).

L = the square-millimeter areas to be counted for the total leukocyte count. The encircled area is the area seen with the 16-mm. objective with the diaphragm almost closed.

E = the areas to be counted for the total red blood cell count. The encircled area is the area seen with the 4-mm. objective.

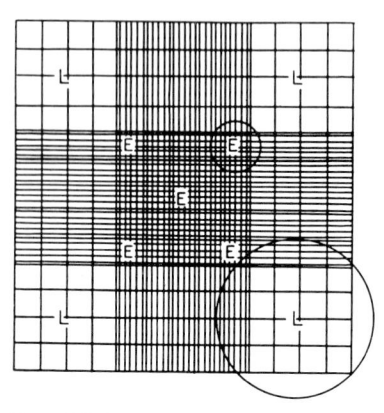

FIG. 20-8. Counting chamber. L, Areas for total leukocyte count; E, areas for total red blood cell count.

Observe the encircled square-millimeter area marked L. It will be noted that closely divided horizontal lines appear at the upper portion of the field, and closely divided vertical lines appear at the left of the field. These lines are easily differentiated from the square millimeter used for counting. These lines identify the square millimeter in the lower left-hand corner as seen through the microscope. The square millimeter in the upper left-hand corner of the illustration may be identified by the horizontal lines at the lower portion of the field and the vertical lines to the right. Each square millimeter may be identified by observing the guidelines. The squares for counting RBCs may be similarly identified.

Method of Counting. Figure 20-9 shows the method used in counting cells. It is of the utmost importance to maintain a certain order when counting in order to assure accuracy and speed. Beginning in the upper left-hand square, count all the cells in one square after the other. Include in the count the cells that touch the upper and left-hand lines, omitting those that touch the right-hand and lower lines. The arrows indicate the direction in which the count should be made. The black-filled cells are the ones that would be counted in the first sweep from left to right. Figure 20–10 illustrates leukocytes in 1 sq. mm.

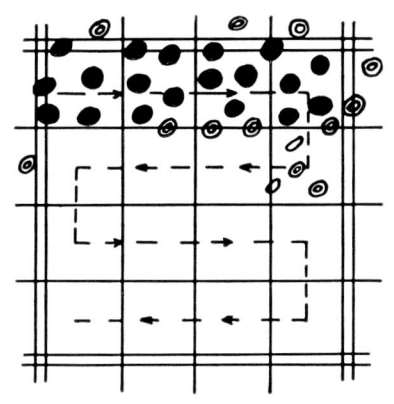

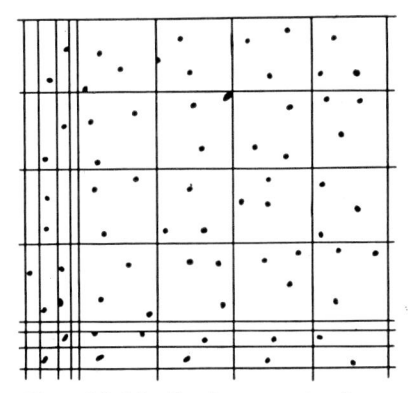

FIG. 20–9. Method of counting cells.

FIG. 20–10. Leukocytes in 1 sq. mm.

Erythrocyte Count. All RBC pipets are made so that if blood is taken to the 0.5 mark and diluted to the 101 mark, the dilution will be 1:200, regardless of the size of the pipet or the shape of the bulb. Blood taken to the 1.0 mark and diluted to the 101 mark will be diluted 1:100. Figure 20–11 shows a red cell pipet.

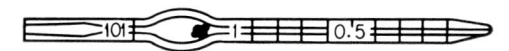

FIG. 20–11. Red blood cell diluting pipet.

MATERIALS AND EQUIPMENT

1. Sterile puncture instrument (preferably a disposable lancet; the Hagedorn needle, automatic lancet, and Bard-Parker No. 12 scalpel blade embedded in a cork are also popular)
2. 70% isopropyl alcohol
3. Cotton sponges
4. RBC diluting pipet

5. RBC diluting fluid
6. Counting chamber and cover glass
7. Microscope

PROCEDURE

1. Cleanse the puncture site with 70% alcohol. Allow the area to dry by evaporation.
2. Puncture the cleansed area with a quick, clean stroke, deep enough (3 to 4 mm.) to cause immediate flow of blood. When puncturing the finger, prick the skin at a right angle to the fingerprint lines. This makes it easier to obtain a drop of blood that will not spread over the finger. Wipe the first drop away with a dry cotton sponge.
3. From a second drop draw blood to exactly the 0.5 mark. Wipe away all blood from the outside of the pipet with dry cotton.
4. Place the pipet in diluting fluid and dilute to exactly the 101 mark. None of the blood must be allowed to escape into the diluting fluid. To avoid air bubbles, keep the pipet exactly vertical during dilution. To avoid blood clots, rotate the pipet between thumb and forefinger while diluting.
5. Place a clean cover slip in the proper position over the ruled areas of the counting chamber.
6. Grasp the pipet between thumb and forefinger. Shake it vigorously for 3 minutes. Do not shake the pipet along its axis. Use a sidewise-rotating (figure-eight) motion. The pipet is shaken in order to distribute the cells evenly throughout the diluting fluid. Figure 20–12 shows the proper method for shaking the pipet.
7. Discard 3 to 5 drops from the pipet (to ensure disposal of the diluting fluid in the pipet stem and ensure the bringing of cells from the bulb to the pipet tip) and immediately touch a drop to the chamber platform so that the drop contacts the edge of the cover slip. The drop will be drawn under the cover glass and over the ruled area by capillary action. The drop must be large enough to cover the entire

LABORATORY TECHNIQUES 307

ruled area but must not spill into the moats on either side. There should be no air bubbles. The cover slip must not be moved after charging. Charging the chamber is illustrated in Fig. 20–13.

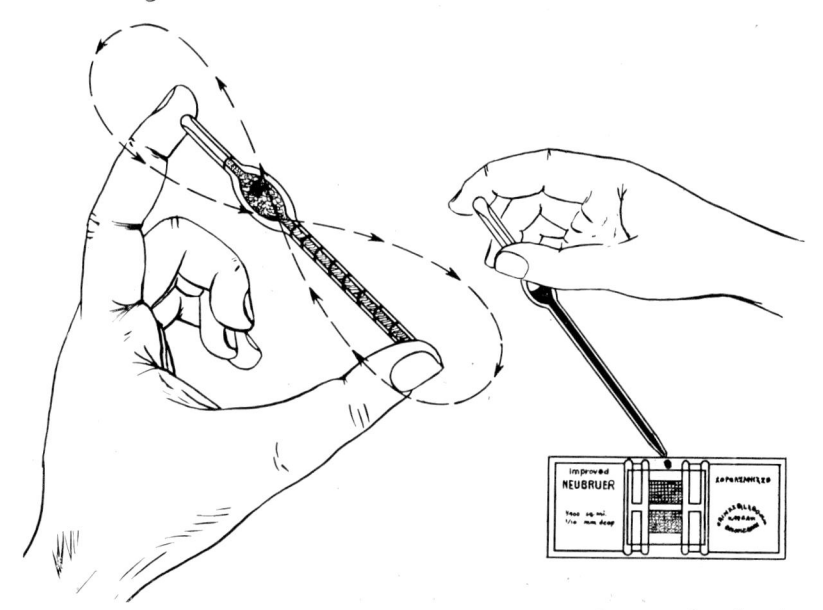

Fig. 20–12. Shaking the pipet.   Fig. 20–13. Charging the chamber.

8. Allow about 2 minutes for all the cells to settle into one plane.
9. Carefully place the chamber on the microscope stage and find the central ruled square under low power (16 mm.). Scan the entire central ruled area to check distribution. If the cells appear equally distributed, move the chamber to center the upper-left secondary square in the microscope field.
10. Switch to high power (4 mm.) and adjust lighting and focus. Count all the RBCs in five secondary squares—the four corner squares and the central square or five squares on a diagonal. The difference between any two squares should not be more than fifteen cells. Total the cells counted.

CALCULATION. Report the number of cells per cubic millimeter.

Total of cells counted $\times$ 5 $\times$ 10 $\times$ 200

$$= \text{RBCs per cubic millimeter}$$

Short calculation: Multiplying 5 × 10 × 200 in the above calculation will yield the figure 10,000; therefore, the following short formula may be used: Cells counted in five secondary squares × 10,000 = cells per cubic millimeter.

Normals:
>Men—4.5 to 6.0 million per cu. mm.
>Women—4.0 to 5.5 million per cu. mm.
>Infants—5.5 to 7.0 million per cu. mm.

Duplicate counts should check within 300,000 cells per cu. mm. When low RBC counts are anticipated the blood may be diluted 1:100 instead of 1:200, the calculation being adjusted accordingly.

DILUTING FLUIDS FOR RBCs. Hayem's solution; 0.85% NaCl; Toison's; Gowers'.

Leukocyte Count. All WBC pipets are made so that if blood is drawn to the 0.5 mark and diluted to the 11 mark, the dilution will be 1:20. If blood is taken to the 1.0 mark and diluted to the 11 mark, the dilution will be 1:10. Figure 20–14 shows a white cell pipet.

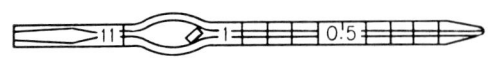

FIG. 20-14. White blood cell diluting pipet.

MATERIALS AND EQUIPMENT. Same as for RBC except that a WBC diluting pipet and WBC diluting fluid are required.

PROCEDURE. Same as for RBC dilution except that blood is drawn to the 0.5 mark in a WBC diluting pipet and diluted to the 11 mark. Count the cells in the four corner primary squares under the 16-mm. objective. If distribution is satisfactory the difference between any two primary squares will be not more than ten cells. Total the cells counted.

CALCULATION. Report the number of cells per cubic millimeter.

Cells counted in four primary squares ÷ 4 × 10 × 20
= cells per cubic millimeter

Short calculation: Multiplying 10 × 20 and dividing by 4 in the above calculation will yield the figure 50; therefore, the following

LABORATORY TECHNIQUES

short formula may be used: Total of cells counted in four primary squares × 50 = cells per cubic millimeter.

Normal:
5,000 to 10,000 WBCs per cu. mm. for both sexes

Unlike the RBCs, which are maintained at fairly constant levels under normal conditions, the WBC count will fluctuate during the day, especially following meals. The WBC count is at its lowest in the basal state.

DILUTING FLUIDS. Turck's solution is probably the most popular. This is a 2% glacial acetic acid in water. A drop or two of aqueous gentian violet added to the diluting fluid will stain the cell nuclei and facilitate counting. 0.1 N hydrochloric acid may also be used for WBC dilutions.

It must be remembered that the red cell diluting fluids do not destroy white blood cells. The white cells may be detected by their size, which is about 12 microns in comparison to the average of 7 microns for the red cells. The white cells are nucleated, and some are granular. The few that may be seen should be excluded from the red cell count. Ordinarily the number of white cells seen while doing a red cell count is so small as to have no appreciable effect on the accuracy of the red cell count.

Hemoglobin Estimation (Sahli hemoglobinometer method)

MATERIALS AND EQUIPMENT
1. Equipment for skin puncture
2. Hemoglobin pipet (20 cu. mm.)
3. Sahli hemoglobinometer (Fig. 20-15)
4. 0.1 (1/10) N hydrochloric acid
5. Distilled water

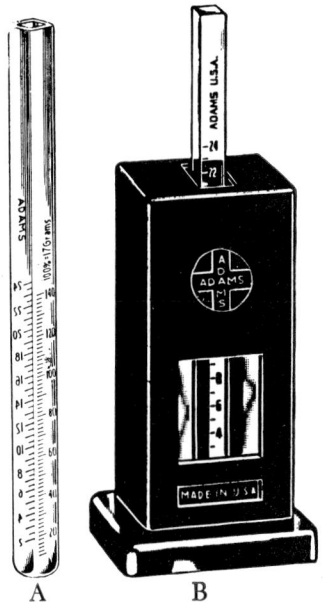

FIG. 20-15. A. Sahli-Adams square hemometer tube. B. Sahli-Adams Plano-Parallel hemometer with tube. (*Clay-Adams Co., Inc.*)

PROCEDURE

1. Place 0.1 N HCl in the graduated hemometer tube to the 10% mark.
2. Puncture the patient's finger (or other site).
3. After discarding the first drop, draw blood to the 20 cu. mm. mark of the hemoglobin pipet. Be sure to wipe all blood from the outside of the pipet with a dry sponge.
4. Place the tip of the pipet in the HCl and gently blow the blood into the acid so that it settles at the bottom. Rinse the pipet several times by drawing up and discharging the clear supernatant acid.
5. Shake the mixture gently to mix the blood and acid thoroughly. Avoid forming bubbles. Let the mixture stand for 10 minutes to allow time for full conversion of the hemoglobin to acid hematin.
6. Dilute the acid hematin with distilled water until its color matches that of the standard. A fine glass stirring rod should be used for mixing during dilution. When the solution appears to match the standard, add 1 more drop of diluent, mix, and examine. If the solution now looks overdiluted, report the previous reading. If the solution still appears to match the standard, take a second reading and proceed as before until overdilution is obtained, reporting the last reading which matched the standard (see Fig. 20–16).
7. Read the hemoglobin per cent from the graduated tube, as well as the grams of hemoglobin per 100 cc. of blood, if the tube bears both graduations (not all hemometer tubes show both).

REPORTING. Since the per cent figure will vary according to the reference standard used, while the amount of hemoglobin measured in grams per 100 cc. of blood remains constant, always report both figures, as well as the standard used.

Example:
$$Hb\ 80\%,\ 12\ Gm.\ (Sahli,\ 15\ Gm. = 100\%)$$

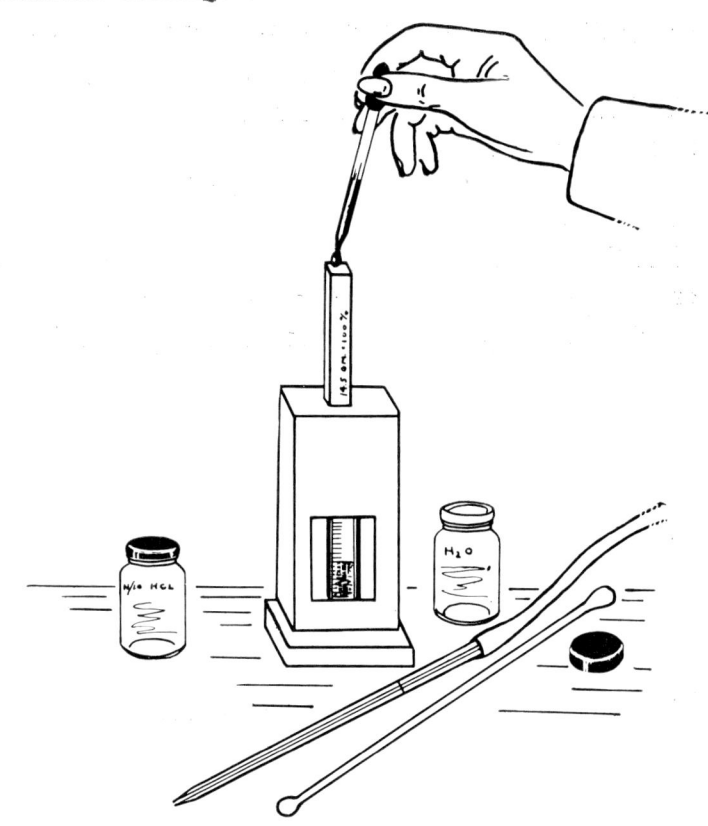

FIG. 20-16. Diluting hemoglobin.

Differential Count Smears

MATERIALS AND EQUIPMENT

1. Equipment for finger puncture
2. Staining rack
3. Wright's stain
4. Distilled water or buffer solution
5. Microslides, 1 by 3 in.

MAKING THE SMEAR

1. Puncture the finger (or other site) as previously described, discarding the first drop of blood.
2. Pick up a small drop of blood, or two small drops side by side, on a clean glass slide by touching the slide to the blood. Do

not touch the finger with the slide, as this will spread the blood on the slide and make it unsuitable for smearing. The blood should be about ¼ in. from the end of the slide, in its center (see Fig. 20–17A).
3. Place the slide on a flat surface (preferable) or hold it between thumb and forefinger.
4. Place the narrow edge of a second slide (called the spreader or pusher) in front of the blood, holding the spreader at about a 25° angle over the blood (see Fig. 20–17B).

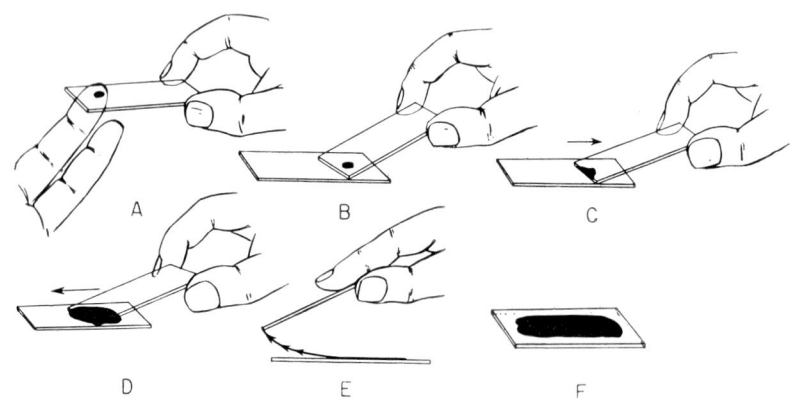

Fig. 20–17. Making a blood smear.

5. Pull the spreader back until it touches the blood. The blood will spread by capillary action. Let the blood spread *almost* to the edges (see Fig. 20–17C).
6. Using a firm, steady movement, push the spreader to the opposite end of the slide (see Fig. 20–17D), finishing the motion by raising the pusher in a smooth, low arc (see Fig. 20–17E). This will yield an ideal smear having a gradation from thick—at the beginning of the smear—to very thin—at the end of the smear (see Fig. 20–17F). In smearing the blood, use a smooth, continuous motion and keep the spreader in firm contact with the smear slide at all times. Pushing the spreader too rapidly will yield a short, thick smear; pushing it too slowly, a long, thin smear.

LABORATORY TECHNIQUES

Important: As soon as the smear is dry, write the patient's name and the date in the beginning, thick part of the smear. Use an ordinary lead pencil. This will provide permanent means of identification. The smear should be stained as soon as possible after it is dry—within a maximum of 24 hours. Beyond this time, cellular changes are such that it is virtually impossible to make satisfactorily stained blood films.

CRITERIA FOR DIFFERENTIAL SMEARS. Smears should be at least 1½ in. long. They should be smooth, with a margin on all sides. If the blood is allowed to spread to the edges of the slide before the smearing is done, the white blood cells tend to migrate to the edges.

About the central half of the smear should be of such thickness that the red blood cells touch each other but do not overlap. This is the area best suited for the differential count.

One end of the smear must be thin enough for a red cell study. In this portion the red blood cells must not touch each other. There should be no streaks, hesitation ridges, or holes. Smears should be thin, because thick smears (1) stain unsatisfactorily, (2) make it impossible to do an RBC study, and (3) make the WBCs small and difficult to identify.

STAINING THE SMEAR

Important: Timing will depend upon the particular lot of stain in use.

1. Place the smear face up on a rack, making sure that the rack is level. (Figure 20–18 illustrates a staining rack and tray.)
2. Completely cover the dry smear with Wright's stain. Leave it for 1 to 3 minutes.
3. Add an equal amount of distilled water or buffer. None must be allowed to fall off the smear. Mix stain and water by gently blowing along the length of the slide. Let it stand for 3 to 6 minutes.
4. Wash by flooding (gently) with tap water from a beaker.
5. The smear should have a lavender-pink color. If it appears purple, hold it under gently running cold water until the

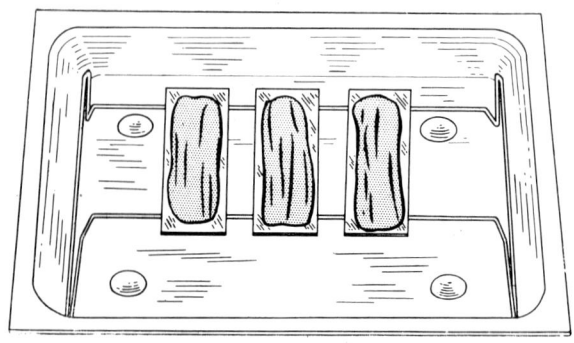

FIG. 20-18. Staining rack and tray. (*Clay-Adams Co., Inc.*)

desired color appears. Let the water strike the slide above the thick portion of the smear and flow down over the smear.

6. Stand the slide on end and allow to dry at room temperature. If the smear must be examined immediately, instead of allowing it to dry it may be blotted, but this is not recommended.

Criteria for a Satisfactorily Stained Smear

1. No precipitated stain on the slide
2. RBCs should be buff-colored
3. Neutrophilic granules should be stained lilac
4. Eosinophilic granules should be stained bright red
5. Basophilic granules should be stained deep blue to black
6. Platelets should be stained purple-blue and be distinct

If the red blood cells appear red and the nuclei of white blood cells appear pale blue to colorless, the stain is too acid. If the red blood cells appear blue, the stain is too alkaline. Varying the timing of the staining procedure will correct these faults.

EXAMINING THE SMEAR. (If the smear is properly prepared, approximately the center half of the smear will be suitable for the differential count of WBCs.) The procedure is as follows:

1. Check the center half of the smear under the 16-mm. objective to be sure the distribution of leukocytes is good. A smear seen to contain aggregates of white blood cells in some spots and sparse numbers of leukocytes in others is unsuit-

LABORATORY TECHNIQUES

able for counting, since distribution has been altered by faulty technique in smearing.
2. Place a drop of immersion oil on the smear and bring the preparation into focus under the oil-immersion objective.
3. Where the total leukocyte count is between 4,000 and 10,000 per cubic millimeter, count and classify at least 100 leukocytes. Be sure to follow a pattern that will cover a representative portion of the smear without duplication. Avoid counting cells at the edges of the smear. They will usually appear distorted and will be out of distribution. Two acceptable patterns to be followed when doing a differential count are illustrated in Figs. 20–19 and 20–20.

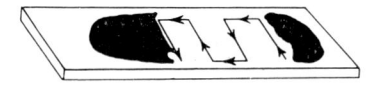

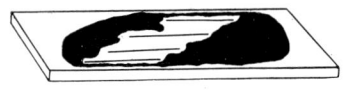

FIG. 20–19. Pattern for counting leukocytes. (Make at least 4 trips across the smear as indicated by arrows.)

FIG. 20–20. Pattern for counting leukocytes. (Count 25 cells along each line.)

4. Shift to the thin portion of the smear and examine several fields of erythrocytes (RBC study). Look for any deviations from normal in size, shape, staining, etc.
5. Report leukocytes in per cent.
6. Report erythrocyte study in standard terms to convey accurate meaning.
7. If nucleated erythrocytes are seen, count them separately while doing the differential leukocyte count and report them in number per 100 WBCs.
8. If neutrophils with toxic granulation are seen, tabulate them separately and report them in per cent.
9. It is of extreme importance that the technician familiarize herself completely with all the normally seen cells, so that she can detect an abnormal cell immediately. The accurate identification of abnormal cells requires much study and experience, but recognizing a particular cell as abnormal is something every technician involved in hematological work

must be able to do. The abnormal cells can be identified by more experienced people in the laboratory, but they must first be recognized and not simply "skipped."

DIFFERENTIAL SMEAR EXAMINATION—SAMPLE REPORT

	Per Cent
Neutrophils	70
Segmented	69
Band	1
Lymphocytes	26
Monocytes	2
Eosinophils	2
Basophils	0
	100

RBC study: marked anisocytosis with predominance of macrocytes

Erythrocyte Sedimentation Rate (Wintrobe-Landsberg Method)

When the determination of the erythrocyte sedimentation rate (ESR) is done, it is absolutely essential that the specific instructions for the particular method being used be followed closely, because a variety of factors influence the rate of sedimentation. Regardless of the method used, the following points should be observed:

1. The syringe and needle must be dry.
2. The needle should be large enough to prevent RBC destruction during aspiration.
3. The specified anticoagulant must be used.
4. The test must be set up within a maximum of 30 minutes after the blood is obtained.
5. All methods are standardized at room temperature (22° to 27°C.). Higher or lower temperatures will increase or retard the ESR.
6. The sedimentation tube should be placed on a steady table and kept from vibrating during the timing interval.
7. The sedimentation tube must be kept absolutely vertical. Even a slight inclination will influence the rate of sedimentation.

MATERIALS AND EQUIPMENT
1. Venipuncture equipment
2. Oxalated tube
3. Hematocrit tube [110 mm. long with a 3-mm. bore; graduated on the left (ESR scale) from 0 to 10 cm. and on the right (packed cell scale) from 10 to 0 cm., with divisions of 1 mm. on both sides] and rack
4. Capillary dropper

PROCEDURE
1. Place exactly 5.0 cc. of venipuncture blood in a prepared oxalated tube. Stopper the tube and invert it repeatedly. (These tubes can be purchased.)
2. With a capillary dropper, fill the hematocrit with blood to the 0 mark of the ESR (left) scale. Place the capillary tip in the bottom of the tube and gradually withdraw it, while expelling blood, until the 0 mark is reached. Avoid the formation of air bubbles.
3. Place the tube in its rack and read the ESR in millimeters at 15-minute intervals for a total of 60 minutes (or as directed).

Normal:
>   Males—0 to 9 mm. in 1 hour
>   Females—0 to 20 mm. in 1 hour

BACTERIOLOGIC SMEARS

To confirm the presence of bacteria and to obtain information regarding the type of organism present in a particular lesion, the physician may prepare smears, which the assistant stains and examines. The material to be stained may be from a lesion on the outer skin of the body, the eye, ear, nose, throat, or other body openings, natural or accidental.

MATERIALS AND EQUIPMENT
1. Clean glass microscope slides, 1 by 3 in.
2. Sterile cotton applicator-swabs

3. Bunsen or alcohol lamp
4. Gram's-stain solutions
   a. Crystal or gentian violet (primary stain)
   b. Gram's iodine (mordant)
   c. 95% ethyl alcohol or 1:1 mixture of acetone and 95% methyl alcohol
   d. Safranine or dilute fuchsin (counterstain)
5. Staining tray with rack support for slides
6. Microscope, lamp, immersion oil

MAKING THE SMEAR. The physician will swab the area from which he desires a smear. After obtaining the material on the swab, he will either make the smear himself or hand the swab to his assistant, who will proceed to make the smear. The procedure is as follows:

1. Grip a clean glass slide between thumb and forefinger, as illustrated in Fig. 20–21. Grip the applicator end of the swab between thumb and forefinger of the other hand.

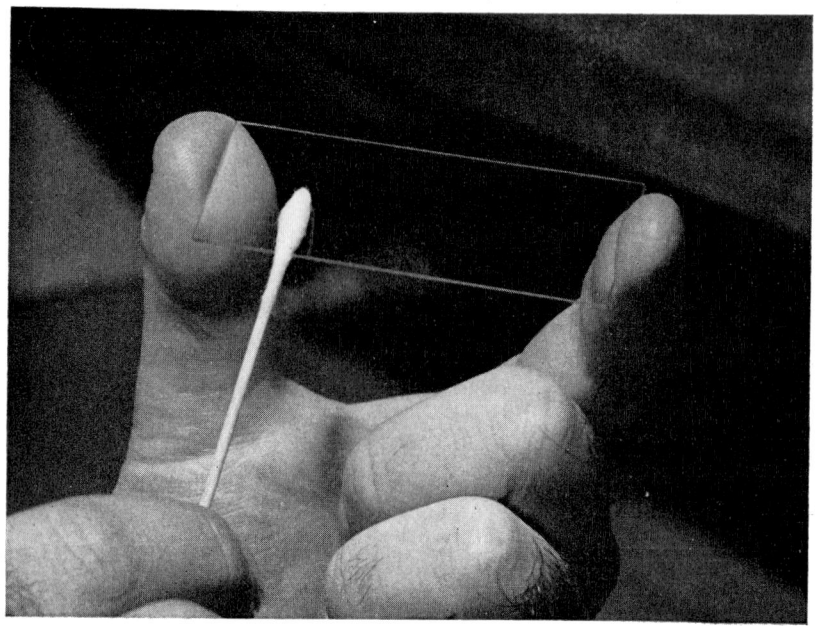

FIG. 20–21. Holding the slide.

LABORATORY TECHNIQUES

2. Place the swab on the surface of the glass slide, about ½ in. from the thumb, so that the swab covers one-half the width of the slide (see illustration).
3. While holding the swab firmly on the slide, roll it towards the forefinger by rotating the applicator end. Stop about ½ in. from the forefinger.
4. Turn the hand holding the slide clockwise. This will bring the clean half of the slide into position for the swab, which is again placed on the slide and rotated along the slide's length (see Fig. 20-22).

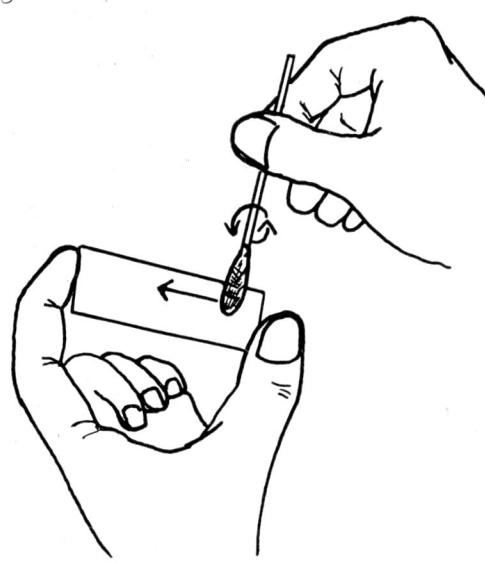

FIG. 20-22. Making the smear.

This procedure is aimed at a transferral of a maximum amount of material from swab to slide with a minimum of disruption and distortion of the elements (tissue cells, blood cells, bacteria) in the process. For instance, if a patient has an infection of the ear caused by streptococci, the physician swabs the lesion and hands you the swab. If you make the smear as described, you will preserve the morphology of the organisms, and when you examine the stained smear you will see cocci in chain formation (streptococci); however, if you just indiscriminately smeared the material on the slide by rubbing the swab over the slide, the end result would probably be quite different. You might see some cocci appearing singly, in pairs, and in groups, and perhaps a few in short chains. You might very easily be at a loss to decide just what type of organism you were looking at. By the same token, tissue and blood cells (red and white) that have been treated with a minimum of manipulation will be easily identified.

5. Allow the smear to dry at room temperature or in a 37°C. incubator. Heat should not be used to speed the drying process, because the heat will cause cell distortion.
6. After the smear is dry, it must be "fixed"; otherwise it will be washed away with the first solution applied. Fixing is accomplished as follows. Hold the slide by the edges of one end between thumb and forefinger, smear side up. Pass the slide through a bunsen or alcohol flame, so that the flame travels along the length of the underside of the slide. This is most easily done by bringing the slide down until the flame hits it close to the fingers and then moving the slide so that the flame travels along its length, always remembering that it is the underside or back of the slide only that is flamed. This should take 1 to 2 seconds and is repeated 3 or 4 times (see Fig. 20-23).

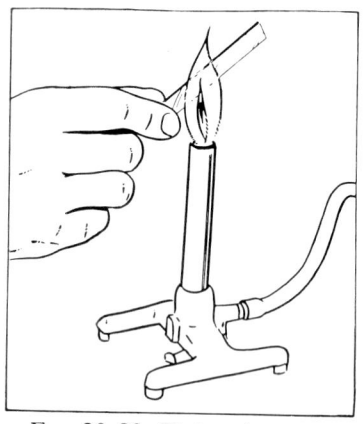

FIG. 20-23. Fixing the smear.

Enough heat must be absorbed by the slide so that when it is placed against the back of the hand, it feels uncomfortably, but tolerably, hot. The object of the fixing procedure is to gel slightly the protoplasm of the cells in the smear and cause them to adhere or become fixed to the slide. Even the minimum amount of heat required to fix a smear will cause some shrinkage and distortion of bacterial and other cells. Excess heat may so distort elements in the smear that the smear is made worthless.

7. Place the slide, smear side up, on a staining rack. In an office

where only an occasional smear is stained, an ashtray across which two applicator sticks have been placed makes a suitable staining tray.

STAINING THE SMEAR (Gram's-stain technique)
1. Cover the smear with crystal or gentian violet. Cover only the smear itself. Do not waste stain by flooding the entire slide. Leave for about 1 minute.
2. Wash the stain off by flooding the smear with water from a beaker or glass.
3. Cover the smear with Gram's iodine. Tilt the slide to allow iodine and water from the washing to run off. Cover again with Gram's iodine. Leave for 1 minute.
4. Wash with water, as above.
5. Decolorize with 95% ethyl alcohol or a 1:1 mixture of 95% methyl alcohol and acetone. This is the critical step in the Gram's-stain procedure. Hold the slide, smear side up, by gripping it with a pair of forceps at one end. Cover it with decolorizer. Tilt the slide to allow the decolorizer to run off. Cover again with decolorizer and tilt; cover and tilt again, always observing the decolorizer as it flows off the slide. When no purple is seen in the washing, immediately wash the smear with water, by either dipping it in water or flooding it from a beaker. The decolorizing should not take more than 10 seconds. Excess decolorizing will render a gram-positive organism gram-negative.
6. Counterstain the smear with safranine or dilute fuchsin for 15 to 30 seconds.
7. Wash by flooding with water.
8. Wipe the *back* of slide and stand it on end to dry in the air. If speed is required, the slide may be gently blotted with a lint-free blotter. This is not recommended, since the smear can be easily rubbed off as long as the slide is wet. When the slide is dry, the smear is fairly permanent.

EXAMINING THE SMEAR. Examine the smear under the oil objective of the microscope. Look for mucus, white blood cells, red blood cells, and bacteria. Use the fine adjustment for detailed study of the bacteria. Be careful to establish the morphology (cocci, bacilli, and spirilla) of the organisms present. Look for groupings:

Cocci—staphylococci (cocci in grapelike clusters); diplococci (cocci in pairs); and streptococci (cocci in chains). Look for details. Are they spherical, lancet-shaped, coffee-bean-shaped? Is there evidence of a capsule (a transparent, envelope-like structure around the bacteria, which does not stain)?

Bacilli—appearing singly, not in any particular grouping, report as such; diplobacilli (bacilli in pairs, end to end); streptobacilli (bacilli in chains). Are they of uniform diameter or do some have thick and thin portions? Are they straight or curved, fine or thick? Do they have rounded, pointed, or squared ends? Are there bands or dark-staining beads (granules) visible? Is there evidence of spore formation or of a capsule?

Spirilla—are there any spiral organisms present? Most spirilla are very difficult to stain, but the borrelia of Vincent's angina (trench mouth) will take a weak gram-negative stain. In the smear, many *Borrelia vincentii* will be seen in each microscopic field, together with a large cigar-shaped gram-negative bacillus, which may have gram-positive bands. Many leukocytes (pus cells) and much mucus will also be seen. Figure 20–24 shows a white blood cell with ingested bacteria. Figure 20–25 shows typical picture in a case of Vincent's angina.

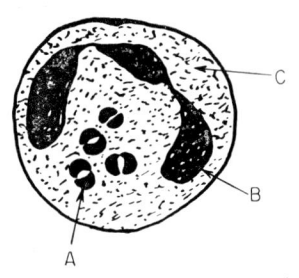

Fig. 20–24. White blood cell with injested bacteria. A, Diplococci; B, cell nucleus; C, cell cytoplasm.

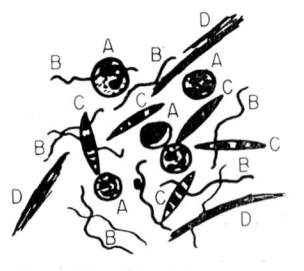

Fig. 20–25. Microorganisms seen in Vincent's angina. A, Leukocytes; B, borrelia; C, fusiform bacilli; D, mucus shreds.

Gram's-stain Reaction. If the bacteria have stained purple to purplish black, they are said to be gram-positive. They have retained the primary stain (crystal or gentian violet) despite the treatment with a decolorizer. If the bacteria have stained red, they are said to be gram-negative. When treated with the decolorizer they gave up the primary dye and then were stained by the counterstain (safranine or dilute fuchsin). A smear made from any given lesion may contain several different species of organism, and some may stain gram-positive; others, gram-negative.

Some gram-positive organisms	Some gram-negative organisms
Staphylococci	Typhoid bacillus
Pneumococci	Dysentery bacillus
Streptococci	Gonococcus
Tubercle bacillus	Whooping cough bacillus
Diphtheria bacillus	Meningococcus

Sample report
Patient's name   Date
Smear from boil on back of neck, stained with Gram's stain.
Results: Many clusters of gram-positive staphylococci seen. Numerous leukocytes and much mucus observed.

Important: The medical office assistant must be aware of the following points:

1. Never identify bacteria by genus and species name on the basis of stained-smear observation alone. Before identification can be made, the organisms must be cultured, and their identification proved. Report only what you see in terms of morphology, grouping, and staining reaction. The physician, on the basis of his experience and examination of the patient, may decide that the gram-negative, coffee-bean-shaped diplococci you saw intracellularly (within white blood cells) are in fact gonococci. He has the right to do so. You do not.

2. Bacteria must be assumed dangerous until proved otherwise; therefore, you must observe all rules for safe handling of con-

taminated articles. The swab that was used for making the smear is considered contaminated. Handle it carefully by the applicator end only. After it is used it must be disinfected by flaming, soaking in a disinfectant (3% Lysol; 5% phenol), or autoclaving before discarding. It is good practice to break the used swab stick by snapping it in two to prevent its reuse. The same applies to tongue blades.

3. Organisms (bacteria) may still be alive after the smear has been fixed.

BIBLIOGRAPHY

Todd, James, Arthur Sanford, and Benjamin Wells: "Clinical Diagnosis by Laboratory Methods," 12th ed., W. B. Saunders Company, Philadelphia, 1953.

21

Special Tests [1]

An important indication of a patient's health is the activity of the thyroid gland, which controls the organism's metabolism. This is determined by means of a test that measures the amount of pure oxygen consumed by a person at complete rest, or the basal metabolic rate, usually abbreviated to B.M.R.

In order to examine the activity of the heart, an electrocardiogram is taken. In this test the impulses of the heart muscles are graphically illustrated by a recording of the electric currents involved. This test is usually referred to as an EKG. The abbreviation originated in Germany, where the test was first developed and was called *Elektrokardiogram*. Organized medicine advocates the use of the abbreviation ECG in this country, and this abbreviation is being increasingly used.

Many doctors who practice a variety of specialties have apparatus in their office for either one or both of these tests, even if they do not have a laboratory. The medical office assistant is expected to perform these tests. This chapter discusses the theory underlying them and gives detailed instruction for handling different types of basal metabolism machines and electrocardiographs. The machines discussed in this section are those manufactured by the Jones Metabolism Equipment Company and the Sanborn Company. The directions given are reproduced from their instruction manuals.

Basal Metabolism Test

The test for the basal metabolic rate (B.M.R.) measures the amount of oxygen consumed by a person at complete rest. The

[1] Based on a manual of medical laboratory techniques by Peter A. Moschetta and Frank O. Waters, Jr.

more oxygen consumed, the more food (fuel) is used up. Inasmuch as the general metabolism, the burning-up process, is controlled largely by the thyroid gland, this test indicates the activity of this gland.

The normal rate is −15 to +15. This means that a person can burn 15 per cent more or 15 per cent less than his calculated norm and still fall within the normal range. A basal metabolic rate of over +15 indicates hyperthyroidism, that is, overactivity of the thyroid gland. Conversely, a figure lower than −15 is indicative of underactivity of the thyroid, called hypothyroidism or myxedema.

The basal metabolism test is a quantitative, not a qualitative, determination, and therefore requires more than ordinary precision in technique. Results with the machine sold under the trademark of Jones Motor-Basal should be within 1 to 4 per cent of the patient's true basal metabolic rate; otherwise the technique is being very crudely performed.

Illustrations that show the technician standing beside the apparatus during the test are misleading. Experienced technicians know that standing at the machine keeps the patient on edge, anticipating what is coming next. The technician should sit at the bedside, just as the doctor does when talking to his patient. Therefore, do not stand or walk about unnecessarily when making the test.

The metabolism room itself should be quiet and closed off from other rooms. The patient should not be made to feel embarrassed, self-consciously aware that he is the center of attention, because embarrassment, fright, worry, or anxiety increase the metabolic rate. A comfortable room temperature should be maintained—neither too warm nor too cool.

The patient is preferably tested in the morning, when all physiologic functions are at low ebb, i.e., near basal. Make certain that the patient has taken no food or drink (especially milk or coffee) for the last 8 hours. Do not withhold water, as this discomfort may increase the metabolic rate. Be sure to ask the patient whether he is taking a sedative or a weight-reducing drug. This point is very often overlooked.

The patient should not be permitted to drowse or sleep during

SPECIAL TESTS 327

the actual test, since this would give a misleading minus or below-basal reading.

Instructions for Operating the Jones Motor-Basal. Figure 21–1 shows a diagram of the Jones Waterless Motor-Basal machine.

PREPARING THE APPARATUS

1. *Tracing sheet.* Adjust tracing sheet on clock plate (1) and insert plate into a slot at front of clock housing (15).
2. *Set pen at air.* Turn three-way valve (breathing valve [31]) parallel to floor, collapse bellows completely, and allow bellows to expand, filling with room air, until pen is at AIR position on tracing sheet. Then turn three-way valve (31) perpendicular to floor to hold bellows fixed in this position.
3. *Oxygen into measuring chamber.* Close needle valve (22) and admit some oxygen into measuring chamber, driving black indicator to about the 20°C. mark on face of pressure gauge (23). (To avoid confusion, remember the difference between the three-way valve and the needle valve.)
4. *Oxygen into bellows.* Open needle valve (22) and admit enough of this unknown quantity of oxygen into bellows to push pen from AIR position to s, M, or L, according to weight of patient. (s—125 lb. or less; M—126 to 174 lb.; L—175 lb. or over.)
5. *Ink pen.* Fill pen (16) with ink and adjust against tracing sheet.
6. *Exact liter into measuring chamber.* Measure off an exact liter of oxygen within measuring chamber by driving black indicator around to position exactly over red temperature indicator on gauge (23).

CONNECTING THE PATIENT. Adjust nosepiece and, after making certain that there is no leakage, insert mouthpiece (10). Ask patient to take one deep breath and then allow breathing to occur naturally.

THE TEST

1. *Start motor blower—take pulse.* Plug in motor blower (7 and 4). Measure patient's pulse.

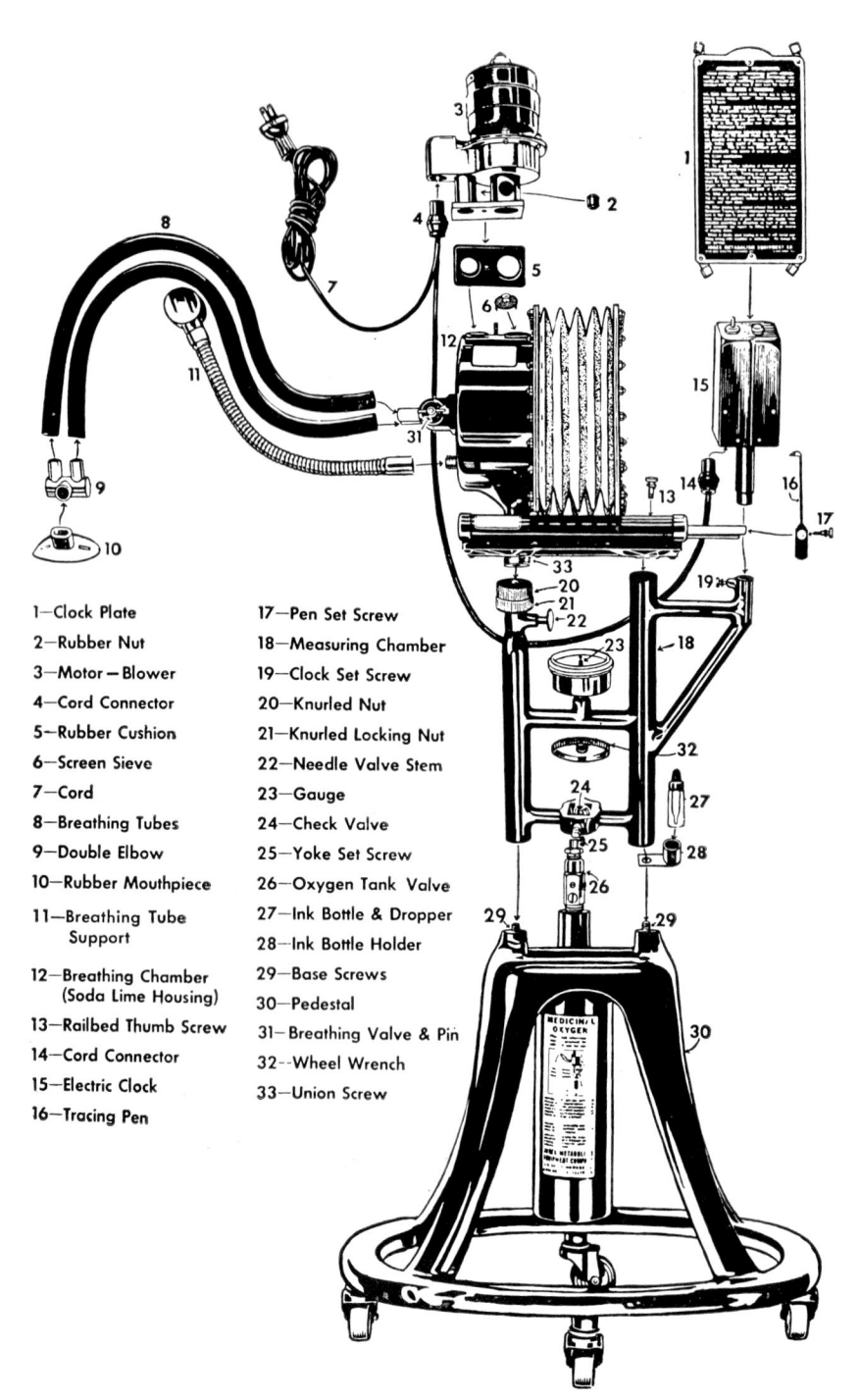

1—Clock Plate
2—Rubber Nut
3—Motor – Blower
4—Cord Connector
5—Rubber Cushion
6—Screen Sieve
7—Cord
8—Breathing Tubes
9—Double Elbow
10—Rubber Mouthpiece
11—Breathing Tube Support
12—Breathing Chamber (Soda Lime Housing)
13—Railbed Thumb Screw
14—Cord Connector
15—Electric Clock
16—Tracing Pen
17—Pen Set Screw
18—Measuring Chamber
19—Clock Set Screw
20—Knurled Nut
21—Knurled Locking Nut
22—Needle Valve Stem
23—Gauge
24—Check Valve
25—Yoke Set Screw
26—Oxygen Tank Valve
27—Ink Bottle & Dropper
28—Ink Bottle Holder
29—Base Screws
30—Pedestal
31—Breathing Valve & Pin
32—Wheel Wrench
33—Union Screw

FIG. 21–1. Diagram of the Jones Waterless Motor-Basal. (*Jones Metabolism Equipment Co.*)

SPECIAL TESTS

2. *Switch breathing into bellows.* At exact end of patient's normal expiration (not forced) turn three-way valve (31) parallel to floor, connecting patient with unknown mixture in bellows.
3. *Start clock.* Start clock (15) to begin tracing.
4. *After A crossing, admit exact liter.* When tracing has definitely crossed within first printed line (see Fig. 21–2) glance at gauge (23) to check liter volume, then open needle valve (22) and admit the exact liter of oxygen to bellows.

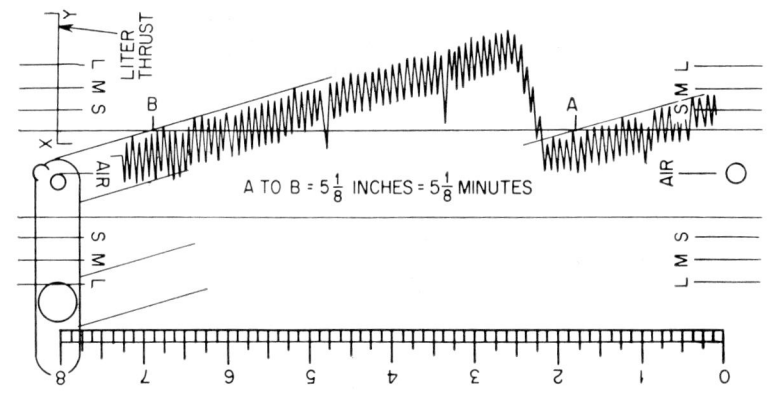

Fig. 21–2. Sample graph of the Jones Waterless Motor-Basal. (*Jones Metabolism Equipment Co.*)

5. *After B crossing, stop test.* When tracing has definitely crossed within first printed line for the second time (see sample graph, Fig. 21–2) the test is over. Pull pen away from sheet, stop clock, stop motor blower, close three-way valve (31), remove mouthpiece, and, after again testing for nose leakage, remove nosepiece. Again, take pulse.

COMPUTING THE RESULTS. With the aid of a protractor, check the tracing and find the time needed to consume an exact liter of oxygen; with the automatic calculator compute the results of the test.

How to determine liter thrust of the pen. The liter-thrust measurement is only made once, to adjust the protractor rules, and is not repeated unless protractor rules are out of adjustment. Do not have the apparatus connected to the patient for this part of the procedure.

1. Measure up liter in usual way.
2. Open breathing valve (31) and pull pen outward until tip is about ¼ in. inside outermost printed base line on tracing sheet; then close breathing valve.
3. Start clock to trace a short line (X—see Fig. 21-2) to mark start of liter thrust.
4. Discharge liter to breathing chamber, making certain black indicator of gauge returns to self-verifying zero mark on gauge dial.
5. Run clock again to trace another line (Y) to mark end of liter thrust. Distance between X and Y is liter-thrust measurement, or expansion of bellows caused by one liter of oxygen, corrected by gauge for variation in temperature, pressure, and aqueous tension.

How to adjust rules of the protractor. To adjust rules or protractor to fit this liter thrust, release the nuts of the short arms of the protractor; set the rules so that the distance from the upper edge of the top rule to the upper edge of the bottom rule is equal to the liter-thrust distance; then tighten the nuts.

How to locate points of crossing of both slopes. Figure 21-2 illustrates the technique for slopes.

1. The upper edge of the upper rule of the protractor should be lined up with the highest regular peaks in the upper graph, in the vicinity of the point of crossing B.
2. At the same time, the short, connecting arms of the protractor must be kept parallel to the ends of the tracing sheet.
3. Also at the same time, the upper edge of the lower rule of the protractor must be lined up with the highest regular peaks in the lower graph, in the vicinity of the point of crossing A.

When the protractor is correctly placed on the tracing, the slope lines are drawn with a sharp-pointed pencil or pen, and the points

SPECIAL TESTS 331

of crossing, A and B, are located at the points where the slope lines *cross* the printed base line—not at point where liter is turned in.

In case the lower rule falls below the tips of the regular peaks, do not draw slope lines to cut off peaks, but push upward on lower rule until it just lines up with tips of peaks, at the same time keeping the upper rule touching the tips of the peaks in the region of B point of crossing. Measure the distance from point A to point B. Record as minutes required to consume 1 liter of oxygen.

Now read off from the automatic calculator (Fig. 21–3) the metabolic rate, according to patient's age, sex, height, and weight

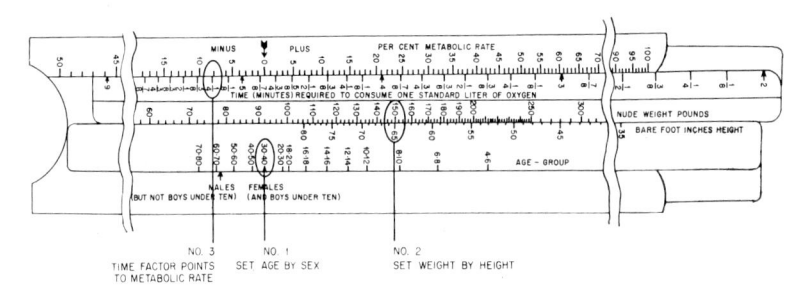

Fig. 21–3. Jones automatic basal metabolism calculator. (*Jones Metabolism Equipment Co.*)

and the time in minutes, as directed by instructions on the back of the automatic calculator, and record all necessary data on the reverse of the tracing sheet.

SPECIMEN TRACINGS. Specimen tracings 1 to 6, Fig. 21–4, illustrate the effects of chance technician errors. Learn to recognize

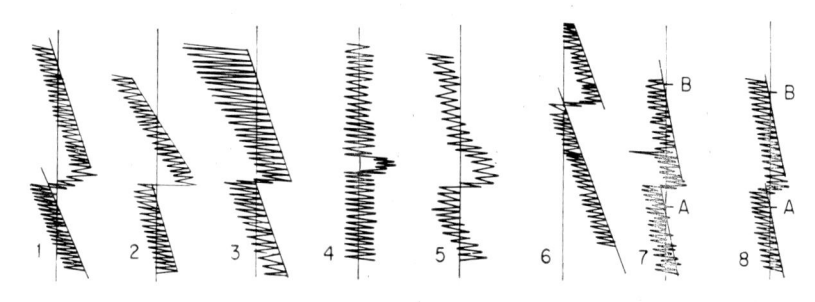

Fig. 21–4. Specimen tracings of the Jones Waterless Motor-Basal. (*Jones Metabolism Equipment Co.*)

and distinguish the unsatisfactory tracing. Do not report an unsatisfactory test. Repeat the test. The following errors can be noted.

1. Indicates one of two errors: either (*a*) patient was not given a moment's preliminary breathing period *into the bellows* before the clock was started; or (*b*) patient had not had sufficient rest (20 to 30 minutes) before the test. The slope lines should be *parallel* to each other.

2. Shows the effect of admitting measured liter of oxygen too abruptly. The sudden hissing noise of escaping oxygen has frightened the patient, thereby causing the metabolic rate to rise. Test will not be accurate.

3. Shows ever-widening depth of respiration, due to failure to change Basal-Lime every 100 tests. Failure of the motor to circulate the air efficiently will cause a tracing of similar appearance.

4. Shows mouth leak or very open nose leak. Patient is breathing room air in and out of faulty nose or mouth connection and is not actually consuming oxygen from the bellows; hence, the vertical tracing.

5. Shows nose leak or slight mouth leak. Note rapid disappearance of liter volume. The curved shape of each slope is characteristic of such leakage.

6. Indicates one of two errors: either (*a*) the bellows was expanded too far at the beginning of the test, and the test, in turn, required much longer than necessary for the first slope to cross the base line and also caused the second slope to extend beyond the tracing sheet; or (*b*) the three-way breathing valve was turned at some time other than at the exact end of an expiration.

Specimen 7 shows correctly drawn slope lines in tracings made by irregular breathers. Place upper protractor edge on the *highest* peaks of the upper graph in the immediate vicinity of the base line (allowing not more than one or two extremely high peaks to pierce this slope line); swing the short arm of the protractor parallel to the short end of the sheet; lower protractor edge should now be lined up with the *highest* peaks in the preliminary or lower graph. Slope lines must be parallel.

SPECIAL TESTS 333

8. Shows results of a test with tracing properly spaced, slope lines properly drawn, nosepiece and mouthpiece adjusted without leakage, patient comfortable and relaxed, test started after a moment's preliminary breathing period into the bellows, and the measured liter admitted just rapidly enough for two or three respirations to occur meanwhile. A is the point where preliminary or lower slope line crosses base line; B is the point where the upper or "liter" slope line crosses base line. The distance between them, measured in inches and directly converted into minutes, represents the time needed by the patient to consume 1 standard liter of oxygen, under exact basal conditions.

Instructions for Operating the Sanborn Metabulator. Figure 21–5 shows a Sanborn Metabulator. Figure 21–6 gives a diagrammatic view of the mechanics of a Sanborn Metabulator. The patient

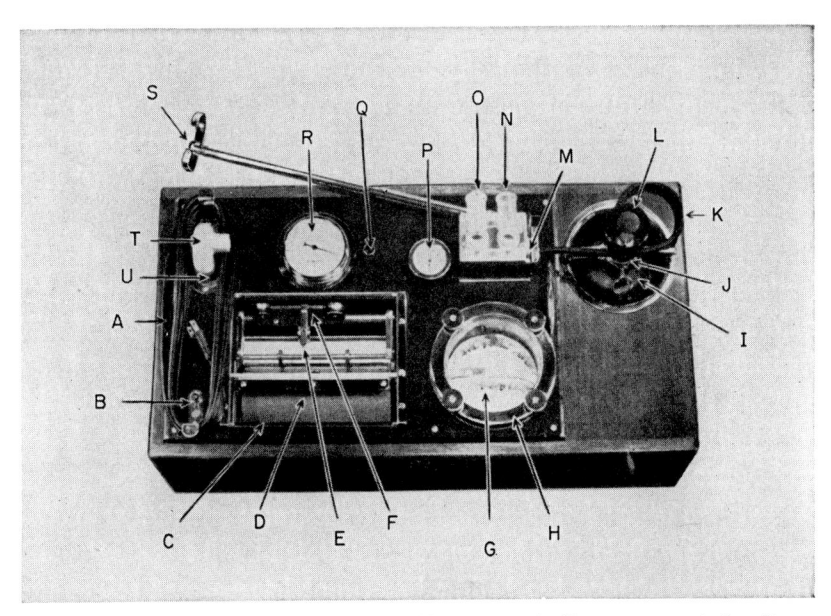

FIG. 21–5. Sanborn Metabulator. A, Power cord; B, motor switch; C, recording compartment; D, roll of recording paper; E, writing stylus; F, bellows carriage; G, Metabolime; H, CO_2 absorption chamber; I, oxygen tank; J, yoke; K, oxygen tube; L, handwheel on oxygen valve; M, breathing valve; N, exhalation outlet; O, inhalation outlet; P, thermometer; Q, pilot light; R, barometer; S, adjustable arm; T, mouthpiece connector; U, breathing tube. (*Sanborn Co.*)

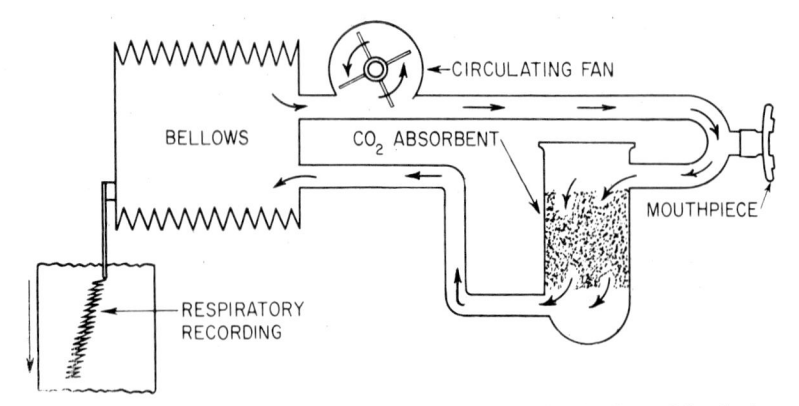

Fig. 21–6. Diagrammatic view of the mechanics of the Sanborn Metabulator. (*Sanborn Co.*)

breathes into a closed circuit in which the air is kept circulating constantly by means of a motor blower. At the beginning of the test the operator fills the bellows by adding pure oxygen, so that the circulating "air" that the patient breathes is an atmosphere rich in oxygen. The carbon dioxide that he produces is extracted from the stream of exhaled air as it passes through the Metabolime chamber, Metabolime being CO_2-absorbent. As the test proceeds, the patient gradually uses up the oxygen in the system, and the bellows slowly shrinks. From the amount of shrinkage during a given time the operator can determine the volume of oxygen per minute that the patient is consuming, and from this figure the basal metabolic rate can be calculated.

PREPARING THE APPARATUS

1. Plug the power cord (A) into the a-c outlet.
2. Place the chromium-plated leak tester in a glass of cold water and allow it to remain there until ready for use.
3. Place a sterilized rubber mouthpiece on the mouthpiece connector (T).
4. Lift the U-shaped, metal mouthpiece connector (T), carrying its long breathing tubes (U) out of the receptacle. Wet the tubes and attach them to the exhalation outlet (N) and the inhalation outlet (O).

SPECIAL TESTS 335

5. Open up the Plexiglas window over the writing stylus (E).
6. Turn the breathing valve (M) to the TEST position, thus connecting the bellows with outside air, and then collapse the bellows by pushing the bellows carriage (F) toward the absorption chamber (H) as far as it will go. If this is not done the patient may become cyanotic and may even faint toward the end of the test. With the bellows in this position, turn the breathing valve (M) back to FILL, thus closing off the bellows.
7. Admit oxygen by carefully turning the handle (L) on the oxygen tank (I) to the left. Continue filling until the writing stylus (E) is about an inch from the top of the paper; then close the valve on the oxygen tank by turning it to the right. The instrument is now ready for the test.

CONNECTING THE PATIENT (see Fig. 21–7)

1. Spread the nose clip and insert it over the nose near the bridge; slide it downward parallel to the patient's face until the pads are against the soft sides of the nostrils (alae nasi). The nose clip should be tight enough so that the patient can

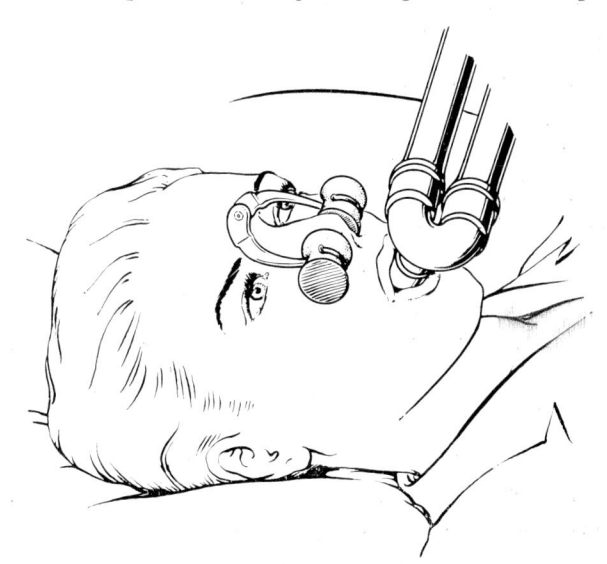

FIG. 21–7. Connecting the patient with the Sanborn Metabulator. (*Sanborn Co.*)

no longer exhale through his nose. Make sure of this by asking him to close his mouth and try breathing out.
2. Adjust the position of the tester and its flexible arms until the rubber mouthpiece is just in front of the patient's mouth, with its long axis pointing across his face.
3. Insert the mouthpiece so that the two small projections lie between the upper and lower teeth and the flange of the mouthpiece lies between the lips and the teeth. Make sure that the lips are not folded under, as this may permit leakage. Pull the lips outward over the flange if necessary.

THE TEST (see Fig. 21-5)
1. Record the temperature on the dial thermometer (P) and the barometric pressure (R). Tap the barometer gently before making the reading.
2. When the patient is breathing room air comfortably, start the record by turning on the motor switch (B). This starts the motor blower and the paper-drive mechanism and turns on the pilot light (Q). The stylus should now be tracing a horizontal line near the top of the record.
3. Observe the breathing of the patient at his diaphragm. At the end of an expiration, flip the breathing valve (M) to the TEST position.
4. Take the leak tester out of the glass of cold water, wipe it dry, and hold it under the nose and at the corners of the mouth, while watching for condensation on the polished surface of the metal. *Do not proceed unless all leaks have been eliminated.*
5. a. Run the test *not less than 6 minutes* and preferably 8 or 10 minutes, unless the bellows become collapsed earlier.
   b. If a duplicate test is desired, turn the breathing valve (M) to the FILL position at the end of the first test, readmit oxygen from the tank as before, and when the bellows has been adequately filled close the valve on the tank and return the breathing valve (M) to the TEST position. If the patient shows any signs of discomfort or reluctance at

SPECIAL TESTS 337

the end of the first test, however, remove the mouthpiece and nose clip and give him a rest before making a second test.
6. When the tests have been completed, throw the breathing valve (M) to the FILL position and disconnect the patient.
7. Pull carefully on the protruding paper (D) in order to bring the remainder of the record out of the machine (release the upper lid of the recording compartment if it is difficult to pull the record out); then bend the paper sharply back over the barometer dial (R) and tear off the protruding portion of paper.
8. Turn the motor switch (B) off.
9. Write the date and the patient's name, height, weight, age, and sex on the record; record the temperature and barometer readings.

COMPUTING THE RESULTS. *Measurement.* Draw a slope line through the top peaks of the record (see A and B, Fig. 21-8, showing some examples of respiration records). The slope line can be drawn through the top, bottom, or middle of the record, as long as it represents the average downward trend. The operator will have to exercise some judgment in deciding what represents the average slope. If the tracing is very irregular, as in Fig. 21-8 (C), it is useless to attempt the placing of any slope line, and the test must be repeated.

Metabulator Scale. A measuring device (Fig. 21-9) will enable the operator to read the oxygen consumption in STP (standard temperature and pressure) cubic centimeters per minute, directly from the record. The device consists of a horizontal bar carrying two slides, each with a vertical hairline lying over a correction scale. One of these scales is for temperature, and the other for barometric pressure. Adjust the sliders so that the hairlines mark the temperature and barometer readings taken during the test. Note that each slider also carries a *horizontal* hairline, lying a little above the upper edge of the long arm of the L. The line on the right-hand slider has a vertical hairline crossing it, and the

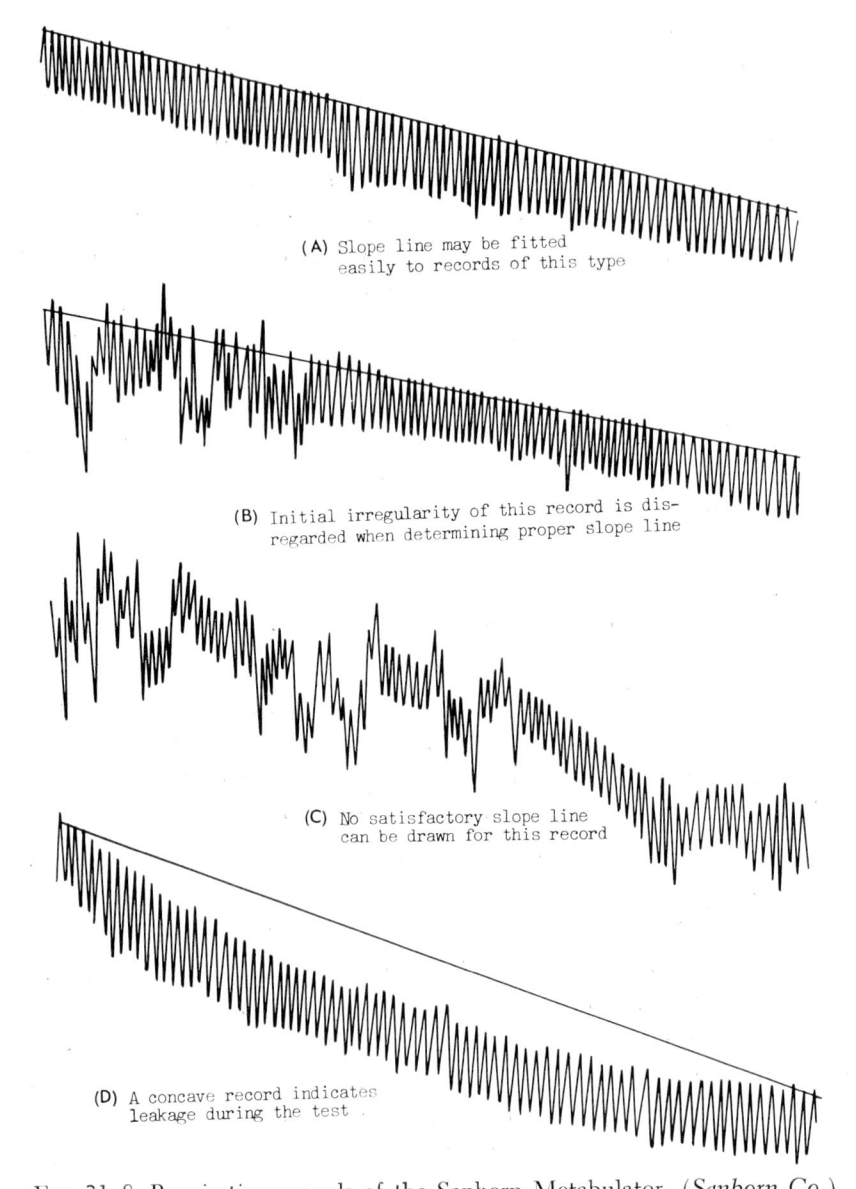

(A) Slope line may be fitted easily to records of this type

(B) Initial irregularity of this record is disregarded when determining proper slope line

(C) No satisfactory slope line can be drawn for this record

(D) A concave record indicates leakage during the test

FIG. 21-8. Respiration records of the Sanborn Metabulator. (*Sanborn Co.*)

SPECIAL TESTS 339

Metabulator scale is to be applied to the respiratory tracing in such a manner that the intersection of these two hairlines on the slider lies exactly over the intersection of the previously drawn slope line and one or other of the horizontal lines printed on the record. When this has been done, adjust the leveling of the L until the horizontal hairline on the *left-hand* slider also coincides with the horizontal line you have chosen. Check the position of the intersection on the right-hand slider again, to be sure that it has not moved, and then read the oxygen consumption directly at the point where the slope line strikes the right-hand margin of the vertical arm of the L. The reading on this latter scale is the patient's oxygen consumption in cubic centimeters per minute, reduced to standard temperature and pressure (STP). Transfer this reading to the record.

Basal Metabolic Rate. To convert the figure for oxygen consumption into a B.M.R., thus indicating to the doctor by how many percentage points the patient's oxygen consumption differs from normal, hold the slide-rule calculator in a good light, directly in front of the eyes, and follow these directions:

1. Adjust the hairline to *oxygen consumption* (corrected to STP).
2. Shift slider to bring *height* under hairline.
3. Reset hairline to actual present *age*, male or female.
4. Move slide to bring *weight* under hairline.
5. Read the basal metabolic rate over B.M.R. arrow.
6. Record the reading on the patient's record.

The Jones Air-Basal Metabolism Unit. An entirely new type of machine for measuring the basal metabolic rate was brought out a few years ago by the Jones Metabolism Equipment Company. This machine does not require special oxygen tanks but utilizes the oxygen in the air. It does away with pressure chamber, valves, oxygen cartridges, barometer, thermometer, and calculations of any kind. The time factor is measured directly on the tracing sheet, and this factor determines the basal metabolic rate, thus reducing the procedure to a few steps.

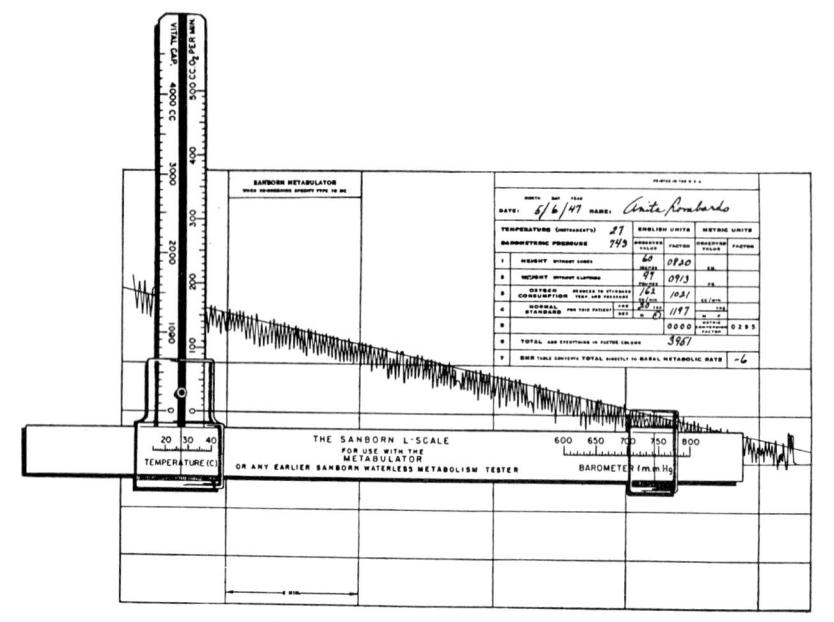

Fig. 21-9. Calculation of the basal metabolic rate with the Sanborn Metabulator. (*Sanborn Co.*)

At present, the majority of physicians are still using the older type of machine, but more and more doctors are acquiring the Air-Basal. A technician who has operated the older machines would have no difficulty in understanding the directions that come with this new machine, which is simpler to operate. Figure 21-10 shows an Air-Basal unit.

Electrocardiography

The assistant will have a better understanding of the significance of the electrocardiogram if she is familiar with the anatomy of the heart. Sketches are therefore shown in Figs. 21-11 and 21-12.

The electrocardiogram, referred to as EKG or ECG, is a graphic representation of the varying body electric currents produced by the heart during the process of contraction. The *electrocardiograph* is an instrument for recording these electrical changes. When the cardiac muscle contracts, the active part becomes electronegative to the inactive part, and an electromotive force is produced, with

SPECIAL TESTS 341

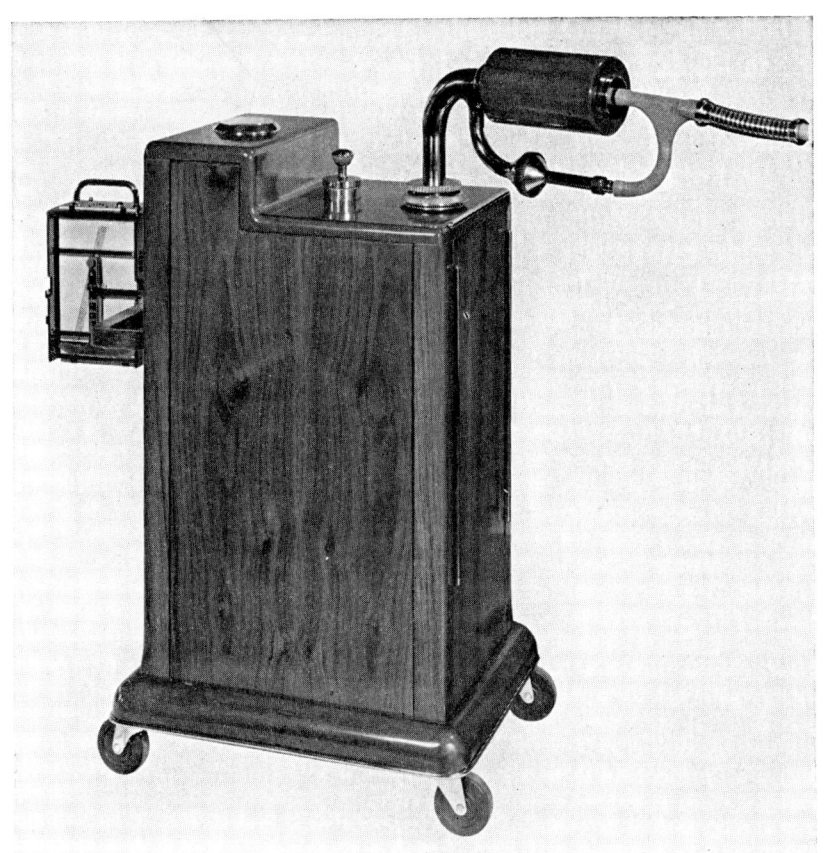

Fig. 21-10. Jones Air-Basal metabolism unit. (*Jones Metabolism Equipment Co.*)

positive and negative potential differences. The electrical potential is led off by the application of electrodes to the patient and then recorded.

A cardiograph record, the electrocardiogram, is composed of a series or pattern of deflections or waves, which are constantly repeated. These waves or deflections are designated by the letters P, Q, R, S, T, and U. Of these, the P, R, and T waves are fundamental and practically always used in the interpretation of the record; the others, Q, S, and U (which are often not present), though important, are used less frequently.

The waves are produced by, and represent, the minute electrical

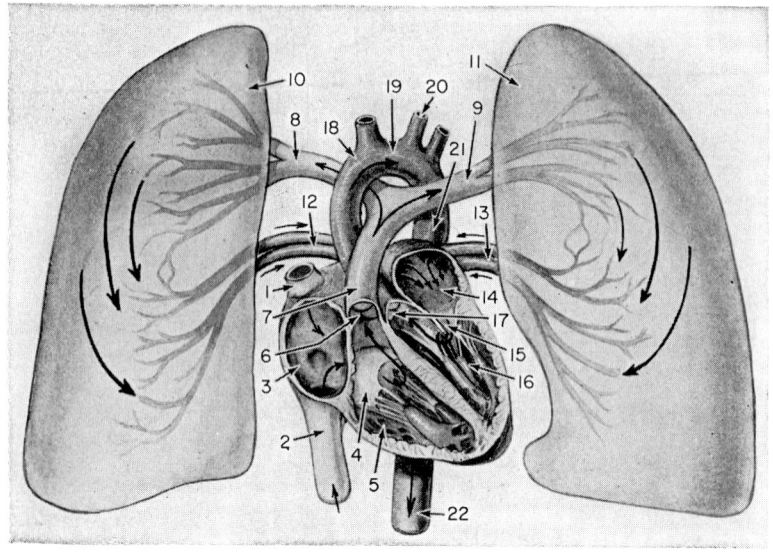

1. Vena cava superior
2. Vena cava inferior
3. Right auricle
4. Tricuspid valve
5. Right ventricle
6. Pulmonary semilunar valve
7. Pulmonary a.
8. Pulmonary a., right
9. Pulmonary a., left
10. Right lung
11. Left lung
12. Pulmonary v., right
13. Pulmonary v., left
14. Left auricle
15. Bicuspid (mitral) valve
16. Left ventricle
17. Aortic semilunar valve
18. Ascending aorta
19. Arch of aorta
20. Left common carotid a.
21. Descending aorta (thoracic)
22. Descending aorta (abdominal)

FIG. 21-11. Anatomy of the heart. (*From Blakiston's New Gould Medical Dictionary*, 2d ed., McGraw-Hill Book Company, Inc., Blakiston Division, New York, 1956.)

voltages generated by the muscular actions of the heart. Ordinarily, the potentials are fractions of a millivolt, and because they are so small, they must be magnified or amplified so that their variations may be readily seen when converted into a permanent graph or record.

The successive contractions of auricles and ventricles are due to the passage of an excitation process, which occurs slightly in advance of each contraction. This impulse starts normally in the sinoauricular (S.A.) node, the "pacemaker." The initial deflection, the *P wave* of the electrocardiogram, is produced by the passage of this impulse through the auricles. From the auricles, the impulse passes to the ventricles by way of the auriculoventricular (A.V.)

SPECIAL TESTS   343

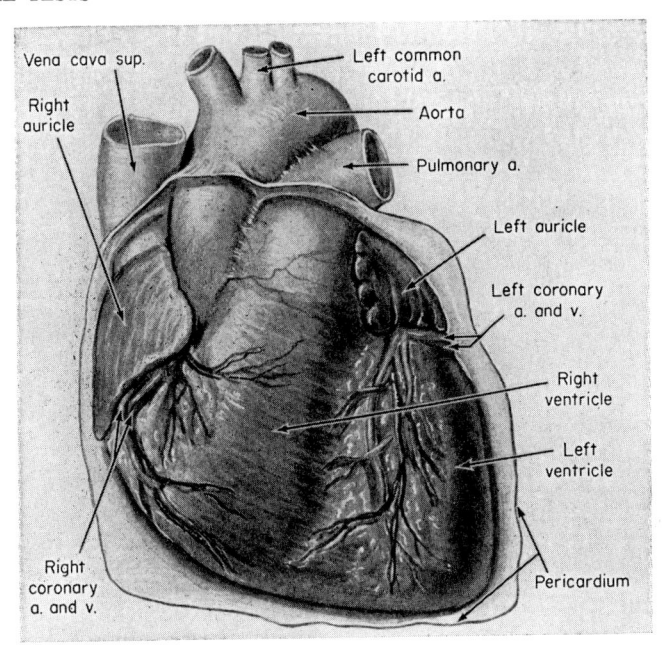

FIG. 21-12. Anterior view of the heart. (*From Blakiston's New Gould Medical Dictionary*, 2d ed., McGraw-Hill Book Company, Inc., Blakiston Division, New York, 1956.)

node, spreading down the bundle of His through its right and left branches to invade the ventricular muscle. This is registered by the *QRS complex*. Normally, the R wave is the most prominent, and the Q and S waves are very small or missing altogether. The final deflection, the *T wave*, occurs as the ventricular excitation subsides. Normally, it is upright in leads 1, 2, 4, and usually in 3. The *U wave* is seen occasionally after the T wave. Its origin is still debatable.

In the following pages the technique of taking electrocardiograms is described with instruments manufactured by the Sanborn Company and the Beck-Lee Corporation. The specific directions given in each case are taken from the instruction manual that accompanies each machine.

Figure 21-13 illustrates the usual direction of electrical currents from the heart when lead 1 is being recorded. Beginning at the left shoulder, the currents pass down the left arm, through the lead wires, through the electrocardiograph, through the right arm and shoulder, and back through the chest to the left shoulder; thus, a complete circuit is made, and the varying phases of each heartbeat are transmitted.

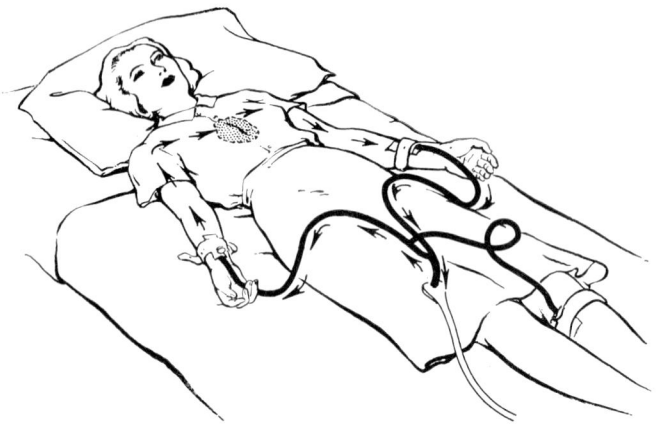

FIG. 21-13. Flow of current. (*Sanborn Co.*)

Figure 21-14 illustrates the position of the heart in relation to the points where the electrodes are attached for the limb leads. This arrangement closely parallels the shape of the heart itself,

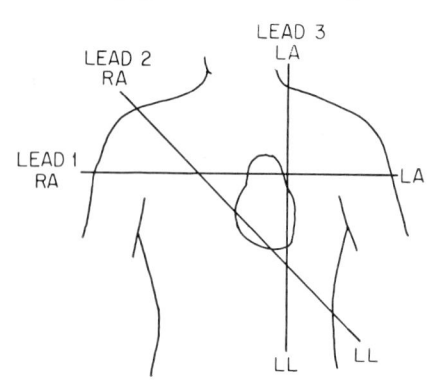

FIG. 21-14. Position of the heart. (*Sanborn Co.*)

which, roughly speaking, takes the form of an inverted triangle within the body.

Figure 21-15 shows the correlation of the EKG with the cardiac cycle.

SPECIAL TESTS 345

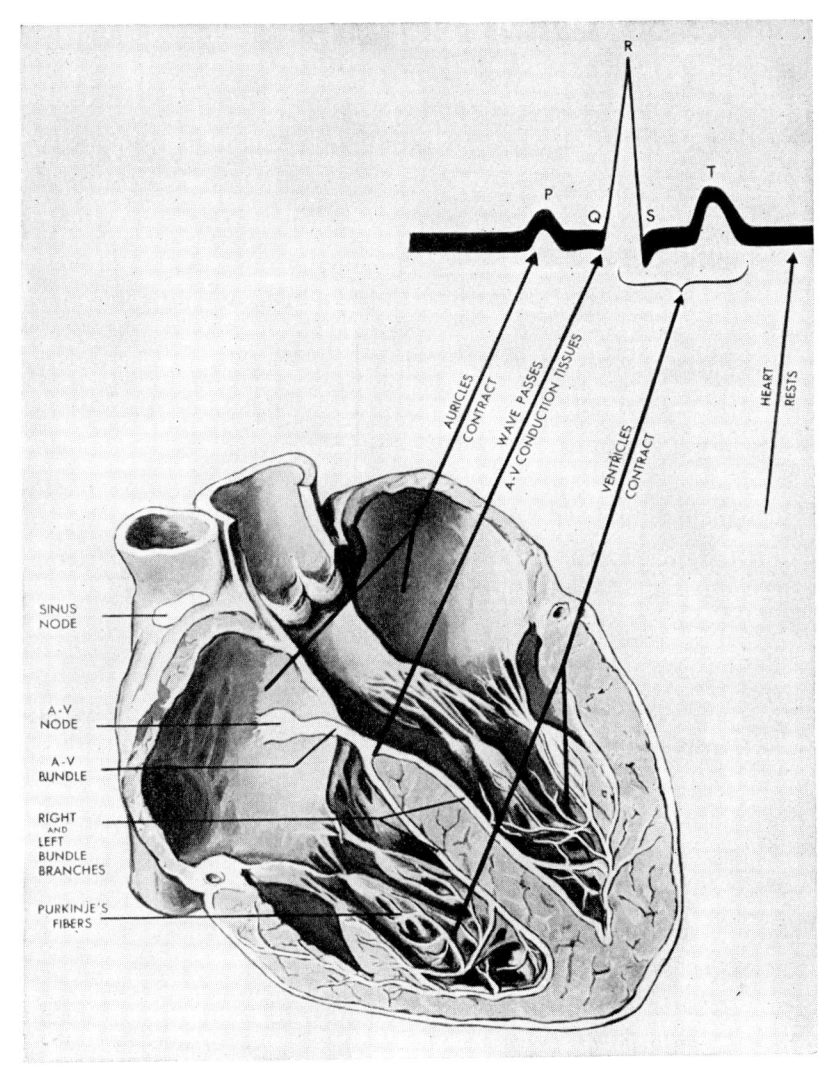

Fig. 21-15. Correlation of the EKG with the cardiac cycle. (*Merck Sharp & Dohme Research Laboratories*)

When the patient is being prepared for an electrocardiogram, it is essential that he be comfortable and completely relaxed. If the patient is chilled, overheated, or ill at ease mentally, the cardiogram will be affected. The patient should not be allowed to talk or move about while the cardiograph is in operation.

Application of the Electrodes. Expose the patient's forearms and the lower portions of the legs. If the precordial leads are to be taken, the chest should also be exposed.

Squeeze about ½ in. of jelly onto the inside, fleshy portion of the right forearm. Using a piece of gauze (not cotton) or a tongue depressor, rub the jelly into the skin until a slight, but definite, reddening of the skin develops. The reddening of the skin indicates that the blood vessels have dilated enough to provide the proper electrical conduction.

Now, attach one end of the strap to one of the rectangular electrodes by slipping the contact post of the electrode through one of the holes near the end of the strap. Squeeze about ½ in. of jelly onto the center of the electrode and place it directly over the reddened area. Fasten it in place by drawing the strap around the arm and slipping the proper hole over the contact post. A tight strap will not provide a better contact; tighten straps just enough to prevent electrodes from moving or slipping.

The left-arm electrode is applied in exactly the same manner as the right-arm electrode. The left- and right-leg electrodes are placed on the inside, fleshy portions of the legs or near the calf. Good contact is essential.

Since there are several locations for application of the chest electrode, the operator must be careful to locate the exact desired position. The physician will determine which chest position or positions to take. Figure 21–16 shows how to locate positions for chest leads.

Important: Care must be taken not to spread the jelly from one position to another.

The recommended positions for precordial or chest leads are:

Lead V_1—The chest electrode is placed in the fourth intercostal space just to the right of the sternum.
Lead V_2—The chest electrode is placed in the fourth intercostal space just to the left of the sternum.
Lead V_3—The chest electrode is placed midway between the positions of leads V_2 and V_4.

SPECIAL TESTS

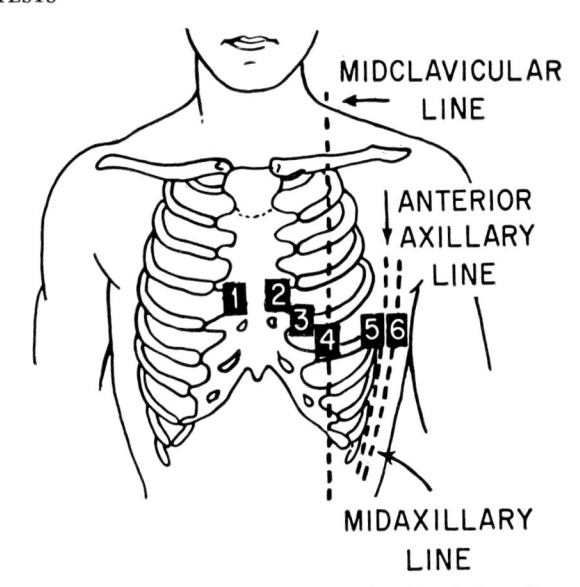

Fig. 21-16. Positions of chest leads. (*Beck-Lee Corp.*)

Lead V_4—The chest electrode is placed on the fifth left intercostal space at the mid-clavicular line.

Lead V_5—The chest electrode is placed on the left anterior axillary line at the level of lead V_4.

Lead V_6—The chest electrode is placed on the left mid-axillary line at the level of V_4.

Electrocardiograph Lead Circuits. The internal wiring of the lead-selector switch automatically combines the potentials of the contacts to be used in any particular lead. These leads have been given certain designations, which, by convention, always indicate certain electrode combinations.

Limb leads:
    Lead 1—right arm and left arm
    Lead 2—right arm and left leg
    Lead 3—left arm and left leg
Precordial leads:
    Lead CR—chest and right arm
    Lead CL—chest and left arm
    Lead CF—chest and left leg

Unipolar leads (exploring electrode listed first and indifferent electrode last):

Lead AVR—right arm and central terminal consisting of combined potentials of the left leg and left arm

Lead AVL—left arm and central terminal consisting of combined potentials of the left leg and right arm

Lead AVF—left leg and central terminal consisting of combined potentials of the right and left arm

Lead V—chest and central terminal consisting of the combined potentials of the right arm, left arm, and left leg, each through equal resistances of 5,000 ohms

Beck-Lee Electrocardiograph (string galvanometer). The principle upon which the Beck-Lee electrocardiograph is built may be observed in the simplified diagram shown in Fig. 21-17. The cardiac current is taken from any two standard points on the patient's body and carried directly to the ends of the gold-plated quartz

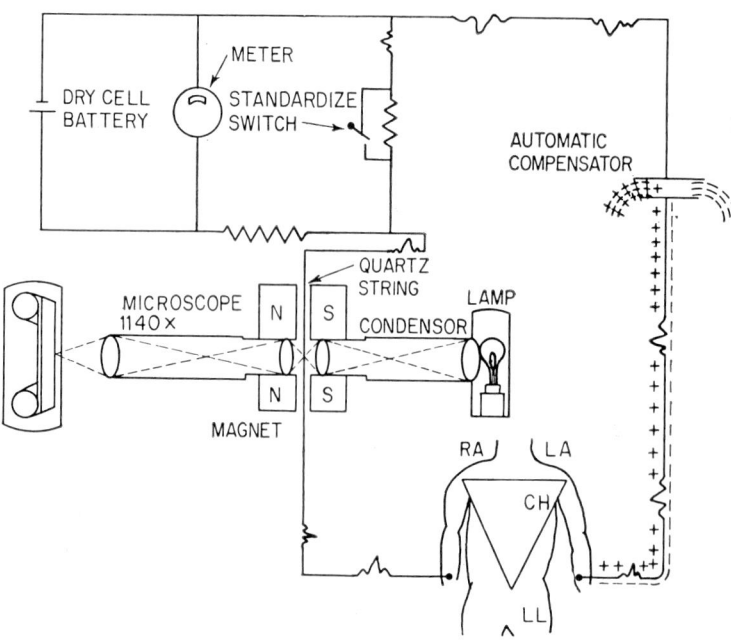

FIG. 21-17. Beck-Lee (string galvanometer) electrocardiograph. (*Beck-Lee Corp.*)

SPECIAL TESTS

string in the Einthoven galvanometer. The changes of the heart current in the circuit thus formed cause the string to move in the magnetic field between the two pole faces of the permanent magnet in the galvanometer.

If a source of light is placed behind and focused on the string, it will cast a moving shadow. Since the string is only 0.00006 in. in diameter, the shadow must be magnified. This is accomplished by an achromatic microscope of 1140X.

The magnified shadow is then cast upon the photographic paper, which is moved in the camera by a constant-speed electric motor. For the purpose of measuring the resulting graph, horizontal lines 1 mm. apart and vertical lines at intervals of 1/25 of a second are simultaneously photographed on the graph.

It will be observed that *no current other than that produced by the heart is involved*. The electricity taken from the wall socket is only employed for the lamp, the film drive, and the independent timing mechanism.

In order that the cardiogram may be compared with a standard, the instrument must be *standardized before each lead is taken*. This standardization is accomplished by passing a current of exactly 1 mv. through the string. On the Beck-Lee instrument, the accuracy of this current is verified by a meter on the control panel.

The tension of the string is then set so that this standardization current causes the string to deflect exactly 1 cm. on the viewing screen. The recording of this important standardization on the graph is illustrated in Fig. 21-18. The control panel is shown in Fig. 21-19.

CALIBRATION (see Figs. 21-20 and 21-21)
1. Turn on the light switch, observing the viewing screen (8). The string shadow will be apparent and will be approximately at the zero line. If the string shadow is not at zero, bring to zero position by turning string-centering knob (4). The flickering observed is due to the time wheel intercepting the light beam.

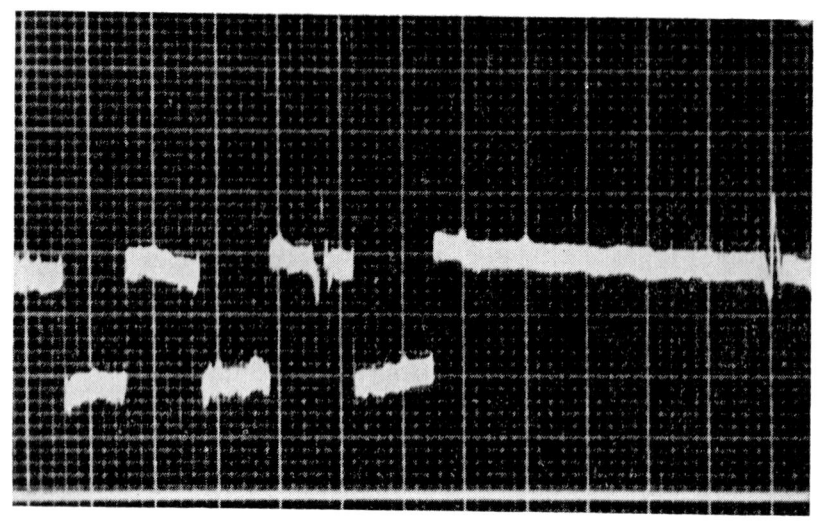

FIG. 21-18. Standardization with the Beck-Lee galvanometer. (*Beck-Lee Corp.*)

2. Turn the lead switch to TEST position. The needle of the meter (3) should now appear at the red line. In the event that the needle of the meter does not appear at the red line when the lead switch is in TEST position, unscrew the inner-compartment knob (21) in the back compartment. An adjustment knob will be found, which should be turned to the point where the needle appears on the red line. If, with this adjustment, it is impossible to bring the needle to the red

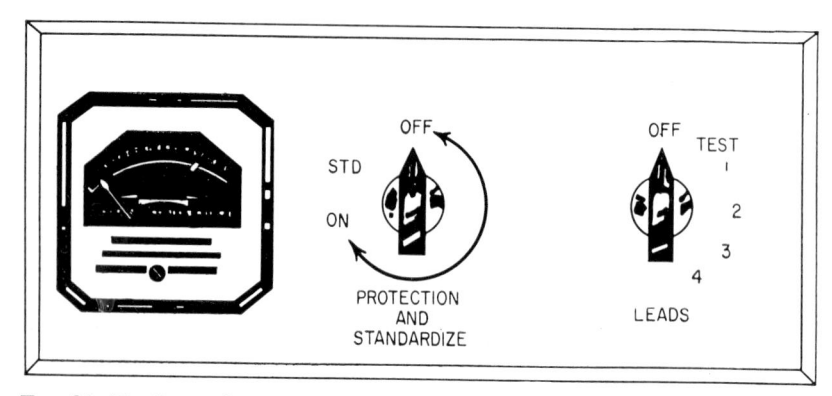

FIG. 21-19. Control panel of the Beck-Lee galvanometer. (*Beck-Lee Corp.*)

SPECIAL TESTS 351

line, the flashlight cell should be replaced with a new one. Screw inner cover back in place and proceed.
3. With the lead switch in TEST position, turn the protection-standardize switch from OFF position around to ON position. From ON position flip the switch to the standardize (STD) position and release, noting on the viewing screen the amount of deflection of the string shadow. Loosen string-tension control knob (2) by turning to the left a slight amount, while measuring the deflection of the string again by flipping the standardize switch. Continue this procedure cautiously until a deflection of 1 cm. is obtained. One centimeter is indicated on the viewing screen by the first long line, marked 1.
4. Return the protection-standardize switch to the OFF position.

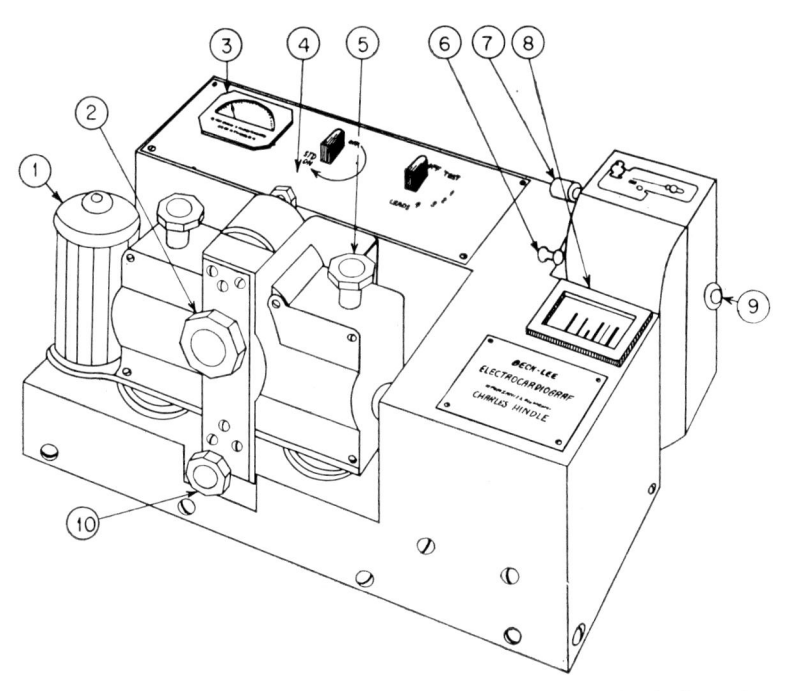

FIG. 21–20. Front view of the Beck-Lee electrocardiograph. *1*, Lamphouse cover; *2*, string-tension control knob; *3*, current meter; *4*, string-centering knob; *5*, microscope-adjustment knob; *6*, camera switch; *7*, camera-locking stud; *8*, viewing screen; *9*, camera-revolution indicator; *10*, carrier-locking knob. (*Beck-Lee Corp.*)

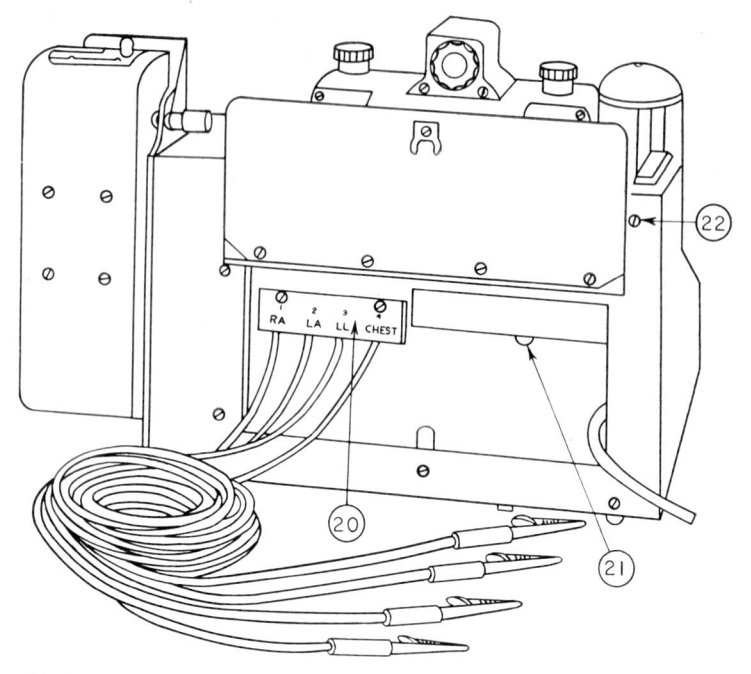

FIG. 21 21. Back view of the Beck-Lee electrocardiograph. 20, Lead-cable indicator; 21, inner-compartment knob; 22, ground post. (*Beck-Lee Corp.*)

TAKING LEAD 1

1. Turn lead switch to position 1.
2. Turn the protection-standardize switch from the OFF position, bringing it around slowly; observe the string shadow and its position to the zero line. If the string shadow deviates greatly (more than ½ cm.) from zero, return the protection-standardize switch to the OFF position. Now bring it to the ON position more slowly, to allow the automatic compensator to take hold.
3. Flip the protection-standardize switch from ON position to STD and release, noting the deflection. If the deflection (not necessarily from the zero line, but simply the total deflection) is 1 cm. or greater, it is indicated that the electrode applications are well made and the skin resistance is 2,000 ohms or less. If a deflection of 1 cm. cannot be obtained, return the protection-standardize switch to the OFF position leaving the

SPECIAL TESTS 353

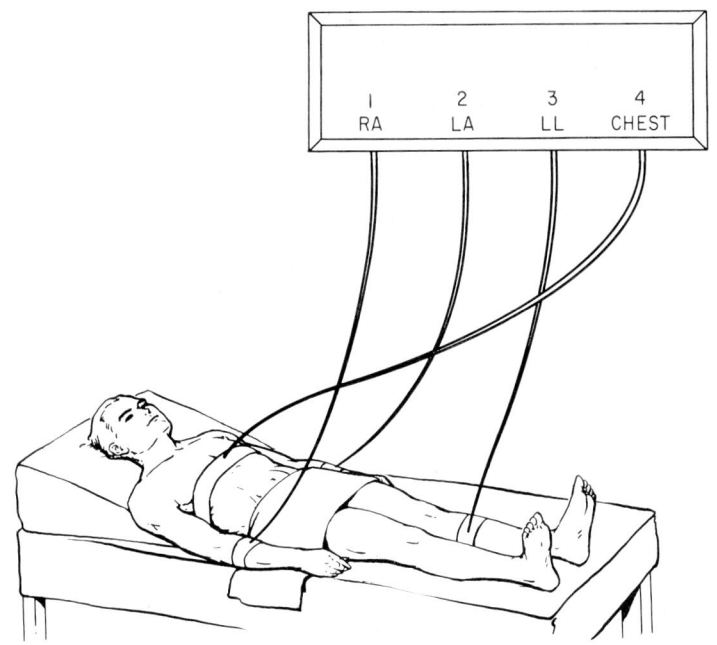

FIG. 21–22. Lead connections of the Beck-Lee galvanometer. (*Beck-Lee Corp.*)

other parts of the instrument as they are. Then reapply the electrodes. After reapplying the electrodes, bring the protection-standardize switch slowly around from OFF position to ON position. If the string shadow wanders from side to side on the viewing screen, turn the protection-standardize switch to OFF position and allow the patient to relax further. Then, when relaxation has been accomplished, bring the protection-standardize switch around slowly to ON position.

4. Flip protection-standardize switch to STD to check for 1 cm. of standardization. If string shadow is not deflected exactly one centimeter, rotate string-tension control knob (2), tightening or loosening the string until 1 cm. of deflection is obtained.
5. Return protection-standardize switch to OFF position.
6. Rotate microscope-adjustment knob (5) to focus the string shadow on the viewing screen to the darkest and sharpest image possible.

7. Bring the protection-standardize switch slowly around to ON position. We are now ready to take the graph.
8. Turn camera switch (6) on. Flip protection-standardize switch to STD *once*. Shut off camera after approximately 8 seconds.
9. Return protection-standardize switch to OFF position. Be sure this is done.

TAKING LEAD 2

1. Turn lead switch to position 2.
2. Flip protection-standardize switch to STD to determine if 1 cm. of standardization is obtained on the screen. Loosen or tighten string-tension control knob (2) until exactly 1 cm. of deflection is observed on the viewing screen.
3. Return protection-standardize switch to OFF position.
4. Focus string shadow with microscope-adjustment knob (5).
5. Return protection-standardize switch to ON position slowly.
6. Turn camera switch (6) on. Flip protection-standardize switch to STD *twice*. Shut off camera after approximately 8 seconds.
7. Return protection-standardize switch to OFF position. Be sure this is done.

TAKING LEAD 3

1. Turn lead switch to position 3.
2. Do steps 2 to 5, as in taking lead 2.
3. Turn camera switch on. Flip protection-standardize switch to STD *three times*. Shut off camera after approximately 8 seconds.
4. Return protection-standardize switch to OFF position. Be sure this is done.

TAKING LEAD 4

1. Turn lead switch to position 4.
2. Do steps 2 to 5, as in taking lead 2.
3. Turn camera switch (6) on. Flip protection-standardize

SPECIAL TESTS

switch to STD *four times*. Shut off camera after approximately 8 seconds.
4. Return protection-standardize switch to OFF position. Be sure this is done.
5. Turn string-tension control knob (2) to the right to tighten string. Turn to STOP position, but do not force. Be sure this is done each time a cardiogram is completed. Turn lead switch to OFF position. Turn off light switch.

DEVELOPING THE CARDIOGRAM
1. Remove camera from the electrocardiograph and take camera into darkroom.
2. Open the camera and remove exposed film. To do this, raise up the slotted take-up spool and slip off the exposed portion of the film. Draw a few inches of film through the cross bar and tear off. Rethread the unexposed portion of the film. Close the camera and lay it aside in a safe place.
3. Place film in developer. The time the film should remain in the developer will vary from 1 to 4 minutes, depending upon the temperature and age of the developer and the number of graphs already passed through it. If a great number of graphs have been passed through the developer in a short time, it will take longer for the following graphs to develop than if the developer had been used fewer times. The density or darkness of the background can be determined by viewing the graph under the red (safe) light from time to time.
4. After it has been determined that the background is of the desired degree of blackness, remove the film from the developer and place it in the water for approximately ½ minute.
5. Remove the film from water and place it in hypo or fixer. It should remain in the hypo for approximately twice the length of time it was in the developer, assuming the fixer is reasonably fresh (if mixed according to directions, approximately four weeks old).
6. Remove film from hypo or fixer and allow it to rinse in clear

water for approximately the length of time it remained in the fixer.
7. Remove film from water and allow it to dry in the air, making sure that the emulsion side is not touched by any other object.

The entire developing process should normally take less than 5 minutes. The chemicals will last longer if covered when not in use.

LOADING THE CAMERA (Fig. 21–23). To remove camera, loosen camera-locking stud and lift camera up and out of the instrument. Take camera into darkroom for loading.

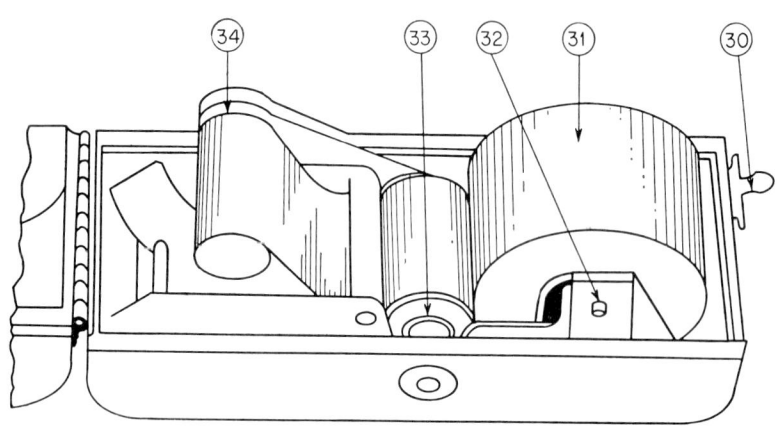

FIG. 21–23. Loading the camera of the Beck-Lee galvanometer. (*Beck-Lee Corp.*)

To load camera, open by sliding knob (30). Remove wooden spool (31) by spreading spring holders (32). Place film on this spool and replace film and spool by spreading spring holders, making certain that the spool is securely held by both holders. The film should be placed so that it unrolls from underneath, with the emulsion side up.

Pass the film over the rubber roller (33) and *under the bar*. Raise up the slotted take-up spool (34) and insert film in the slot. Rotate take-up spool one or two revolutions, so that the emulsion side of the film is on the *outside*. Push down take-up spool and

SPECIAL TESTS

close and lock the cover of the camera. In replacing the camera on the electrocardiograph, the small stud on the side of the camera near the bottom should be inserted into the slotted receptacle on the side of the camera mount. The camera-locking stud is then tightened until the camera is secure.

Cardi-all. This direct-writing instrument is shown in Fig. 21–24.

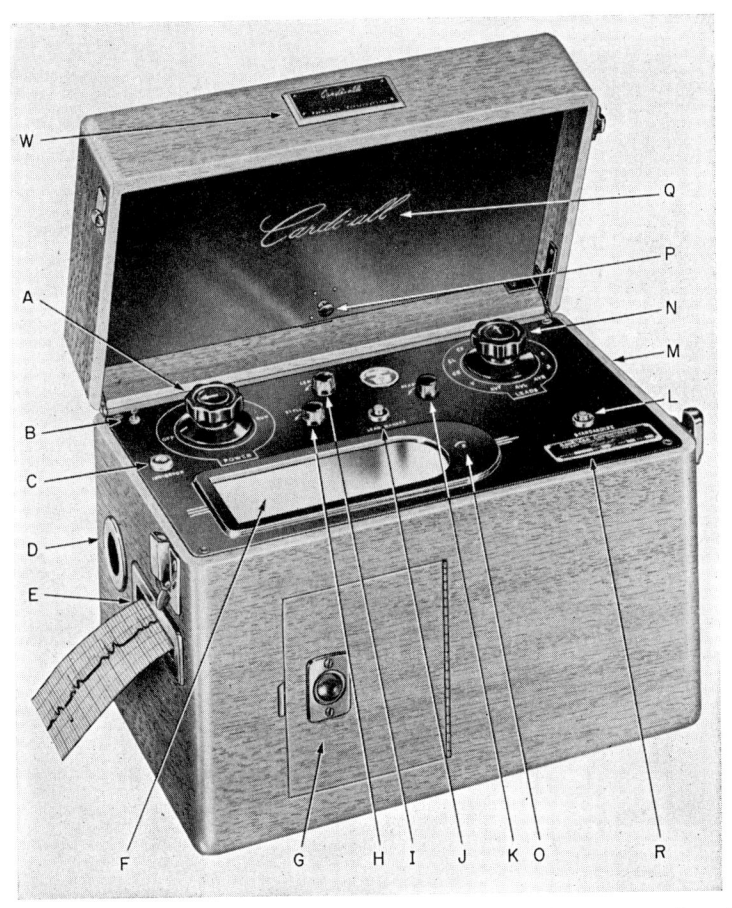

FIG. 21–24. Cardi-all direct-writing instrument. A, Power-control switch; B, grounding post; C, ground indicator; D, line-cord receptacle; E, paper-exit slot; F, record-viewing window; G, paper-loading door; H, stylus-heat control; I, stylus-centering control; J, lead-marker button; K, sensitivity control; L, standardization button; M, lead-cable receptacle; N, lead-selector switch; O, window lock; P, compartment-door knob; Q, accessory compartment; R, serial-number plate; W, window plate. (*Beck-Lee Corp.*)

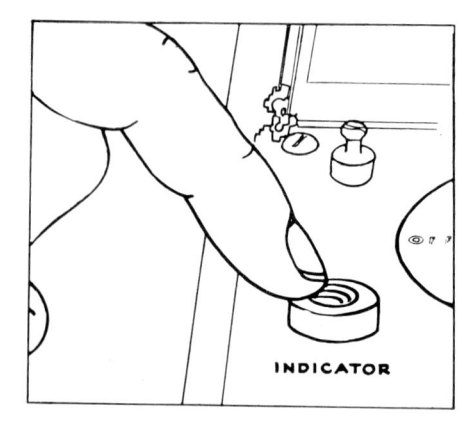

Fig. 21-25. Ground indicator on the Cardi-all. (*Beck-Lee Corp.*)

PREPARING THE APPARATUS

1. Insert the line cord (D) so that the ground indicator lamp (C) does not glow when only the ground indicator ring is touched. (See Fig. 21-25.)
2. Turn the power-control switch (A) to ON and allow 2 full minutes for warm-up. This time should be utilized to prepare the patient.

CONNECTING THE PATIENT

1. Connect the four limb leads to the patient.
2. Connect the four tips of the lead cable to the electrodes, according to their markings.

THE TEST

1. Bring the stylus to the center of the record with the centering control (I). Turn the lead-selector switch (N) to lead No. 1 and the power-control switch (A) to RUN. Adjust the stylus heat (H) to proper operating temperature (width of one small division).
2. With power-control switch (A) on RUN, adjust the sensitivity control (K) so that 1-cm. (10 small divisions) deflection is obtained when the standardization button (L) is depressed.

SPECIAL TESTS 359

3. With the power-control switch (A) in the ON position, connect the patient lead cable to the instrument (M).
4. Turn the power-control switch (A) to RUN, depress the standardization button (L), and mark the lead with the lead-marker stylus by depressing the lead-marker button (J). Allow approximately 6 in. of recording paper to run out.
5. Return the power-control switch (A) to ON and turn the lead-selector switch (N) to lead No. 2.
6. Turn the power-control switch (A) to RUN and again standardize and mark the lead. The remainder of the leads are recorded by repeating steps 4 and 5.
7. When the precordial leads are recorded, the power-control switch (A) *must* be in the ON and not RUN position when the electrode is removed from the patient.
8. When all the desired leads are recorded, remove the patient cable from the instrument and turn the power-control switch (A) to OFF.
9. Remove the lead wires from the electrodes and remove the electrodes from the patient. Wash the electrodes and lead tips in warm (not hot) water and wipe dry with a soft cloth.

THE COMPLETED RECORD. Compare your record with Fig. 21–26. Note the even-level base line and the sharpness of the record. Each lead should show the standardization deflection and the lead marking.

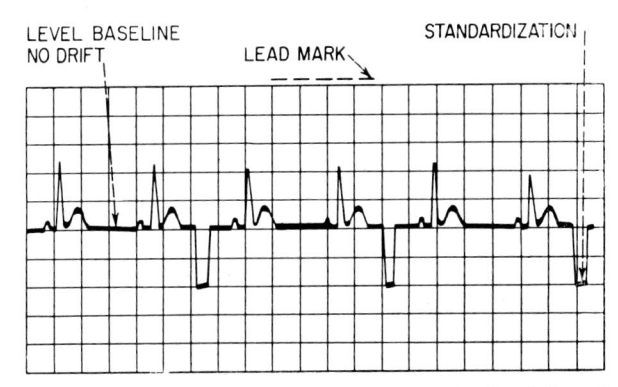

FIG. 21–26. Completed record on the Cardi-all. (*Beck-Lee Corp.*)

CHANGING THE RECORDING PAPER (see Fig. 21-27)
1. Turn the paper-loading lever upward (counterclockwise) as far as it will go. Do not force.
2. Remove the cardboard core of the exhausted roll of paper from the paper roll shaft.
3. Unroll about 8 in. of paper from the new roll. Holding the roll in the right hand, slide it on the paper roll shaft as far as it will go, and at the same time guide the end of the unrolled length of paper with the left hand to left and underside of the silver paper-tension stud and into the paper-loading slot.

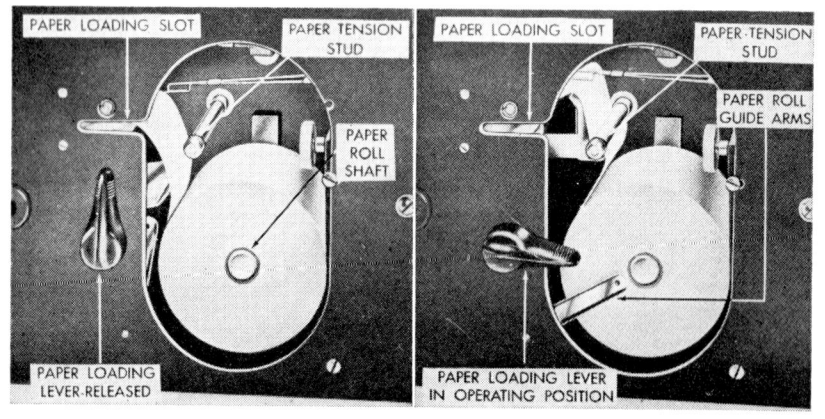

Fig. 21-27. Loading the paper of the Cardi-all. (*Beck-Lee Corp.*)

4. Be sure that the roll of paper is put all the way on the paper roll shaft.
5. Be certain that enough paper has been fed into the paper loading slot so that it extends an inch or two to the left of the paper-drive roller.
6. Release the paper-loading lever by turning downward.
7. Turn power-control switch to RUN and allow a few inches of paper to run out. Make sure the paper passes freely under the tension stud.

Viso-Cardiette. A different type of electrocardiograph is the Viso-Cardiette, shown in Fig. 21-28.

SPECIAL TESTS

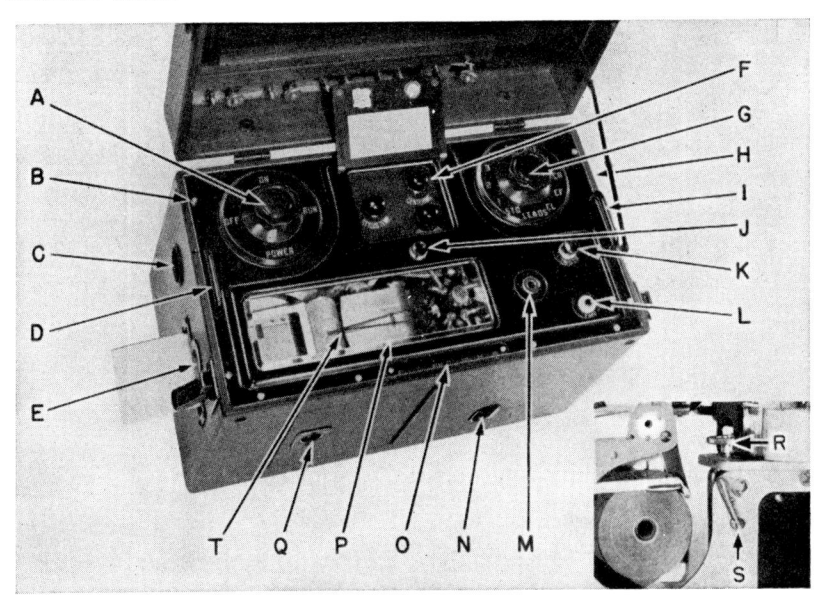

FIG. 21-28. Viso-Cardiette. A, Power switch; B, ground-wire lug; C, power-cord socket; D, lifting handles; E, paper-discharge slot; F, control box; G, lead-selector switch; H, patient-cable socket; I, lifting handles; J, lead-marker button; K, instomatic switch; L, 1-mv button; M, grounding disk; N, independent time marker; O, serial number; P, viewing window; Q, paper-drive door; R, stylus-pressure adjustment; S, galvanometer-lifting lever; T, writing arm. (*Sanborn Co.*)

PREPARING THE APPARATUS. Plug in power cord at C and check proper grounding by touching the grounding disk (M) with the index finger. Be certain that no other part of the body touches the instrument; otherwise this check will be valueless. If the grounding disk glows, rotate the power cord one-half turn. If the instrument is properly grounded the neon lamp in the grounding disk (M) will not glow when touched by the finger. (See Fig. 21-29 for ground indicator.)

CONNECTING THE PATIENT. Turn power switch (A) to ON and prepare the patient (see first part of

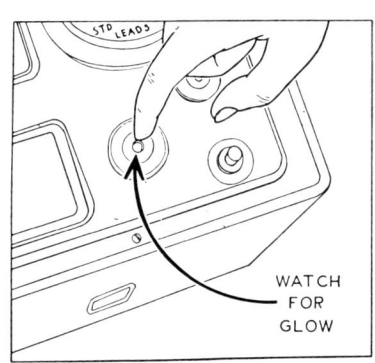

FIG. 21-29. Checking the grounding of the Viso-Cardiette. (*Sanborn Co.*)

this section, Electrocardiography). The lead tips are marked RA for right arm, LA for left arm, RL for right leg, LL for left leg, and C for chest. Connect the tips of the leads to the electrodes and plug the patient cable into its receptacle (H).

THE TEST
1. Turn lead-selector switch (G) to STD.
2. Locate the stylus-temperature control in the control box (F) and turn the power switch (A) to RUN. Lower and raise the stylus temperature (by turning the knob to the left and then to the right) until you reach the point at which the top and bottom edges of the base line on the record become sharply outlined. The width of the line should be no more than one of the smallest boxes.
3. Now adjust the position of the writing arm approximately to center by means of the centering knob in the control box (F).
4. Adjust the sensitivity. Observe the writing arm (T), while the 1 mv button at the right-hand end of control box (F) is being depressed and released rapidly, and adjust the sensitivity control (F) until the deflection sweeps through ten of the small squares (two large squares) on the recording paper. Be sure to measure deflections from one edge of the base line to the same edge of the deflection line. If the vertical portions of the standardizing deflections are not visible, increase the stylus temperature until they are.
5. Turn the power switch (A) to ON. Push the instomatic switch (K) and, holding it in position, turn the lead-selector switch (G) to lead 1. Keep the instomatic switch (K) depressed for a second longer and then release it.
6. Start the record by turning the power switch (A) to RUN.
7. Mark the lead by briefly pressing the lead-marking button (J) once for lead 1, twice for lead 2, and so on.
8. Register the sensitivity of the instrument directly on the record by depressing the 1-mv button (L) briefly between two heartbeats. This calibration of the actual record should

SPECIAL TESTS 363

be repeated in each lead, but the sensitivity control itself should not be disturbed.
9. Allow the record to run for about 8 or 10 seconds, so that you have 8 or 10 in. of record for later examination.
10. Stop the record by turning the power switch (A) from RUN to ON. You are now ready to record lead 2.
11. Push and hold the instomatic switch (K) and turn lead-selector switch (G) to lead 2. Release the switch after a second.
12. Observe writing arm movement. Turn power switch (A) to RUN. Mark the lead. Register the sensitivity (standardize). Run about 8 or 10 in. of the record. Follow this same procedure for lead 3 and, if the physician directs, for the augmented unipolar (AV) limb leads, etc.

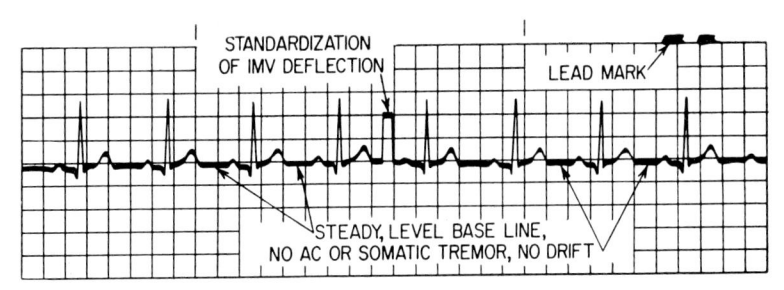

FIG. 21-30. Sample tracing of the Viso-Cardiette. (*Sanborn Co.*)

RECORDING CHEST LEADS AT MULTIPLE LOCATIONS. If the recording of chest leads is to be done from more than one position on the chest wall, some manipulation or shifting of the chest electrode will be necessary. To avoid disturbing the Viso-Cardiette amplifier, thus keeping it ready for immediate recording of each chest-electrode location, and also to protect the stylus ribbon against possible damage while the chest electrode is shifted, the instomatic switch (K) is provided with a protective locking feature.

LEAD MARKING. With the growing multiplicity of leads being recorded, it is suggested that a code system be utilized for marking the various leads.

Example:

> Lead 1—one dash
> Lead 2—two dashes
> Lead 3—three dashes
> Lead AVR—one dash and one dot
> Lead AVL—one dash and two dots
> Lead AVF—one dash and three dots
> Lead V_1—one dot
> Lead V_2—two dots
> etc.

CHANGING RECORDING PAPER. Power switch should be turned off.
1. Open the paper-drive door (Q) in front of cabinet.
2. Open galvanometer viewing window (P) by pressing from below through paper-drive door or by turning knob at end.
3. Swing galvanometer tilt handle (A, Fig. 21-31) one-half turn counterclockwise.
4. Raise tension plate by pressing up on thumb latch (B). Continue pressing up firmly until you hear, and see, the black roller-guide plate (C, Fig. 21-31) snap up.
5. Remove remaining paper (while still pressing up on thumb latch) by (a) turning the roll counterclockwise, to bring unrolled paper back onto the roll; and (b) sliding out.
6. Grasp new roll of paper in hand so roll unwinds when turned in clockwise direction.
7. Lift tension plate (B, Fig. 21-31) and slide paper roll onto spindle, pushing against the spring as far as the roll will go. Release tension plate and check that tension-plate apron is at outside of the roll, not riding on the roll. Now turn roll

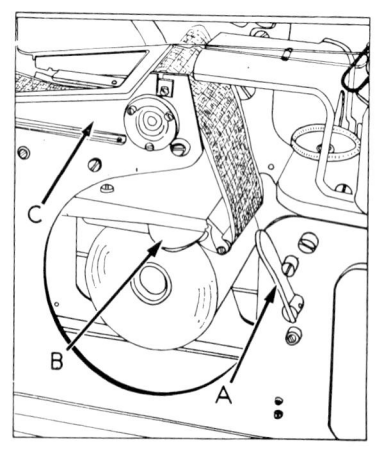

FIG. 21-31. Loading the paper of the Viso-Cardiette. (*Sanborn Co.*)

SPECIAL TESTS 365

clockwise so that an inch or two of the paper with unprinted side up projects beyond tension plate toward galvanometer magnets (Fig. 21–32).
8. With left hand, rotate roll of paper on spindle clockwise, while guiding end of paper up and over horizontal writing platen (Fig. 21–33) with the right hand.
9. With the left hand (working from the top, through the open viewing window) place the edge of paper underneath the roller-guide plate, which is in the raised position (Fig. 21–33).

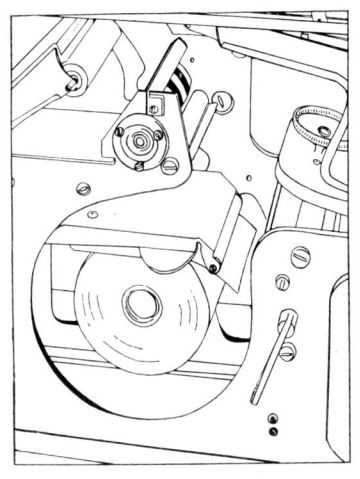

FIG. 21–32. Loading the paper of the Viso-Cardiette. (*Sanborn Co.*)

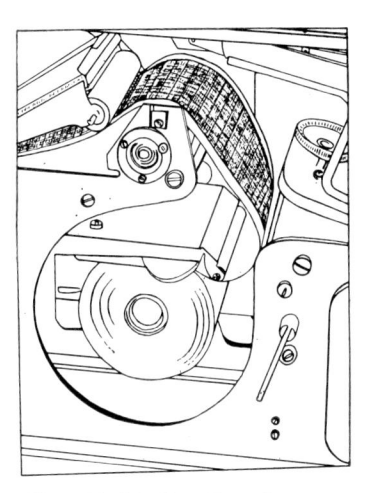

FIG. 21–33. Loading the paper of the Viso-Cardiette. (*Sanborn Co.*)

10. Inspect the paper throughout its exposed length to make sure it is smooth and even.
11. Press the roller-guide bar firmly down until it snaps into position.
12. Turn power switch to ON.
13. While paper is moving, press and hold forefinger against the roll of paper to take up slack. This *must* be done if proper operation is to be obtained. Use fingers also, if needed, to guide paper through and out the discharge slot.

The paper should now feed through smoothly and evenly. If it does not, repeat steps as necessary.
14. Rotate galvanometer tilting handle clockwise one-half turn.
15. Close viewing window.

APPENDIX

Medical Terminology

Knowledge of medical terminology is a requisite for the medical assistant. If her duties include taking dictation of medical histories, she must know not only how to write medical terms in shorthand but also how to spell these terms—in any case she needs enough familiarity with the terminology to enable her to find a term in a medical dictionary. Even if the assistant does not take dictation, she should know what the doctor means when he uses a medical term or what a certain term means when she comes across it in the medical literature. The doctor will certainly expect his assistant to know the meanings of the most comon terms and abbreviations, especially those of his own specialty.

COMMON ABBREVIATIONS

āā equal parts of each
a.c. before meals
ad lib. at will
alt. dieb alternate days
alt. hor. alternate hours
b.i.d. twice a day
B.M.R. basal metabolic rate
C. centigrade
cc. cubic centimeter
coq. boil
d.d. let it be given to
dil. dilute
div. divide
dr. dram (drachm), drams (drachms)
d.t.d. give of such a dose
EEG electroencephalogram
EKG electrocardiogram
extr. extract
F. Fahrenheit
fl. fluid
fl.oz. fluidounce
f.pil. let pills be made
fract.dos. in divided doses
ft. let there be made
ft. pulv. let a powder be made
Gm. gram, grams
gr. grain, grains
gt. drop
gtt. drops
I.Q. intelligence quotient

min. minim, the sixtieth part of a fluidram, a drop
mm. millimeter
N.A.D. no appreciable disease
noct. at night
N.P.N. nonprotein nitrogen
N.Y.D. not yet diagnosed
O.D. right eye
O.L. left eye
o.m. every morning
o.n. every night
O.S. left eye
ov. ovum
oz. ounce
p.a. in equal parts
p.c. after food; after meals
q.d. four times a day
q.h. every hour
q.2h every second hour
q.3h. every third hour
q.i.d. four times a day
q.s. as much as is sufficient
℞ take
S. or Sig. give the following directions
stat. immediately
syr. syrup
t.i.d. three times a day
tr. tincture
W.r. Wassermann reaction

ANALYSIS OF MEDICAL TERMINOLOGY

Nonmedical persons are often appalled by the formidable and specialized vocabulary used by the medical profession to describe illnesses and operations. A study of the medical vocabulary, however, will show that it is made up largely of many variations of prefixes or suffixes and word elements. The actual number of words or parts of words that the medical assistant should know, therefore, is not so great as one would expect.

The prefixes, suffixes, and word elements and their meanings should be studied diligently, for with a little practice in analyzing the component parts of medical terms, the assistant will soon learn to figure out their meanings. For example, the word **gastrostomy**, meaning an opening into the stomach, is a combination of the word elements *gastro-*, stomach, and *-stomy*, opening; **atypical**, meaning not typical, is readily understandable when the assistant knows that it is made by adding the prefix *a-*, meaning not, to *typical*, a common word in her vocabulary. Some other examples of how words are made and their literal meanings are:

gastrectomy (*gastr-* + *-ectomy*), surgical removal of the stomach
tonsillitis (*tonsil* + *-itis*), inflammation of a tonsil
neuritis (*neur-* + *-itis*), inflammation of a nerve
hyperesthesia (*hyper-* + *esthesia*), increased sensation
anesthesiology (*an-* + *esthesio-* + *-logy*), the study of loss of sensation
hypoacidity (*hypo-* + *acidity*), decreased acidity

Commonly Used Prefixes, Suffixes, and Word Elements

In the following list the position of the hyphen with the word element indicates the more common form; but it should be remembered that a word element may be used before or after another word element or as the word which carries the meaning when it is used with a prefix or a suffix.

For euphony, a vowel or a consonant may be added or dropped between the elements of a word.

a- without, not
ab- from away
ad- to, toward
adeno- gland, glandular
aesthesio- sensation, perception
-al characterized by
-algia pain
ambi- both
amphi-, amph- on both sides, around
an- not, without
ana- up, back, again
andro-, andr- man, male
ante- before
antero- front
anti- against
-ase enzyme
auto- self
bi-, bis- twice, double
bili- bile
bio- life
blast- germ cell
brachy- short

brady- slow
cata- down, lower, under
-cele swelling, tumor
cephal-, cephalo- head
chromo- color
-cide causing death
circum- around, about
co-, com-, con- together, with
-coele, -cele chamber, ventricle
contra- against, counter
-cyst bladder, bag
-cyte cell
dacryo-, dacry- tears, lacrimal apparatus
dactylo-, dactyl- finger
de- down, from
dextro- to the right
di- double, twice
dia- through, apart
diplo- double, twin
dis- apart, away from
dorsi-, dorso- to the back, back
dys- difficult, painful

e- out of, from
ec- out of
ecto- outside
-ectomy surgical removal of
-emia blood
-en in, into
endo- within
entero- intestine
ento- within, inner
epi- upon
erythro- red
esthesio-, aesthesio- sensation, perception
ex-, exo- outside, out of
extra- outside of, beyond
-fuge driving away
gastro-, gastr- stomach
-genetic, -genic producing, origin
-genous kind
glyco- sugar
-gram tracing, picture
-graph instrument for recording
gyno-, gyn- woman, female
hemi- half
hemo-, haemo-, hem-, hemato- blood
hepato- liver
hetero- other, unlike
homo- same, like
hyper- over, increased
hypo- under, decreased
hystero- uterus
-iasis condition of
-ic, -ical pertaining to
in- into
in- not
infra- below, beneath
inter- between, among
intra- within, into
intro- into
-itis inflammation
juxta- near, nearby
-kinesis, -kinetic motion
latero- side
leuko-, leuco white
levo- to the left
lith- stone, calculus
-logy study of, science of
-lysis setting free
macro- large
mal- bad
-malacia softening
mega-, megalo- large
melano- black
meso- middle
meta- beyond, change
-meter measure
micro- small
mono- one, single

multi- many, much
myo- muscle
neo- new
neuro-, neur- nerve, nervous system
ob- against
-odynia pain
-oid like, resembling
olig-, oligo- few, less than normal
-oma tumor
opistho- backward
ortho- normal, straight
-osis condition, state, process
-ous full of
pan- all, every
para- apart from, beside, next to
patho- disease
-pathy, -pathia disease of, feeling
-penia lack
per- through
peri- around
-phage consuming
-plastic molded
-plegia paralysis
pleuro- side, rib
pluri- more, several
poly- many
post- after
pre- before
pro- in front of
proto- first
pseudo- false
pyo- pus
pyro- fever, fire
quadri- four
re- back, again
retro- backward, back of
-rrhagia sudden flow
-rraphy suture of
-rrhea flow
-scopy inspection or examination of
semi- half
steno- contracted, narrow
stereo- firm, solid
-stomy opening
sub- less, under
super- above, excessive
supra- above, upon
sym-, syn- with, together
tendo-, teno- tendon
-tomy incision of, cut
trans- across, through
tri- three
-trophy nutrition
-tropy a turning
ultra- beyond, excess
-uria urine
ventro- to the front, abdomen

369

VOCABULARY OF MEDICAL TERMS

The following vocabulary lists are arranged according to medical specialties to help the student familiarize herself with the terms she is most likely to encounter in her particular position. Obviously such an arrangement must be arbitrary, as many terms might be included under several headings, and practically all terms belong to the field of general medicine. In order to avoid needless duplication, very few general medical words are repeated. The General Medicine list and the list of prefixes, suffixes, and word elements should therefore be used for terms not found in specialty lists.

There are acceptable variant spellings for many medical terms, and it is well for the assistant to be able to recognize them. Some of these variant spellings appear in the lists, but preferred spellings are used in the text.

Capitalization likewise may vary; for example, trademarked drug names and terms derived from proper nouns are sometimes capitalized.

The definitions are as simple as seems consistent with clarity. Details and technical elaborations are omitted, since the object is to give the reader only a general idea of the meaning of each term, not to teach her medicine.

Pronunciation is shown with most words, because it may be unfamiliar to the student. Many medical terms are anglicized derivatives from Greek and Latin, so pronunciation may vary. Since there is no one authority for pronunciation, only that most generally used is shown. The pronunciation and syllabication here may differ from that shown in some dictionaries.

To indicate pronunciation, words are respelled within parentheses. The general rule is: a vowel at the end of an accented syllable is long; a vowel within an accented syllable ending in a consonant is short; and a vowel standing alone in a syllable is usually long. The long *i* is always marked ī. A long mark (¯) or a short mark (˘) is used over a vowel when it is an exception to the general rule.

The symbol ~ is used to indicate that the entry word is to be repeated.

General Medicine

abdomen (ab-do′men), the part of the body between the chest and the pelvis.
abduct (ab-dukt′), to draw away from the middle line.
aberration (ab-er-a′shun), deviation from the usual or normal course.
abiosis (ab-e-o′sis), without life.
ablution (ab-lu′shun), a washing or cleansing.
abrasion (ab-ra′zhun), a rubbing or scraping off of the skin.
abrasive, something that causes an abrasion.
absorption, the process of assimilating by suction or chemical action.
accretion (ak-re′shun), accumulation.
acetabulum (as-et-ab′u-lum), a cup-shaped cavity in the hip bone.
acetonuria (as-et-o-nu′re-ah), excretion of acetone in the urine.

acetylcholine (as-et-il-ko′lēn), a substance produced in the body.
Achilles tendon (ak-il′ēz), the tendon attached to the heel bone.
acidity, the state of being acid.
acidosis, decrease of the normal alkalinity of the blood.
acromion (ak-ro′me-on), the end of the spine of the shoulder blade.
ACTH (adrenocorticotropic hormone), a hormone used as remedy in various conditions.
acute, (1) showing severe symptoms and a rapid development. (2) sharp.
adduct (ad-ukt′), to draw toward the middle line.
adenitis (ad-en-i′tis), inflammation of a gland.
adenopathy (ad-en-op′ath-e), any disorder of a gland.

adrenal (ad-re'nal), (1) near the kidney. (2) a gland on the upper part of the kidney.
adrenalin (ad-ren'al-in), an extract from the adrenal gland.
agranulocytosis (ag-ran-u-lo-sī-to'sis), reduction in the number of granular leukocytes.
albumin (al-bu'min), a protein.
albuminuria (al-bu-min-u're-ah), presence of albumin in the urine.
alimentary (al-im-en'ta-re), pertaining to nutrition.
alimentation (al-im-en-ta'shun), the process of giving or taking nourishment.
alkali (al'ka-lī), a compound capable of neutralizing acids.
alkaloid (al'kal-oid), pertaining to alkali.
alkalosis (al-kal-o'sis), abnormal increase of the alkaline state of the blood.
allergic (al-er'jik), pertaining to allergy.
allergy, a tendency of an individual to react with pathological manifestations to otherwise harmless substances.
amebiasis (am-e-bī'a-sis), infected with amebae.
amebic dysentery (am-e'bik), dysentery due to amebae.
ampoule, a small glass container for hypodermic solutions.
anabolic (an-ab-ol'ik), pertaining to constructive metabolism (opposite of catabolic).
analysis, resolution into component elements.
anamnesis (an-am-ne'sis), the past medical history of a patient.
anaphylaxis (an-af-il-ak'sis), increased susceptibility or decreased resistance to a drug, protein, or toxin after taking the substance.
anemia, lack of blood or of sufficient red blood cells.
anesthesia (an-es-the'ze-ah), absence of feeling or sensation.
aneurysm (an'u-rizm), dilatation of part of an artery.
angiectasis (an-je-ek'tas-is), dilatation of a vessel.
angiitis (an-je-ī'tis), inflammation of a vessel.
angina (an-ji'nah), any disease accompanied by attacks of feelings of suffocation.
angiostenosis (an-je-o-sten-o'sis), narrowing of a blood vessel.

anhydremia (an-hī-dre'me-ah), deficiency of water in the blood.
anodyne (an'o-dīn), (1) relieving pain. (2) a medicine that eases pain.
anorexia (an-o-rek'se-ah), lack or loss of appetite.
ante mortem (an'te mor'tem), before death.
antibiosis (an-ti-bi-ō'sis), association of two or more organisms in which one is destroyed.
antibiotic (an-ti-bī-ot'ic), pertaining to destruction of life. At present used to designate certain substances used as remedy to destroy infectious microorganisms.
antidote (an'te-dōt), a remedy for poisoning.
antigen (an'te-jen), a substance that under certain conditions produces antibodies in the organism.
antipyresis (an-te-pī-re'sis), the application of remedies against fever.
anuresis, anuria (an-u-re'sis), deficient urine; cessation of urine.
apnea, apnoea (ap-ne'ah), temporary cessation of respiration; asphyxia.
aqua, water.
aqueous (a'kwe-us), watery, containing water.
arteriosclerosis (ar-te-re-o-skle-ro'sis), a hardening of the arteries.
arteriospasm (ar-te're-o-spazm), spasm of an artery.
arteritis (ar-te-rī'tis), inflammation of an artery.
artery, any one of the vessels through which the blood passes from the heart to the various parts of the body.
arthritis (ar-thrī'tis), inflammation of a joint.
articulate, to unite as for a joint.
ascites (as-ī'tēz), a collection of fluid in the abdominal cavity.
aspirator, an instrument used for removing fluids or gases from a cavity by suction.
assimilation, the absorption of food; constructive metabolism.
asthenic (as-then'ik), weak or feeble.
asthma (az'mah), a condition characterized by attacks of difficulty in breathing with coughing and a feeling of suffocation.
astragalus (as-trag'al-us), a bone in the ankle.

atelectasis (at-el-ek'tas-is), insufficient expansion of the lungs of the new born; lack of air in the lung tissue.

athermic (ah-ther'mik), without heat or rise of temperature. (Also applied to mild short waves.)

atlas, the first cervical vertebra.

aureomycin (aw-re-o-mī'cin), antibiotic substance.

auscultation (aws-kul-ta'shun), the act of listening for sounds in the body for determining from these sounds the condition of the organs below and for the detection of pregnancy.

autointoxication, poisoning by some toxins produced within the body.

autopsy (aw'top-se), examination of a body after death.

avitaminose, avitaminosis (ah-vi-tam'in-ōs, ah-vi-tam-in-o'sis), any disease due to a lack of vitamins.

axilla, armpit.

bacteriemia (bak-tē-rĭ-ē'me-ah), bacteria in the blood.

balneology (bal-ne-ol'o-je), the science of spas and their therapeutic use.

benign (be-nīn'), not malignant, recurrent, or fatal.

beriberi, a disease due to vitamin deficiency.

bilirubin (bil-e-roo'bin), a red pigment in the bile.

biopsy (bī'op-se), examination of living tissue removed from an organism.

botulism, a disease caused by food poisoning.

bronchiectasis (brong-ke-ek'tas-is), dilatation of the bronchi or of a bronchus.

bronchopneumonia (brong-ko-nu-mo'ne-ah), inflammation of the bronchi and lungs.

Buerger's disease (bur'gerz), a disease of the arteries and veins of the leg, often leading to gangrene.

bursa (ber'sah), a sac or pouch filled with fluid in places in the body where there would otherwise be friction.

cachectic (kak-ek'tik), characterized by cachexia.

cachexia (kak-ek'se-ah), a condition a profound ill health, wasting, and malnutrition due to some devastating disease.

caduceus (ka-du'she-us), emblem of the medical profession—the staff of Mercury entwined with two serpents.

caffeine (kaf'e-in), a stimulant, found especially in coffee and tea.

calcaneum, calcaneus (kal-ka'ne-um, kal-ka'ne-us), the heel bone.

calcification, hardening of the tissues by a deposition of calcium salts.

capitulum (kap-it'u-lum), the rounded head of a part.

caput (kap'ut), any head or knob.

carpus, the wrist.

catabolic (kat-ab-ol'ik), pertaining to or due to catabolism.

catabolism (kat-ab'o-lizm), destructive metabolism.

catharsis (kath-ar'sis), a cleansing or purging.

catheter (kă'the-ter), a rubber, metal, or glass tube for introduction into a cavity through a narrow passage.

cavern, a cavity due to disease, especially in the lung caused by tuberculosis.

cavity, a hollow or space within the body or any of its organs.

cecum (se'kum), the intestinal pouch at the head of the colon.

celiac (se'le-ak), pertaining to the abdomen.

cervix, the neck, any necklike part.

chemotherapy (kem-o-ther'ap-e), the treatment or prevention of disease by chemicals injected into the body to cause destruction of the disease agent without harming the patient.

chloromycetin (klor-o-mī'se-tin), antibiotic agent.

chlorosis (klo-ro'sis), a form of anemia in young women.

cholagogue (ko'lag-og), (1) causing increased flow of bile. (2) a medicine that increases the production of bile.

cholesterol (ko-les'ter-ol), a substance found in all animal fats and oils.

chondroma (kon-dro'mah), a tumor consisting of cartilaginous tissue.

chondrosarcoma (kon-dro-sar-ko'mah), a malignant chondroma.

chromosome (kro'mo-sōm), a particle into which a portion of the cell nucleus splits up prior to division; assumed to be the determinant of species and of sex.

circulation, the movement of fluids in blood and lymph vessels.

cirrhosis (sir-o'sis), a pathologic change in the connective tissues of an organ, particularly the liver.

GENERAL MEDICINE

clavicle (klav'ik-el), the collarbone.
clysis (klī'sis), administration of an enema.
coagulation, formation of a clot.
  electric ~, the congealing of tissue through the application of an electric current by means of a needle.
coagulum (ko-ag'u-lum), a clot or curd.
coccyx (kok'siks), the last bone of the spinal column.
collapse, (1) complete prostration and depression. (2) pathological falling or breaking down of the walls of any part or organ.
colorimeter (kol-or-im'et-er), an instrument for comparing a color with a standard.
coma, complete unconsciousness.
complication, a disease occurring at the same time as another disease.
concatenation (kon-kat-in-a'shun), the connection between nerve cells by means of the nerve fibers.
congenital, existing at or from birth.
congestion (kon-jes'chun), excessive collection of fluid in tissues.
constriction, compression of a tubular part.
convulsion, a violent involuntary contraction of muscles.
cortisone (cor'tĭ-sōn), an adrenal cortex hormone, now used extensively as remedy in many conditions.
costa, a rib.
costal, pertaining to a rib or ribs.
counterirritant, producing an irritation to relieve an internal congestion.
creatine (kre'at-in), a substance found in the blood.
crepitus, bony (krep'it-us), a sound heard when fragments of a fractured bone rub against one another.
cyanosis (sī-an-o'sis), a state in which the skin turns bluish owing to insufficient oxygen in the blood.
cytobiology (sī-to-bī-ol'o-je), the biology of cells.
cytology (sī-tol'o-je), the study of cells.
defervescence (def-er-ves'ens), the abatement of fever.
deficiency disease, any disease due to lack of vitamins or minerals.
degeneration, deterioration of the condition of the body tissues.
delirium (de-lir'e-um), a disturbance in orientation, usually of short duration, due to fever, disease, or intoxication.
depletion, the process of emptying a vessel, such as bloodletting.
desiccant (des'sik-kant), a drying-up remedy.
diabetes (dī-ab-e'tes), a disease marked by increased secretion of urine.
diabetes mellitus. (See **Endocrinology**, page 387.)
diaphoresis (dī-af-or-e'sis), perspiration; especially, excessive perspiration.
diaphragm (dī'af-ram), the muscle between the abdominal cavity and the chest.
diathermy (dī'ath-er-me), the production of heat in the tissues by means of high-frequency currents.
dietotherapy (dī-et-o-ther'a-pe), treatment by diet.
diuresis (dī-u-re'sis), increased secretion of urine.
diuretic, (1) increasing the flow of urine. (2) a medicine that increases the flow of urine.
dosage, the measurement of doses of medicines.
dropsy, a pathological collection of serous fluid in the cellular tissues or in a cavity of the body.
ductus (duk'tus), any passage, canal, or duct.
dullness, a nonresonant sound heard on percussion.
dysentery (dis'en-ter-e), inflammation of the intestines causing pain in the abdomen and frequent bloody stools.
dyspnea, dyspnoea (disp-ne'ah), difficult or labored breathing.
edema (e-de'mah), swelling due to a collection of fluid in the tissues of the body.
electrodesiccation, destruction by high-frequency current.
embolism (em'bo-lizm), an obstruction in an artery by air, fat, or a blood cot.
emetic (e-met'ik), causing vomiting.
empirical (em-pir'ik-al), based on experience; not knowing the cause.
empyema (em-pī-e'mah), pus in a cavity of the body, especially the chest.
endemic, in a certain locality. Applied to a disease that appears regularly among certain groups.
enzyme (en'zīm), a ferment formed within living organisms that is capa

ble of transforming other chemical compounds.

eosinophilia (e-o-sin-o-fil′e-ah), the presence of an abnormal number of blood cells that are easily stained by the dye, eosin.

epithelium (ep-ith-e′le-um), the covering of the surface of the skin and of mucous membranes.

erysipelas (er-is-ip′el-as), an acute, contagious disease, due to a streptococcus, marked by chills, fever, and inflammation of the skin.

erythrocyte (er-ith′ro-sīt), a red blood corpuscle.

etiology (e-te-ol′o-je), the study of the cause of a disease.

exacerbation (eks-as-er-ba′shun), increased severity of a symptom or a disease.

excitation, an act of irritation or stimulation.

expectorant (eks-pek′to-rant), an agent promoting the ejection of sputum.

exudate (eks′u-dāt), a substance thrown out or discharged.

exudation (eks-u-da′shun), a substance thrown out; the act of discharging a substance.

febrile (feb′ril), pertaining to fever; feverish.

femur (fe′mur), the thigh bone.

fibula (fib′u-lah), the outer, thinner bone of the leg.

follicle (fol′ik-el), a small secretory sac or gland.

foramen (for-a′men), an opening, especially in a bone.

fossa (fos′ah), a pit, depression, or furrow.

geriatrics (je-re-at′riks), the study of old age and treatment of its diseases.

gerontology (jer-on-tol′o-je), same as geriatrics.

glossa (glos′ah), the tongue.

glossitis (glos-ī′tis), inflammation of the tongue.

glycosuria (gli-ko-su′re-ah), the presence of sugar in urine.

gustation (gus-ta′shun), the sense of taste.

habitus (hab′it-us), physical make-up.

hectic, applied to a feverish flush.

hemacytometer (hem-a-sī-tom′et-er), an instrument for counting blood corpuscles.

hematemesis (hem-at-em′es-is), the vomiting of blood.

hematology (hem-at-ol′o-je), the science of the composition and function of the blood.

hematuria (hem-at-u′re-ah), blood in the urine.

hemoglobin (hem-o-glo′bin), the main constituent of matter in the red blood corpuscle.

hemoglobinemia (hem-o-glo-bin-e′me-ah), the presence of hemoglobin in blood plasma.

hemoglobinometer (hem-o-glo-bin-om′-et-er), an instrument for determining the amount of hemoglobin in the blood.

hemoglobinuria (hem-o-glo-bin-u′re-ah), the presence of hemoglobin in the urine.

hemophilia (hem-o-fil′e-ah), a congenital tendency to hemorrhage due to deficient clotting of the blood.

hemoptysis (hem-op′tis-is), the spitting of blood.

hemorrhage (hem′or-ej), a bleeding.

hemothorax (hem-o-tho′raks), an accumulation of blood in the chest.

hepatic (hep-at′ik), pertaining to the liver.

hepatitis (hep-at-ī′tis), inflammation of the liver.

hepatization (hep-at-iz-a′shun), the transformation of tissue into a liverlike substance.

hernia (her′ne-ah), the protrusion of a part of an organ or tissue through an abnormal opening.

heterogenous (het-er-o-je′nus, or het-er-og′e-nus), derived from various sources, of varied origin.

hiatus (hī-a′tus), any gap, fissure, or opening.

hilus (hī′lus), a depression at the point where vessels and nerves enter.

Hippocratic (hip-o-krat′ik), pertaining to or described by Hippocrates, famous Greek physician of the fifth century B.C.

histamine (his′tam-in), a chemical substance used for therapeutic purposes.

histology (his-tol′o-je), the study of the minute structure of body tissues.

homeostasis (ho-me-os′tas-is), the state of or tendency to stability and equilibrium in the organism.

GENERAL MEDICINE

homogeneous (ho-mo-je′ne-us), having the same origin or the same characteristics of all parts.

hormone (hor′mōn), a chemical substance produced in one organ which, when carried to another organ by the circulation, stimulates the latter organ to functional activity.

humerus (hu′mer-us), the bone of the upper arm.

hydronephrosis (hī-dro-nef-ro′sis), an accumulation of urine in the kidney due to an obstruction.

hydrophobia (hī-dro-fo′be-ah), rabies in human beings.

hydrops (hī′drops), dropsy.

hydrothorax (hī-dro-tho′raks), the presence of fluid in the chest.

hypercalcemia (hī-per-kal-se′me-ah), excessive amount of calcium in the blood.

hyperglycemia (hī-per-glī-se′me-ah), excess of sugar in the blood.

hyperglycosuria (hī-per-glī-ko-su′re-ah), extreme glycosuria.

hyperpyrexia (hī-per-pī-reks′e-ah), very high fever.

hypertrophy (hī-per′trof-e), the abnormal enlargement or excessive growth of an organ or part.

hypnotic (hip-not′ik), a drug that causes sleep.

hypochondrium (hī-po-kon′dre-um), the region at each side of the abdomen below the lowest rib.

hypochromia (hī-po-kro′me-ah), a form of anemia characterized by increased pallor of the red blood cell center.

hypodermic (hī-po-der′mik), applied or administered underneath the skin (as an injection).

hypoglycemia (hī-po-glī-se′me-ah), deficiency of sugar in the blood.

hypoglycemic (hī-po-glī-se′mik), characterized by or causing hypoglycemia.

icteric (ik-ter′ik), pertaining to jaundice.

icterus (ik′ter-us), jaundice.

idiosyncrasy (id-e-o-sin′kras-e), an individual and peculiar way of reacting to some substance or stimulus.

ilium (il′e-um), part of the hipbone.

immune, protected against a particular disease.

immunity, the condition of being immune.

immunology (im-u-nol′o-je), the science or study of immunity.

indicatio causalis (in-dik-a′she-o kaws′a-lis), an indication regarding the treatment of a disease based on its cause.

indication, a sign or condition that points to the proper treatment of a disease.

infiltration, a penetration of tissues by fluids; the condition due to such effusion.

influenza, an infectious, sometimes epidemic disease; the grippe.

innervation, the supply of nerves to the different parts of the body and the impulses sent through these nerves.

insulin, a hormone produced in the pancreas; also an extract from the pancreas gland of animals used in the treatment of diabetes.

intermittent fever, fever that alternates with periods of normal temperature.

intumescence (in-tu-mes′ens), a swelling.

ionization, medical (ī-on-iz-a′shun), a form of treatment in which chemical ions are introduced into the body tissues by means of an electric current. It is called also iontophoresis, iontherapy, galvanoionization and ionic medication.

ischemia, ischaemia (is-ke′me-ah), local anemia due to disturbed circulation.

jaundice (jawn′dis), a disease characterized by yellow discoloration of the skin and eyes (icterus).

jennerization (jen-er-iz-a′shun), vaccination.

lavage (lah-vahzh′), irrigation of an organ.

leukemia (lu-ke′me-ah), a fatal disease with great increase in the number of leukocytes in the blood.

leukocyte (lu′ko-sīt), the white blood cell.

leukocytosis (lu-ko-sī-to′sis), an increase in the number of leukocytes (white blood cells) in the blood.

localization, the determination of the location of any pathological process.

lumbago (lum-ba′go), pain in the lumbar region.

lumbar (lum′bar), pertaining to the loins.

lymph (limf), the fluid in the lymphatic vessels.

lymph capillaries (kap'il-er-ēs), the smallest lymphatic vessels.
lymphangitis (lim-fan-ji'tis), inflammation of a lymphatic vessel.
lymphocyte (lim'fo-sīt), a variety of white blood corpuscle.
lymphocytosis (lim-fo-si-to'sis), excess of lymphocytes in the blood.
macroblast (mak'ro-blast), an abnormally large red blood cell.
macrocyte, a large red blood cell.
macrocytosis (mak-ro-si-to'sis), an abnormally large amount of giant red blood cells.
macroscopy (mak-ros'ko-pe), examination with the naked eye.
malaria (mal-a're-ah), a disease characterized by fever and chills, caused by a blood parasite.
malignant (mal-ig'nant), tending to cause death.
malingering (mal-in'ger-ing), the feigning of illness or injury.
malpractice, injurious medical treatment due to negligence.
manometer (man-om'et-er), an instrument for measuring the pressure of liquids or gases.
materia medica (mat-e're-ah med'ik-ah), that branch of medicine which deals with the study and use of drugs.
mediastinal (me-de-as'te-nal), pertaining to the mediastinum.
mediastinum (me-de-as-te'num), the space between the lungs.
medication, (1) a medicine. (2) the administration of remedies.
megaloblast (meg'al-o-blast), an abnormally large red blood corpuscle.
membrane, a thin sheet or layer of tissue that lines a surface or separates a space or organ.
meninges (men-in'jēz), the three membranes that envelop the brain and the spinal cord.
meningitis (men-in-ji'tis), inflammation of the meninges.
metabolism (met-ab'o-lizm), the physical and chemical processes by which living organisms produce the necessary energy to maintain life.
metacarpus, the bones between the wrist and the fingers; the palm of the hand.
metastasis (met-as'tas-is), the spread of a malignant growth (cancer) to other parts of the body.

metatarsus (met-ah-tar'sus), the bones of the foot between the instep and the toes.
modality, a form of application of a treatment.
monocyte (mon'o-sīt), a large leukocyte.
monograph (mon'o-graf), a long article on one subject.
morbid, diseased.
moribund (mor'ib-und), dying.
morphinism (mor'fin-izm), the habit of taking morphine.
morphology (mor-fol'o-je), the study of the forms and structure of organisms.
mucosa (mu-ko'sah), the mucous membrane.
mucus (mu'kus), the viscid (sticky) secretion of the mucous membranes.
myelocyte (mi'el-o-sīt), a marrow cell.
nausea, tendency to vomit.
necrology (nek-rol'o-je), statistics or reports on mortality.
necropsy (nek'rop-se), a post-mortem examination; autopsy.
nephritis (nef-ri'tis), inflammation of the kidneys.
nephrosis (nef-ro'sis), any degenerative disease of the kidneys.
neurovascular (nu-ro-vas'ku-lar), both nervous and vascular.
nocturnal (nok-tur'nal), pertaining to the night.
node (nōd), a swelling or knoblike eminence.
nodule (nod'yul), **nodulus**, a small node.
normoblast (nor'mo-blast), a red blood corpuscle present in certain pathological conditions.
noxious (nok'shus), harmful; poisonous.
occlusion (ok-kloo'zhun), the closing of an opening or passage.
oliguresis, oliguria (ol-ig-u-re'sis, ol-ig-u're-ah), decreased secretion of urine.
oral, pertaining to the mouth.
organ, any part of the body that performs a special function.
organotherapy (or-gan-o-ther'ap-e), the treatment of disease by the administration of animal organs or their extracts.
oscillograph (os-il'o-graf), an instrument for recording changes in blood volume.
osteitis (os-te-i'tis), inflammation of the bone.
osteoarthritis (os-te-o-ar-thri'tis), inflammation of the bones and joints.

osteology (os-te-ol'o-je), the study of bones.
osteomyelitis (os-te-o-mī-el-ī'tis), inflammation of the bone marrow, or of the marrow and the bone.
osteoporosis (os-te-o-po-ro'sis), a condition in which a bone has become abnormally porous.
outpatient, a patient who does not stay in the hospital wards but visits the hospital clinic for treatment.
palpable, something that can be felt.
palpation, the act of feeling by hand during an examination.
pancreas (pan'kre-as), a gland behind the stomach that produces a digestive ferment and insulin.
pancreatitis (pan-kre-at-ī'tis), inflammation of the pancreas.
pandemic, affecting a wide area or a large part of the population.
papilla (pap-il'ah), a small cone-shaped swelling.
parenchyma (par-en'kim-ah), the functional elements of an organ as distinguished from its connective tissue.
parenteral (par-en'ter-al), by way other than through the alimentary tract—for instance, by injection.
parietal (pa-rī'e-tal), pertaining to the walls of an organ or part.
parotid (pa-rot'id), near the ear.
parotis (pa-ro'tis), the salivary gland below the ear.
paroxysm, an intense attack, a spasm.
patella, the knee cap.
pathogenesis (path-o-jen'es-is), the development of a disease.
pathognomy (pa-thog'no-me), the interpretation of the signs and symptoms of a disease.
pathologic, pathological, pertaining to pathology; diseased.
pathology, the science that deals with the nature of disease.
pellagra (pel-ah'grah), a disease affecting the skin and nervous system, due to deficiency of certain vitamins.
pelvis, the basinlike bone at the end of the trunk.
penicillin (pen-i-cīl'lin), antibiotic agent.
percussion, a diagnostic method consisting of striking the body with short, sharp blows.
perforation, a hole made through a part due to injury or disease.

periarticular, around a joint.
periosteum (per-e-os'te-um), a membrane covering the bones.
periphery, the surface of a body.
peritoneum (per-it-o-ne'um), the membrane lining of the abdominal walls.
peritonitis (per-it-o-nī'tis), inflammation of the peritoneum.
petechia (pe-te'ke-ah), a small spot under the skin due to subcutaneous bleeding.
phagocyte (fag'o-sīt), a cell that destroys bacteria or harmful matter in the body by absorption or ingestion.
pharyngitis (far-in-jī'tis), inflammation of the pharynx.
phlebitis (fle-bī'tis), inflammation of a vein.
photomicroscopy (fo-to-mi-cro'sco-pe), photography of minute objects.
photospectrometer, an apparatus for chemical analysis by use of the spectrum.
phrenectomy, phrenicectomy (fren-ek'to-me, fren-is-ek'to-me), removal or resection of the phrenic nerve.
phthisis (thī'sis), (1) a wasting away. (2) pulmonary tuberculosis; consumption.
plasma, the fluid part of the blood.
plethora (pleth'o-rah, or ple-tho'rah), an abnormally large amount of blood in the body.
pleura (plu'rah), the membrane that envelops the lungs and lines the inner chest walls.
pleurisy (plu'ris-e), inflammation of the pleura.
pneumonia (nu-mo'ne-ah), inflammation of the lungs.
pneumothorax (nu-mo-tho'raks), air or gas in the pleural cavity. **artificial ~**, the injection of nitrogen gas into the chest in order to collapse and thereby immobilize one lung; a form of treatment in pulmonary tuberculosis.
poikilocytosis (poi-kil-o-sī-to'sis), the presence of malformed or oversized red blood corpuscles in the blood.
polycythemia, polycythaemia (pol-e-sī-the'me-ah), excess of red corpuscles in the blood.
polydipsia (pol-i-dip'se-ah), excessive thirst.
polyuria (pol-e-u're-ah), excessive secretion of urine.

post mortem, after death; an autopsy.
prognosis, a prediction regarding the probable development of a disease and the prospects regarding recovery.
prophylactic, preventing or protecting from disease; a remedy that prevents disease.
prophylaxis, prevention of disease; a medicine that prevents disease.
prostration, extreme exhaustion.
protein (pro'te-in), one of a class of important compounds containing carbon, nitrogen, hydrogen, oxygen, and sulphur, found in all organisms.
protoplasm, the essential substance of the cell body and the nucleus of the cell.
protuberance, a projecting part.
pruritus (pru-rī'tus), an itching.
pseudohypertrophy (su-do-hī-per'trof-e), a nonpathologic enlargement of a body part.
purgative, a medicine that causes evacuation of the bowels.
purpura (pur'pu-rah), a condition marked by the formation of purple spots due to hemorrhages in the skin.
purulent (pu'ru-lent), containing pus; caused by pus.
putrefaction, decay or decomposition due to microorganisms.
pyemia, pyaemia (pī-e'me-ah), a general poisoning of the system resulting in the formation of abscesses in the parts of the body where the bacteria lodge.
pyknic (pik'nik), being of short and stocky build.
pyothorax (pī-o-tho'raks), accumulation of pus in the chest; empyemia.
pyrexia (pī-rek'se-ah), fever.
quartan, a fever that returns every third or fourth day.
quinsy, an inflammation of the throat with abscesses around the tonsils.
rabies, an infectious fatal disease of certain animals such as dogs and wolves and communicable to man by a bite of an infected animal; sometimes called hydrophobia in human beings.
radial, radiating or spreading from a center, as a pain.
radioactive isotopes. (See **Radiology,** pages 409–411, for all terms relating to radioactivity.)
radius, the outer bone of the forearm.
râle (rahl), a rasping sound in the lungs.

recrudescence (re-krew-des'sense), a new attack or outbreak of a disease.
regeneration, new growth or restoration of injured tissue.
remission, a temporary improvement.
respiration, the act of breathing.
reticulocytosis (rĕ-tic-u-lo-cī-to'sis), an excess of a certain kind of red blood cell, the reticulocyte.
retroperitonitis (rĕ-tro-per-it-o-nī'tis), inflammation of tissues behind the peritoneum.
rheumatism, an inflammation of the muscles, joints, or nerves.
rheumatoid, resembling rheumatism.
Rh factor, an antigenic substance found in the red blood cells of 85 per cent of the population. This is called Rh positive. If an Rh negative individual receives a transfusion of Rh positive blood, an antibody reaction might occur. Subsequent transfusions of Rh positive blood would then prove disastrous. (See also **Pediatrics,** pages 407–408.
sacrum, the lowest bone of the spine, forming the pelvis.
salvarsan (sal'var-san), an arsenical compound used in protozoan infections, especially syphilis.
scapula, the shoulder blade.
sciatic (sī-at'ik), pertaining to the hip.
sciatic nerve, the hip nerve that runs down the back of the thigh.
sciatic syndrome (sin'drōm), a combination of symptoms involving the sciatic region.
sciatica (sī-at'ik-ah), an inflammation of the sciatic nerve.
scurvy, a disease due to vitamin C deficiency.
secretion, the fluid product of cells, including the glands.
sedative (sed'at-iv), a remedy that has a quieting effect.
sedimentation rate, reaction, or **test,** a test to determine the degree of rapidity of the sinking of red blood cells in a mass of drawn blood, as an indication of the presence of an infection.
seizure, an attack, as of a disease or of convulsions.
senescence (sen-es'ens), the process of aging.
sepsis, a poisoning of the system.
septicemia (sep-ti-se'me-ah), a patho-

GENERAL MEDICINE

logic condition due to bacteria and their poisons in the blood.
serous (se′rus), pertaining to, producing, or containing serum.
serum, (1) the clear, watery component of any animal fluid separated by coagulation from its more solid constituents. (2) blood serum from animals rendered immune to a particular disease by inoculation with bacteria.
shingles, a virus infection characterized by a series of small blisters along the root of a nerve and generally associated with pain in that region.
siderosis (sid-er-o′sis), (1) a disease of the lungs due to the inhalation of iron particles. (2) abnormally large amounts of iron in the blood.
spasm, a sudden, violent, involuntary muscular contraction.
spasmophilia (spaz-mo-fil′e-ah), a tendency to spasms or convulsions.
sphincter (sfink′ter), a ringlike muscle around a natural opening, which contracts and closes the latter; usually, the sphincter at the anus.
sphygmomanometer (sfig-mo-man-om′-et-er), an instrument for determining the blood pressure.
spirochaete, spirochete pallida (spi-ro-ke′tah pal′id-ah), the micro-organism causing syphilis.
spirochetosis (spi-ro-ke-to′sis), an infection with any of the spirochetes.
splanchnic (splank′nik), pertaining to the viscera.
spleen, a large glandlike organ on the left side of the abdomen.
splenic (splen′ik), pertaining to the spleen.
splenomegalia, splenomegaly (sple-no-meg-a′le-ah, sple-no-meg′al-e), enlargement of the spleen.
spondylitis (spon-dil-i′tis), inflammation of a vertebra.
sputum, anything that is expectorated.
stasis (sta′sis), a stoppage of the blood circulation.
sternum, the breast bone.
stethoscope, an instrument for listening to the sounds in the body.
stoma (sto′mah), an opening.
stomatitis (sto-ma-ti′tis), inflammation of the mouth.
streptococcemia (strep-to-kok-se′me-ah), streptococci in the blood.
streptomycin (strep-to-mi′sin), antibiotic agent.
streptosepticemia (strep-to-sep-te-se′me-ah), septicemia due to a streptococcus.
stride, a grating, shrill sound.
stroma, the connective tissue which forms the structure of an organ.
stupor, lack of consciousness.
subacute, less than acute.
sudation, the act of sweating; excessive perspiration.
sulcus, a groove, especially a groove of the brain.
sulfadiazine (sul-fa-di′a-zin), anti-infectious agent of the sulfanilamide group.
sulfa drugs, an abbreviation for the group of sulfanilamide substances.
sulfanilamide (sul-fa-nil′a-mid), a substance with strong antibacterial effect, usually called sulfa.
sulfathiazole (sul-fa-thi′a-zol), anti-infectious agent of the sulfanilamide group.
suppuration (sup-u-ra′shun), the formation or discharge of pus.
suppurative, forming or discharging pus.
susceptibility, the state of being easily affected by a disease agent, or of not being immune.
sympathicus (sim-path′e-kus), the sympathetic nervous system.
symptomatology (simp-tom-at-ol′o-je), the study of symptoms.
symptom-complex, see **syndrome.**
syncope (sin′ko-pe), a fainting spell.
syndrome (sin′drom), the sum of various symptoms occurring together.
syphilis (sif′il-is), a contagious venereal disease.
syringe, an instrument for injecting liquids.
systemic (sis-tem′ik), pertaining to the body as a whole.
tampon (tam′pon), a plug made of cotton, gauze, or a sponge.
tarsus, the instep.
temple, the flat sides of the forehead.
temporal, pertaining to a temple.
terramycin (ter-ra-mi′sin), antibiotic agent.
tetanic (te-tan′ik), pertaining to or producing tetanus.
tetanus, (1) a continuous contracture of a muscle (2) lockjaw.

therapeutics (ther-ap-u′tiks), the application of remedies in the treatment of diseases; the art of healing.
therapy, treatment of disease.
thorax, the chest.
thrombo-angiitis (throm-bo-an-je-ī′-tis), inflammation of blood vessels; Buerger's disease.
thrombocyte (throm′bo-sīt), a blood platelet active in blood clotting.
thrombophlebitis (throm-bo-fle-bī′tis), inflammation of a vein or veins accompanied by formation of a blood clot.
thrombosis (throm-bo′sis), the formation of a thrombus, that is, a blood clot.
thrombus (throm′bus), a blood clot in an artery or vein.
tibia, the inner and larger bone of the leg below the knee.
tincture (tink′tur), a medicinal solution, generally with an alcoholic base.
tolerance, the ability to endure the effects of a drug.
tonic, an agent which produces or restores a normal state of tension.
torticollis (tor-ti-kol′is), a contraction of the cervical muscles resulting in a contortion of the neck.
toxemia (tok-se′me-ah), a general poisoning of the blood following a local infection.
toxin, a poison produced by bacteria.
trauma (traw′mah), an injury.
traumatic, pertaining to or caused by an injury.
trichinosis (trik-ĕ-no′sis), an infection caused by eating trichina-infested pork.
trophic, pertaining to nutrition.
tubercular, pertaining to the tubercle bacillus or its effects.
tuberculosis, an infectious disease caused by the tubercle bacillus.
tuberculous, pertaining to tuberculosis.

tumor, a swelling, an enlargement, or a new growth.
typhoid, resembling typhus.
typhoid fever, abdominal typhus.
typhus, typhus fever, a contagious fever.
typing of blood, determining the type of the blood of both donor and recipient before a blood transfusion in order to ascertain whether the blood of both is compatible.
ulcer, a sore.
ulna (ul′nah), the outer bone of the forearm.
ulnar, pertaining to the ulna, the ulnar nerve, or the ulnar artery.
uremia (u-re′me-ah), the presence of toxic substances in the blood.
vagus (va′gus), the pneumogastric nerve.
varicose, abnormally dilated or swollen, usually said of a vein.
vascular, pertaining to, or consisting of vessels.
vasoconstrictor (va-so-kon-strik′tor), nerves which produce constriction of the blood vessels.
vasomotor (va-so-mo′tor), regulating the contraction and dilatation of the blood vessels. Anything that controls the muscles of vessels.
vegetative, (1) pertaining to growth and nutrition. (2) functioning automatically or unconsciously.
venereal (ve-ne′re-al), relating to sexual intercourse.
venipuncture, the puncture of a vein for therapeutical purposes.
venter, the stomach or abdomen.
vertebra, one of the bones of the spinal column.
vesicle (ves′ik-el), a small blister.
virulence, the quality of producing infection.
viscera (vis′er-ah), plural of viscus.
viscus (vis′kus), any organ in one of the four cavities of the body.

Surgery

abscess, a localized accumulation of pus.
adenocarcinoma (ad-en-o-kar-sin-o′mah), a cancer in a gland.
adenoma, a tumor in a gland.
adenosarcoma, a cancerous adenoma.

adhesion, the formation of tissue by which parts are abnormally connected.
anastamosis (an-as-to-mo′sis), the development of a connection between the passages of two vessels or intestines by surgery or disease.

SURGERY

anesthetic, a drug that produces loss of feeling or sensation.
anesthetist, one trained in the administration of anesthetics.
angioma (an-je-o'mah), a tumor consisting of blood vessels.
angulation, the development of angular bends in the intestines.
antisepsis, use of measures to prevent infection.
antiseptic, (1) something that prevents infection. (2) a substance that destroys germs.
aperture, an opening or outlet.
appendectomy, removal of the appendix.
appendicitis, inflammation of the appendix.
appendix vermiformis, vermiforma, the worm-shaped sac attached to the cecum.
applicator, an instrument for applying remedies locally.
asepsis, absence of bacteria.
astringent, causing shrinking of mucous membranes.
Burow's solution, a solution used for dressings.
cancer, a malignant tumor.
cannula, a small tube.
capsulectomy, surgical removal of a capsule.
carcinogenic, producing cancer.
carcinoma, cancer, malignant tumor.
caries, decay of a bone.
catgut, a ligature prepared from sheep's intestine.
caustic, corrosive or searing.
cautery, the searing of a part by the application of a hot iron or wire.
ceco-ileostomy (se-ko-il-e-os'to-me), the operation of making an outlet from the ileum through the abdominal wall.
cellulitis, inflammation of cellular tissue.
chloroform, a volatile liquid used to produce anesthesia.
cholecystectomy (ko-le-sis-tek'to-me), removal of the gall bladder.
cholecystostomy (ko-le-sis-tos'to-me), the operation of making an outlet from the gall bladder through the abdominal wall to permit discharge of its contents.
cholelithotomy (ko-le-lith-ot'o-me), removal of gallstones by surgical means.
cicatrix (sik'at-riks), a scar.

circumcision, removal of the foreskin.
claudication, difficulty in walking; **intermittent** ∼, pain in the legs on walking, associated with a vascular disturbance.
cocainization, the process of anesthetizing by the use of cocaine.
colectomy, resection of the colon.
colotomy, the surgical creation of an opening into the colon.
compression, the process of pressing together.
cyst, a sac that contains a fluid.
cystectomy, removal of a cyst.
débridement (dā-brēd'mang), the cleaning of a wound of all foreign matter and dead tissue.
decapsulation, removal of a capsule, especially of the capsule of the kidney.
decompression, relieving pressure.
decubitus (de-ku'be-tus), a pressure sore.
deposit, a collection of any abnormal matter in the body.
desiccation, the drying up of a diseased part by applying an electric current by means of a needle electrode.
disinfection, the destruction of disease-producing germs.
diverticulitis, inflammation of a pouch or pocket (diverticulum).
drainage, a method of permitting the gradual discharge of fluids (pus).
duodenocholedochotomy (du-o-de'no-ko-led-o-kot'o-me), the operation of establishing a connection between the duodenum and the gall bladder.
duodeno-enterostomy (en-ter-os'to-me), the surgical formation of an outlet from the duodenum into the small intestine.
effusion, the oozing of a fluid.
electrodesiccation, same as desiccation.
enchondroma (en-kon-dro'mah), a tumor composed of cartilaginous tissue.
enterostomy, the surgical creation of an outlet from the intestines through the abdominal wall.
erosion, an eating or wearing away; a superficial destruction of the skin or mucous membrane.
evisceration (e-vis-er-a'shun), removal of the viscera.
excision, the cutting out or removing of a part.
exostosis, formation of a bony growth.
extirpation, excision.

extradural, outside the dura mater.
extravasation, an effusion of blood or other fluid into the tissues.
fibroma, a fibrous tumor.
flap, a partly loosened piece of skin or flesh.
fulguration, same as desiccation.
furuncle, a boil.
furunculosis, the development of many boils.
graft, a piece of tissue for transplantation.
granulation, "proud flesh."
granuloma, a tumor composed of granulation tissue.
hematoma (hem-at-o'mah), a tumor consisting of blood.
hernia, the condition in which a part of an organ or tissue protrudes through an opening; a rupture.
hiatus, any gap or opening.
hypernephroma, a malignant tumor of the adrenal gland.
implantation, the surgical introduction of living tissue into the body.
incarcerated, held fast, hemmed in, confined.
induration, hardened tissue.
inguinal (in'gwin-al), pertaining to the groin.
inguinal hernia, protrusion of a loop of the intestines into the inguinal canal.
iodoform, a substance used as a local antiseptic.
jejunostomy (jej-u-nos'to-me), the operation of making an outlet from the jejunum through the abdominal wall.
keloid, excessive scar formation.
laminectomy (lam-in-ek'to-me), excision of the lamina of a vertebra.
lancet, a small, pointed, two-edged knife used in surgery.
laparotomy (lap-ar-ot'o-me), an incision into the abdominal wall.
ligation, the act of tying up a blood vessel.
ligature, (1) a thread of silk or catgut for tying a blood vessel. (2) the process of applying a ligature.
lipoma, a tumor composed of fat.
lithotomy, the surgical removal of a stone, generally from the bladder; cystotomy.
lymphadenitis (lim-fad-en-i'tis), inflammation of the lymph glands.

lymphangioma (lim-fan-je-o'mah), a tumor composed of lymph vessels.
lymphosarcoma, a malignant tumor consisting of lymph glands.
metastasis (met-as'tas-is), the spread of a malignant growth (cancer) to other parts of the body.
myeloma (mī-el-o'mah), a tumor composed of marrow cells.
myoma (mī-o'mah), a tumor composed of smooth muscle tissue.
narcosis, unconsciousness induced by a drug; same as general anesthesia.
necrosis, death of a circumscribed part of tissue.
neoplasm, a new growth, a tumor.
nephrectomy, excision of the kidney.
nephrolithotomy (nef-ro-lith-ot'o-me), the surgical removal of a stone from the kidney.
nephrotomy, incision into the kidney.
nodulus, a small swelling or elevation.
onychia (o-nik'e-ah), inflammation of the matrix of the nail.
osteoma (os-te-o'mah), a tumor consisting of bonelike tissue.
otoplasty, plastic surgery of the external ear.
papilloma, a tumor of the skin, composed of hypertrophied tissue.
paracentesis (par-a-cen-te'sis), the tapping of a cavity to draw off fluid.
paronychia (par-on-ik'e-ah), an abscess on the last finger joint.
periostitis, inflammation of the periosteum.
peritonitis, inflammation of the peritoneum.
phagocytosis, destruction of microorganisms by phagocytes.
phlebitis, inflammation of a vein.
puncture, a hole made by a pointed instrument.
reduction, the setting of a fracture or dislocation; replacement of a hernia.
resection, cutting out part of an organ.
sarcoma, a malignant tumor.
scalpel, a small, straight knife.
scirrhus (skir'us), a hard cancer.
septic, pertaining to sepsis or putrefaction.
sterile, free from bacteria; aseptic.
strangulation, constriction or compression of a passage, strong enough to interfere with circulation.
strumectomy, excision of a goiter.

suturation, the process of suturing.
suture (su'tur), the surgical stitches for joining the edges of a wound.
sympathectomy (sim-path-ek'to-me), excision of part of a sympathetic nerve.
tampon, a plug made of cotton, gauze, or a sponge.
teratoma, a congenital tumor containing parts of a fetus.
thoracoplasty (tho-rak'o-plas-te), plastic surgery of the chest.
thrombo-angiitis (throm-bo-an-je-i'tis), inflammation of the inner coat of an artery, accompanied by thrombosis.
thyroidectomy (thi-roi-dek'to-me), the surgical removal of the thyroid gland.
tourniquet (toor'ne-ket), an appliance to stop bleeding by compressing the blood vessels.
transfusion, the transfer of blood from the veins of one person to those of another; the injection of blood or blood plasma.
transplantation, the grafting of skin or other tissue either from another part of the same person or from someone else.
trauma (traw'mah), a wound or injury, or the resulting condition.
tumor, a swelling or an enlargement.
ulceration, the development of an ulcer.

Cardiology

anacrotic (an-ak-rot'ik), pertaining to anacrotism.
anacrotism, a form of pulse irregularity.
aneurysm (an'u-rizm), a local dilatation of the walls of an artery.
angina pectoris (an-ji'nah pek'to-ris), acute pain in the heart region and a feeling of suffocation, due to spasm or hardening of the coronary arteries.
aorta (a-or'tah), the main artery, coming from the left ventricle of the heart.
aortitis (a-or-ti'tis), inflammation of the aorta.
aortosclerosis (a-or-to-skle-ro'sis), hardening of the walls of the aorta.
apex (of the heart) (a'peks), the rounded lower end of the heart.
apex beat, the beat of the heart against the chest wall.
apex murmur, a murmur over the apex of the heart.
apoplexy (ap'o-plek-se), sudden paralysis and loss of consciousness.
arrhythmia (ah-rith'me-ah), an abnormal, irregular rhythm of the heart beat. The different types of arrhythmia are sinus arrhythmia, extra systole, heart block, auricular fibrillation, auricular flutter, pulsus alternans, and paroxysmal tachycardia.
arteriosclerosis (ar-te-re-o-skle-ro'sis), hardening of the arteries.
atheroma (ath-er-o'mah), degenerative process in the walls of the larger arteries.
atrium (a'tre-um), an auricle of the heart.
auricle (aw'rik-l), the chambers of the heart on each side above the ventricle.
auriculoventricular (aw-rik-u-lo-ven-trik'-u-lar), pertaining to an auricle and a ventricle.
auricular, pertaining to an auricle.
bradycardia (brad-ik-ar'de-ah), abnormally slow pulse.
cantering rhythm, a heart rhythm similar to the cantering rhythm of a horse.
capillary, the minute hairlike blood and lymph vessels.
cardiac, pertaining to the heart.
cardiopathy (kar-de-op'ath-e), any disorder or disease of the heart.
carotid (kar-ot'id), the main artery on each side of the neck.
Cheyne-Stokes' respiration (chain'-stōks'), an abnormal form of breathing.

compensation, the counterbalancing by the heart of any defect of structure or function.

coronary (kor′o-na-re), pertaining to the arteries that supply the heart muscles.

cyanosis (sī-an-o′sis), blueness of the skin due to insufficient oxygen in the blood.

decompensation, failure to compensate cardiac disfunction.

depressant, (1) diminishing functional activity. (2) a medicine that decreases functional activity.

diastole (dī-as′to-le), the period of dilatation of the heart as opposed to systole, which is the period of contraction.

dicrotic pulse (dī-krot′ik), a double beat in the pulse.

digitalis, a drug used to stimulate the action of the heart muscle.

dilatation, the state of being expanded or increased in size beyond the normal dimensions.

edema, cardiac (e-de′mah), swelling of the body tissues due to heart disease.

effort syndrome, symptoms of breathlessness, dizziness, pain in the chest region, and palpitation due to exertion; called also "soldier's heart."

EKG, ECG, abbreviation for electrocardiogram.

electrocardiogram (e-lek-tro-kar′de-o-gram), a graphic tracing of the electric current produced by the action of the heart muscle.

electrocardiograph, an instrument for taking electrocardiograms.

embolism (em′bo-lizm), the obstruction of a blood vessel by a foreign body, such as a clot, air, or oil.

endarteritis (end-ar-ter-ī′tis), inflammation of the innermost coat of an artery.

endocardial (en-do-kar′de-al), within the heart.

endocarditis (en-do-kar-di′tis), inflammation of the endocardium.

endocardium, the lining membrane of the heart.

exocardial (eks-o-kar′de-al), outside the heart.

extrasystole (eks-tra-sis′to-le), a premature contraction of the heart.

fibrillation (fi-bril-a′shun), a condition in which the muscle fibers of the heart contract individually instead of the muscle as a whole.

flutter, atrial or **auricular** (a′tre-al, aw-rik′u-lar), an irregular action of the heart.

heart block, an abnormal mechanism in which the ventricle beats independently from the auricle.

hypertension, high blood pressure; essential ∼, high blood pressure without discoverable cause.

hypotension, low blood pressure.

infarct (in′farkt), local deterioration of tissue due to an obstruction in the supplying blood vessel.

insufficiency, cardiac, inadequate function of the heart.

mitral (mī′tral), pertaining to the mitral valve (between the left auricle and the left ventricle).

murmur, aortic, an abnormal sound indicating a pathologic condition of the aortic valves.

myocarditis (mī-o-kar-di′tis), inflammation of the heart muscles.

myocardium, the heart muscle.

oligocardia (ol-e-go-kar′de-ah), same as bradycardia.

palpitation, unduly strong beating of the heart.

pancarditis (pan-kar-di′tis), general inflammation of the heart.

pericarditis (per-e-kar-di′tis), inflammation of the pericardium.

pericardium (per-e-kar′de-um), the sac holding the heart.

phlebitis (fle-bi′tis), inflammation of a vein.

plethysmograph (ple-thiz′mo-graf), an instrument for measuring changes in the volume of organs due to alteration in the blood supply.

presystolic (pre-sis-tol′ik), before or at the beginning of the systole.

pulsate, to beat or throb.

quinidine (kwin′id-in), a substance used to influence the action of the heart.

stenocardia (ste-no-kar′de-ah), same as angina pectoris.

stenosis (ste-no′sis), a narrowing or constriction of any passage or opening; **aortic** ∼, narrowing of the aortic opening of the heart or the aorta itself.

stethoscope (steth′o-skōp), an instrument for listening to the cardiac and arterial sounds.

strophanthus (stro-fan′thus), a drug for the stimulation of heart action.

syncope anginosa (sin′ko-pe an-jī-no′-sah), a state of collapse due to closure of the coronary arteries.

systole (sis′to-le), the period when the heart contracts.

tachycardia (tak-e-kar′de-ah), abnormally rapid heart action.

thrombosis (throm-bo′sis), the development or formation of a thrombus.

thrombus, a blood clot in a vein or artery.

tricuspid, the heart valve between the right auricle (atrium) and the right ventricle.

valve, a fold in a canal or passage that allows the flow of its contents in one direction only; especially in those leading from and to the heart chambers.

vasoconstriction (va′so-), constriction of blood vessels.

vasodepressor, causing depression of the circulation.

vasodilatation, dilatation of a blood vessel.

vasodilator, (1) inducing dilatation of the blood vessels. (2) a nerve or drug that produces dilatation of the blood vessels.

vasospasm (va′so-), spasm of the blood vessels.

ventricles, the two lower cavities of the heart from which the blood is pumped into the arteries.

Dermatology

acne, an inflammation of the sebaceous glands, ordinarily called pimples.

acnitis, a skin inflammation, with pus discharge, that leaves pits in the skin.

alligator skin, same as ichthyosis.

alopecia (al-o-pe′se-ah), pathological total or partial baldness.

athlete's foot, a fungus infection between the toes.

aurantiasis cutis (aw-ron-tī′as-is ku′tis), yellow discoloration of the skin.

bulla, a large blister.

callosity, hard skin.

callous (adj.), like a callus.

callus (n.), any callosity.

carbuncle, an extensive inflammation of subcutaneous tissue.

chancre, primary sore in syphilis.

chancroid, a soft venereal sore not caused by syphilis.

chloasma (klo-as′mah), discoloration of the skin.

cicatrix (pl. cicatrices), a scar.

clavus, a horny thickening of the skin; a corn.

corium, the layer of skin under the epidermis.

corneum, the uppermost stratum of the epidermis.

cutaneous, pertaining to the skin.

cuticle, the epidermis.

cutis, the true skin or derma.

depilatory, an agent for removing hair.

derma, the skin.

dermatitis, inflammation of the skin.

dermatophytide (der-mat-of′it-īd), the skin eruptions caused by a fungus growth.

dermatophytosis, a skin disorder caused by a fungus, such as athlete's foot.

dermatosis, any skin disease.

desquamation (des-kwa-ma′shun), peeling.

ecchymosis (ek-im-o′sis), an effusion of blood and the discoloration of the skin caused by it.

eczema (ek′ze-mah), a skin disease marked by a watery discharge and the formation of scales.

electrolysis, removal of hair by a galvanic current.

epidermis, the outer layer of the skin.

epilation, the removal of hair.

epithelioma (ep-ith-e-le-o′mah), a cancer of the skin.

eruption, a rash of any kind.

erythema (er-ith-e′mah), redness of the skin due to dilatation of the capillaries from a variety of causes, e.g., sunburn.

exanthem, exanthema (eks-an′them), any skin eruption.

excoriation (eks-ko-re-a'shun), a scaling of the upper layers of the skin.
exfoliation, the process of scaling.
favus, a contagious disease of the skin.
follicle, a very small secretory gland.
folliculitis, inflammation of a follicle.
furuncle, a boil.
furunculosis (fu-run-ku-lo'sis), a condition characterized by the development of boils.
herpes, an inflammation of the skin characterized by the formation of small blisters.
herpes simplex, fever blisters.
herpes zoster, shingles.
hidradenitis (hī-dra-den-ī'tis), inflammation of a sweat gland.
hidrosis (hī-dro'sis), excessive sweating.
hives, a skin disorder marked by reddish wheals with itching or stinging sensation; urticaria. (Often a sign of allergy.)
hyperkeratosis (hī-per-ker-at-o'sis), hypertrophy (excessive development) of the horny layer of the skin.
ichthyosis (ik-the-o'sis), a disease characterized by dry scales.
idrosis (id-ro'sis), any defective function of the sweat glands.
impetigo, an inflammatory skin disease.
intertrigo (in-ter-trī'go), a skin rash caused by chafing.
Kahn's test, a test for determining the presence of syphilis.
keratoma, a tumor of the corneous layer of the skin.
keratosis, an abnormal horny growth.
leukoderma (lu-ko-der'mah), the formation of white patches on the skin; vitiligo.
lues, syphilis.
lupus (lupus vulgaris), a tuberculous disease of the skin.
lymphogranuloma (lim-fo-gran-u-lo'-mah), a venereal disease.
macule (mak'ul), any abnormally colored spot on the skin.
malpighian (mal-pig'e-an), pertaining to the stratum malpighii.
melanoleukoderma (mel-an-o-lu-ko-der'-mah), blotched or spotted skin.
nevus, a mole.
onychia (o-nik'e-ah), inflammation of the root of the nail.
onychomycosis (o-nik-o-mī-ko'sis), ringworm of the nails.

pachydermia (pak-id-er'me-ah), thickening of the skin.
papule, a pimple.
parapsoriasis (par-ah-so-rī'as-is), a condition resembling true psoriasis.
patch test, a method of identifying the cause of dermatitis by applying to the healthy skin patches soaked in a solution of the substance suspected of being the irritant.
pediculosis (pēd-ik-u-lo'sis), being infested with lice.
pemphigus (pem'fig-us), a disease marked by the development of blisters.
pigment, coloring matter in living organisms.
pigmentation, discoloration produced by a pigment.
pityriasis (pit-ir-ī'as-is), the formation of scaly patches.
prurigo (pru-re'go), a disorder of the skin accompanied by chronic itching.
pruritus (pru-rī'tus), itching, usually without visible lesions.
psoriasis (so-rī'as-is), a skin disease marked by the appearance of red, scaly patches.
purpura (pur'pu-rah), a disease marked by blood extravasation under the skin causing purple spots.
pustule, pimples containing pus.
ringworm, a contagious skin disease due to fungus infection.
rosacea (ro-za'se-ah), reddening and thickening of the skin on the face caused by alcoholism.
scabies, an infectious disease of the skin caused by a parasite, the itch mite.
scleroderma, a disease of the skin marked by the formation of hardened, pigmented patches.
sclerodermatitis, sclerodermitis, inflammation and hardening of the skin.
scratch test, a test to determine the sensitivity to a substance. The procedure consists in rubbing a solution of the substance into a scratch on the skin.
sebaceous glands (se-ba'shus), glands located in the skin that secrete a greasy substance.
seborrhea (seb-o-re'ah), a disease of the sebaceous glands characterized by an abnormally increased discharge of their secretion.
shingles, a skin condition marked by the development of blisters.

slough (sluf), devitalized tissue that is thrown off by living tissue.
squama (skwa'mah), a scale.
stratum malpighii, a layer of the epidermis.
sycosis (sī-ko'sis), an inflammation of the hair follicles.
syphilid, syphilide, pertaining to the skin lesions caused by syphilis.
syphilis, a contagious venereal disease.
trichomycosis (trī-ko-mī-ko'sis), a parasitic infection of the hair.
trichosis (trī-ko'sis), any disease of the hair.
urtica (er'tik-ah), a wheal.
urticaria (er-tik-a're-ah), nettle rash or hives.
varioliform, resembling smallpox marks.
venereal (ve-ne're-al), pertaining to diseases such as syphilis or gonorrhea.
verruca (ver-oo'kah), a wart.
vesicle, a blister.
vitiligo, a skin disease marked by the formation of smooth, light-colored patches; same as leukoderma.
vulgaris, common (as in lupus vulgaris).
Wassermann test or **reaction**, a test to determine the presence of syphilis.
wheal, a long white or red raised mark on the skin.
xeroderma (ze-ro-der'mah), a pathological dryness of the skin.
yaws, a tropical disease with skin lesions.
zoster. (See herpes zoster.)

Endocrinology

acromegaly (ak-ro-meg'al-e), excessive enlargement of the tissues of hands, feet, and face, due to a glandular disorder.
Addison's disease, a disease due to hypofunction of the suprarenal glands.
adenitis (ad-en-ī'tis), inflammation of a gland.
adenopathy (ad-en-op'ath-e), any disease of a gland.
adiposity (ad-ip-os'it-e), obesity.
adrenal gland, a gland on top of the kidney.
adynamia (ad-i-na'me-ah), loss of normal powers; decreased vitality.
amenorrhea (a-men-o-re'ah), absence or abnormal cessation of menstruation.
anorexia (an-o-rek'se-ah), loss of appetite.
asthenic (as-then'ik), weak or feeble.
basal metabolism, see **metabolism**.
Basedow's disease, toxic goiter.
calory (*pl.* calories), (1) the unit of heat necessary to raise the temperature of 1 gram of water 1 degree centigrade (the small calory). (2) the unit of heat needed to raise the temperature of 1 kilogram of water 1 degree (the large calory, used in the study of metabolism).
castration, removal of the sex glands.
climacterium, the menopause.
constitution, the physical make-up or disposition of an individual.
cortico-adrenal (kor'te-ko-ad-re'nal), pertaining to the adrenal cortex.
cretinism (kre'tin-izm), a disorder marked by defective physical development and idiocy, ascribed to lack of activity of the thyroid gland.
diabetes, a disease marked by increased secretion of urine.
diabetes insipidus, a disease marked by the passage of large amounts of urine without excretion of sugar.
diabetes mellitus, a disease of metabolism marked by an abnormal amount of sugar in the blood and the passage of urine containing sugar.
diathesis (di-ath'es-is), a predisposition to a particular disease.
endocrine, pertaining to the ductless glands.
endocrinopathy (en-do-krin-op'ath-e), any disease due to the disordered function of any of the endocrine glands.
ergosterol (er-gos'te-rol), a substance that when irradiated becomes an antirachitic agent.
eunochoid (u'nuk-oid), (1) pertaining to a condition of impaired masculinity. (2) a pathologic condition of a physiologically inactive testicle.
eunuch (u'nuk), a male person who has been castrated.
exophthalmic goiter (eks-of-thal'mik goi'ter), a disease marked by protrusion

of the eyeballs and an enlarged thyroid gland.

exophthalmos, exophthalmus (eks-of-thal'mus), abnormal protrusion of the eyeballs.

flushes, transient redness of the face and neck such as occurs during the menopause.

gigantism (ji-gan'tizm), abnormal overgrowth, ascribed to a disease of the anterior lobe of the hypophysis.

glucatonia (glu-kat-o'ne-ah), reduction of blood sugar following insulin injections to a degree that pathologic signs appear; insulin shock.

glycogen (gli'ko-jen), a carbohydrate formed in the liver and transformed into sugar when needed by the organism.

glycosuria (gli-ko-su're-ah), the presence of sugar in urine.

goiter, enlargement of the thyroid gland.

gonad (gon'ad), a gland serving the reproductive system, an ovary or a testis.

Graves' disease, a form of goiter.

hirsutism (her'sut-izm), abnormal hairiness, especially in women.

hormone, the secretion of endocrine glands.

hyperadrenalism (hi-per-ad-re'nal-izm), excessive function of the adrenal glands.

hyperinsulism, abnormally increased production of insulin.

hyperpituitarism (hi-per-pit-u'it-ar-izm), excessive activity of the pituitary gland.

hyperthyroidation, hyperthyroidism (hi-per-thi-roi-da'shun, hi-per-thi'roi-dizm), overactivity of the thyroid gland.

hypoadrenalism (hi-po-ad-re'nal-izm), deficient functioning of the adrenal glands.

hypoglycemia (hi-po-gli-se'me-ah), abnormally low amounts of sugar in the blood.

hypoglycemic (hi-po-gli-se'mik), characterized by or causing hypoglycemia.

hypogonadism (hi-po-go'nad-izm), dysfunction of the gonads.

hypomenorrhea (hi-po-men-o-re'ah), scanty menstrual flow.

hypo-orchidia (hi-po-or-kid'e-ah), deficient endocrine activity of the testes.

hypo-ovarianism (hi-po-o-va're-an-izm), deficient endocrine activity of the ovaries.

hypophysis (hi-pof'is-is), the pituitary gland, located in a depression of the sphenoid bone and attached to the brain.

hypopituitarism (hi-po-pit-u'it-ar-izm), deficient function of the pituitary gland.

hypothyroidism (hi-po-thi'roi-dizm), deficient activity of the thyroid gland.

infantilism (in-fant'il-izm), a condition marked by retarded mental development, underdeveloped sexual organs, and at times stunted growth.

insulin, the hormone produced by the pancreas.

lipodystrophia, lipodystrophy (lip-o-dis-tro'fe-ah), a disturbance of fat metabolism.

lipomatosis (lip-o-ma-to'sis), the presence of fatty deposits.

menopause (men'o-pawz), the period when menstruation normally ceases; change of life.

menorrhagia (men-o-ra'je-ah), abnormally excessive menstrual flow.

metabolism, the physiological processes by which the cells of an organism produce chemical changes in order to build up new living matter and to supply the energy necessary to maintain life.

metabolism, basal, the minimal energy expended to maintain all organic functions.

migraine, very severe headache, sometimes combined with nausea.

multiglandular, affecting many glands.

myxedema (miks-e-de'mah), a disease marked by dropsylike swellings, due to deficient activity of the thyroid gland.

neurasthenia (new-ras-the'ne-ah), weakness of the nervous system.

obesity, the condition of being excessively fat.

oligohypermenorrhea (ol-ig-o-hi-per-men-o-re'ah), abnormally prolonged intervals between the menstrual periods with excessive flow.

oligohypomenorrhea (ol-ig-o-hi-po-men-o-re'ah), abnormally prolonged intervals between the menstrual periods with scanty flow.

oligomenorrhea (ol-ig-o-men-o-re'ah), abnormally prolonged intervals between the menstrual periods.

ovary, the female sex gland in which the egg (ovum) is developed.

pancreas, a gland behind the stomach that produces a digestive ferment and insulin.

parasympathetic (par-ah-sim-path-et′ik), a part of the autonomic nervous system.

parathyroid (par-ah-thī′roid), (1) situated beside the thyroid gland. (2) any one of the four small glands situated on the surface of the thyroid gland.

perisplenitis (per-is-ple-nī′tis), inflammation of the capsule of the spleen.

pineal body or **gland** (pī′ne-al), a small gland at the base of the brain.

pituitary (pit-u′it-a-re), pertaining to the pituitary body (gland).

pituitary body or **gland,** same as hypophysis.

polyglandular, involving many glands.

polymenorrhea (pol-e-men-o-re′ah), abnormally frequent menstruation.

progeria (pro-je′re-ah), premature senility.

spleen, a large glandlike organ on the upper left side of the abdomen.

splenitis, inflammation of the spleen.

splenomegaly (sple-no-meg′al-e), enlargement of the spleen.

splenoptosis (sple-nop-to′sis), dropping down of the spleen.

struma, goiter.

sugar tolerance test, the administration of a sugar test meal to determine the state of carbohydrate metabolism.

sympathicus, the sympathetic nervous system.

testis, the male sexual gland.

testosterone (tes-tos′ter-ōn), a male hormone.

thymus gland (thī′mus), a ductless gland between the upper part of the thorax and the lower part of the throat which atrophies or disappears in adults.

thyroaplasia (thī-ro-ap-la′ze-ah), underdevelopment of the thyroid gland and its function.

thyroid body or **gland,** a ductless gland in front of and on each side of the trachea.

thyrotoxicosis (thī-ro-toks-e-co′sis), any form of hyperthyroidism.

virilism (vir′il-izm), (1) masculinity. (2) the development of masculine traits in a woman.

Gastroenterology

achlorhydria (ah-klor-hī′dre-ah), lack of hydrochloric acid in the gastric juice.

aerophagia (a-er-o-fa′je-ah), the swallowing of air.

alimentary canal, the channel through which food passes from the mouth to the anus.

alimentation, the act of giving or taking food.

amebiasis, intestinal (am-e-bī′as-is), the condition of having amebae in the intestines.

antacid (ant-as′id), a substance that reduces acidity.

antiperistalsis (an-te-per-is-tal′sis), peristaltic motion toward the stomach instead of toward the rectum.

appendix vermiformis, the worm-shaped sac opening into the cecum.

Ascaris (as′kar-is), as intestinal parasite.

bile (bīl), the secretion of the liver; gall.

biliary (bil′e-a-re), pertaining to bile.

cardiospasm, contraction of the cardiac sphincter of the stomach.

cecum (se′kum), the pouch in the intestines into which open the ileum, the colon, and the appendix vermiformis.

chlorhydria (klor-hī′dre-ah), an excess of acid in the gastric juice.

cholangitis (ko-lan-ji′tis), inflammation of the bile ducts.

cholecystitis (ko-le-sis-ti′tis), inflammation of the gall bladder.

choledochus (ko-led′o-kus), the bile duct.

clysma (kliz′mah), an enema.

clyster (klis′ter), an injection into the rectum; an enema.

colic (kol′ik), (1) pertaining to the colon. (2) sharp abdominal pain; a cramp.

colitis, inflammation of the colon.

colon, that part of the large intestine extending from the cecum to the rectum.
colonic, pertaining to the colon.
constipation, infrequent, insufficient, or difficult evacuation of the bowels.
coprostasis (kop-ros′tas-is), collection of feces in the intestines.
costive (kos′tiv), constipated.
costiveness, constipation of the bowels.
crepitus (krep′it-us), the act of expelling flatus from the bowels.
defecation (def-ek-a′shun), evacuation of fecal matters from the bowels.
diarrhea (di-ar-e′ah), abnormal frequency of evacuation and liquidity of stool.
digestion, the conversion of food into chemical substances that can be absorbed and assimilated by the body.
distention, the state of being extended, enlarged, or bloated.
diverticulitis (de-ver-tik-u-li′tis), inflammation of a diverticulum.
diverticulosis, the presence of a diverticulum, particularly of the intestine.
diverticulum, a pouch or pocket, especially in the intestines.
duodenal (du-o-de′nal), pertaining to the duodenum.
duodenum, the first portion of the small intestine.
dyspepsia (dis-pep′se-ah), a disturbance of digestion.
enteritis (en-ter-i′tis), inflammation of the small intestines.
entero-anastomosis (en-ter-o-an-as-to-mo′-sis), the operation of uniting two parts of the intestine so as to establish a connection.
enterocolitis (en-ter-o-ko-li′tis), inflammation of the small intestine and the colon.
enteroptosis (en-ter-op-to′sis), relaxation and descent of the intestine.
enterospasm, a spasm of the intestine.
epigastric (ep-e-gas′trik), pertaining to the epigastrium.
epigastrium, the epigastric region; the part over or in front of the stomach.
eructation (e-ruk-ta′shun), belching.
esophagitis (e-sof-ag-i′tis), inflammation of the esophagus.
esophagoscopy (e-sof-ag-os′ko-pe), the inspection of the esophagus by means of a tubular instrument.
esophagospasm (e-sof′ag-o-spazm), spasm of the esophagus.
esophagostenosis (e-sof′ag-o-sten-o′sis), narrowing of the size of the esophagus, due to scars or spasms.
esophagus (e-sof′ag-us), the gullet; a canal leading from the pharynx to the stomach.
evacuation, emptying of the bowels.
fecal (fe′kal), pertaining to feces.
feces (fe′sez), the excrement discharged from the bowels.
flatulence (flat′u-lens), air or gas in the stomach or intestines.
flatus (fla′tus), gas in or expelled from the intestines.
gall bladder, the pear-shaped sac on the lower surface of the liver, which contains the bile.
gastralgia (gas-tral′je-ah), pain in the stomach.
gastrasthenia (gas-tras-the′ne-ah), decreased function of the stomach.
gastrectasis (gas-trek′tas-is), dilatation of the stomach.
gastric, pertaining to the stomach.
gastritis, inflammation of the stomach.
gastrocolic, pertaining to the stomach and the colon.
gastroenteric, pertaining to the stomach and the intestines.
gastroptosis (gas-trop-to′sis), descent of the stomach.
gastroscopy (gas-tros′ko-pe), examination of the stomach.
gingivitis (jin-jiv-i′tis), inflammation of the gums.
glossitis (glos-i′tis), inflammation of the tongue.
hepatic, pertaining to the liver.
hyperchlorhydria (hi-per-klor-hi′dre-ah), abnormally increased secretion of hydrochloric acid.
hypochlorhydria (hi-po-klor-hi′dre-ah), abnormally low production of hydrochloric acid.
hypotonic (hi-po-ton′ik), reduced tonus (of the stomach); also called "gastric motor insufficiency."
ileum (il′e-um), the lower part of the small intestine.
ileus (il′e-us), vomiting of fecal matter, due to intestinal obstruction, accompanied by colic.
indigestion, disturbed or disordered digestion.

intestine, the tube that leads from the stomach to the anus.
jejunum (je-ju′num), the small intestine following the duodenum.
lavage (lah-vahzh′), irrigation or washing out of the stomach or the bowels.
lingua (ling′gwah), tongue, in Latin.
megacolon (meg-a-ko′lon), an abnormally large colon.
melena (me-le′nah), black stool due to the presence of blood.
mesenteric (mes-en-ter′ik), pertaining to the mesentery.
mesentery (mes′en-ter-e), the folds of tissue that lead from the intestines to the posterior walls of the abdominal cavity and contain the blood and lymph vessels.
mucous colitis (mu′kus ko-li′tis), a condition marked by the passing of mucous material from the colon.
nausea, tendency to vomit.
oral, pertaining to the mouth.
pancreas (pan′kre-as), a gland behind the stomach producing digestive ferments.
pancreatitis (pan-kre-at-i′tis), inflammation of the pancreas.
pepsin, a digestive ferment in the gastric juice.
peristalsis (per-is-tal′sis), the movements of the bowels by which its contents are propelled toward the rectum.

pylorospasm (pi-lor′o-spasm), spasm of the pylorus.
pylorus (pi-lo′rus), the opening of the stomach into the duodenum.
regurgitation (re-gur-jit-a′shun), the casting up of undigested food.
sigmoid (sig′moid), the S-shaped part of the large intestine connecting with the rectum.
sigmoiditis (sig-moi-di′tis), inflammation of the sigmoid.
stasis (sta′sis), an abnormal arrest or retardation of a flow. **ileal** ∼, delayed movement of the contents of the intestines through the ileum; **intestinal** ∼, delayed movement throughout the intestinal tract.
stomatitis (sto-ma-ti′tis), inflammation of the mouth.
tympanites (tim-pa-ni′tes), distention of the abdomen due to gas.
ulcer, a sore.
ulceration, the formation of an ulcer.
ulcus (ul′kus), an ulcer, generally of the stomach.
ventriculus (ven-trik′u-lus), the stomach.
ventro-, relating to abdomen.
viscera, abdominal (vis′er-ah), the organs contained in the abdominal cavity.
volvulus (vol′vu-lus), twisting of the bowels, resulting in intestinal obstruction.

Gynecology and Obstetrics

abdominal gestation or **abdominal pregnancy,** a condition in which the fetus is lodged in the abdominal cavity instead of in the uterus; extra-uterine pregnancy.
ablatio placentae (ab-la′she-o pla-sen′-ta), premature detachment of the placenta.
abort, to cause to miscarry.
abortion, expulsion of the fetus before it is able to live.
abortive, (1) causing abortion. (2) incomplete.
afterbirth, expulsion of placenta with umbilical cord.
amenorrhea (a-men-o-re′ah), absence or abnormal cessation of the menses.
anteflexion, a curving forward.

ante partum, before delivery or childbirth.
anteversion, the tilting forward of the uterus.
areola (ar-e′o-lah), the dark circle around the nipple.
Aschheim-Zondek test, a test for the determination of pregnancy.
Caesarean section, delivery of the fetus by cutting through the abdominal and uterine walls.
cervix, cervix uteri, the narrow end of the uterus.
climacteric, the period when the body undergoes profound changes, such as puberty and the menopause.
climacterium (kli-mak-ter′e-um), the menopause.

clitoris (klī'to-ris), an organ of the female corresponding to the penis in the male.

colostrum, the milky fluid from the breasts a few days before or after childbirth.

colpitis (kol-pī'tis), inflammation of the vagina.

colporrhaphy (kol-por'af-e), the operation for narrowing the vagina.

conception, the fertilization of the human ovum resulting in pregnancy.

conization, the cutting or burning out of a cone of the endocervical tissue.

contraception, the act of preventing pregnancy.

corpus luteum (loo'te-um), a yellow body formed at the spot of the ruptured ovum.

curet, curette, a scoop or scraper for removing diseased tissue, e.g., from the interior of the uterus.

curettage, application of a curet.

cycle, ovarian, the menstrual rhythm.

decidua (de-sid'u-ah), the membrane produced in the uterus during pregnancy, which envelops the ovum.

dysmenorrhea (dis-men-o re'ah), painful menstruation.

eclampsia (ek-lamp'se-ah), an attack of convulsions during pregnancy or delivery.

ectopic, abnormal position; **ectopic pregnancy,** pregnancy outside the uterus.

embryo, the child in the uterus during the first few weeks.

emesis (em'e-sis), vomiting.

encephalotomy (en-sef-al-ot'o-me), the removal of the brain of a fetus in order to make delivery possible.

endometritis (en-do-me-trī'tis), inflammation of the membranous lining of the uterus.

estrogen (es'tro-jen), an ovarian hormone.

extrauterine, outside the uterus.

fallopian tubes, the tubes connecting the ovaries with the uterus.

fecundation, impregnation or fertilization.

fetal, relating to a fetus.

fetus, the embryo after the third month.

fibrosis uteri, the growth of fibroid tissue in the uterus.

flushes, transient redness of the face and neck occurring during the menopause.

forceps, an instrument with two blades or pincers and handles; used to extricate the fetus in cases of difficult labor.

fornix, anterior, the space between the neck of the uterus and the anterior wall of the vagina.

Friedman test, a test for the determination of pregnancy.

funiculus, the umbilical cord.

galactophoritis (gal-ak-tof-or-ī'tis), inflammation of the milk ducts.

gestation, the period of pregnancy.

graviditas, gravidity, pregnancy.

hypo-ovarianism, deficient function of the ovaries.

hysterectomy, the removal of the uterus.

hysterosalpingostomy (his-ter-o-sal-ping-os'to-me), the operation of making a connection between the uterus and a fallopian tube after removing a portion of the tube.

intrauterine, within the uterus.

involution, (1) the return of the uterus to its former size after childbirth. (2) the deterioration due to senility (menopause).

labia (la'be-ah), a lip.

labia majora, the outer folds of the vulva.

labia minora, the inner folds of the vulva.

laceration, tearing of the perineum.

lactation, the secretion of milk.

leukorrhea (lu-kor-re'ah), a white vaginal discharge.

lutein (lu'te-in), a hormone secreted by the corpus luteum.

mammary glands, the milk-producing glands in the breast.

mastitis, inflammation of the mammary glands.

menopause, the period when menstruation normally ceases; change of life.

menorrhagia (men-o-ra'je-ah), excessive menstrual flow.

menorrhalgia (men-o-ral'je-ah), painful menstruation.

menses, the monthly bleeding of women.

metritis (me-trī'tis), inflammation of the uterus.

metrorrhagia (met-ro-ra'je-ah), an abnormal uterine bleeding.

GYNECOLOGY AND OBSTETRICS

multigravida, a woman who has often been pregnant.
multipara, a woman who has given birth to several children.
obstetrics, the branch of medicine dealing with pregnancy and childbirth.
oligohypermenorrhea (ol-ig-o-hī-per-men-o-re'ah), abnormally prolonged intervals between the menstrual periods with excessive flow.
oligohypomenorrhea, abnormally prolonged intervals between the menstrual periods with scanty flow.
oligomenorrhea, abnormally prolonged intervals between the menstrual periods.
oophorectomy (o-of-o-rek'to-me), removal of an ovary or the ovaries.
oophoritis (o-of-o-rī'tis), inflammation of an ovary.
orificium, the opening of the uterus into the vagina.
osteomalacia (os-te-o-mal-a'se-ah), softening of the bone.
ovarian, pertaining to an ovary or the ovaries.
ovariectomy, removal of an ovary or the ovaries.
ovary (pl. **ovaries**), the female sex gland in which the egg is produced.
ovulation, the formation and discharge of an egg (ovum) from the ovary.
ovum, the female reproductive cell or egg.
parametritis, inflammation of the tissue around the uterus.
parametrium, the tissues connecting the uterus with the walls of the pelvis.
parturition, the act of childbirth.
partus, labor, or childbirth.
pelvis, the basinlike bone at the end of the trunk, supporting the spinal column and resting on the lower extremities.
perimetritis (per-e-me-trī'tis), inflammation of the perimetrium.
perimetrium (per-e-me'tre-um), the peritoneal covering of the uterus.
perineum (per-e-ne'um), the region between the anus and the genital organs.
periodicity, the regular interval at which the menses occur.
pessary, an appliance inserted in the vagina to support the uterus.

placenta, the organ within the uterus which nourishes the embryo.
pluripara, a woman who has borne several children.
polymenorrhea, menstruation at abnormally short intervals.
postnatal, after birth.
postpartum, after confinement.
pregnancy, the condition of being with child.
premature, a child born before the full term but living.
prenatal, before birth.
presentation, the part of the fetus which is delivered first.
primipara, a woman who is pregnant for the first time.
prolapse of uterus, the downward displacement of the uterus.
pruritus vulvae, itching around the vulva.
pseudocyesis (su-do-sī-e'sis), simulated pregnancy.
pseudopregnancy, the presence of symptoms simulating pregnancy.
puerpera (pu-er'per-ah), a woman in childbed.
puerperal, pertaining to childbirth.
pyosalpingitis (pī-o-sal-pin-jī'tis), inflammation of a fallopian tube with presence of pus.
retroversion of uterus, the tipping backward of the uterus.
salpingitis (sal-pin-jī'tis), inflammation of a fallopian tube.
salpingo-oophorectomy (sal-pin'go-o-of-o-rek'to-me), surgical removal of an oviduct and ovary.
salpingo-oophoritis (sal-pin'go-o-of-o-rī'tis), **salpingo-ovaritis,** inflammation of a fallopian tube and an ovary.
salpinx, a uterine tube.
speculum, an instrument for dilating a passage or cavity of the body to facilitate examination.
sterility, inability to reproduce, to have children.
superinvolution, excessive involution; reduction of the size of the uterus after childbirth to less than its former size.
suppository, an easily melted, medicated preparation, usually cone-shaped, for insertion into the vagina or rectum.
umbilicus, the navel.

uterus, the womb; the organ in which the fetus is developed.
vagina, the canal in the female extending from the vulva to the cervix uteri.
vaginismus, painful spasm of the vagina.
vaginitis, inflammation of the vagina.
version, the turning by hand of the fetus in delivery.
viable (vī′ab-l), capable of living.
vulva, the external genitals of the female.

Medical Laboratory

acetonuria (as-e-to-nu′re-ah), abnormal amount of acetone in the urine.
achromatic, not producing any color; difficult to stain.
acid, (1) a substance having a sour taste. (2) a compound of replaceable hydrogen combined with another element. If active, acid has the ability to turn blue litmus paper red.
acid-fast, pertaining to bacteria that, when stained, cannot be decolorized by acid.
acidophil (as-id′o-fil), (1) easily stained by acid dye. (2) thriving in acid media.
aerobic (a-er-o′bik), unable to live without oxygen.
agar-agar, gelatin of various seaweeds used in making culture media.
agglutination, a joining together; especially, the clumping together of bacteria by the action of certain antitoxins.
agglutinin, a substance found in immune serum.
albumin, the simple protein present in most animal and vegetable tissues.
albuminuria (al-bu-me-nu′re-ah), presence of albumin and other proteins in the urine, usually a result of kidney disease.
alkali, a strongly basic substance which neutralizes acids and turns red litmus paper blue.
amorphous (ă-mor′fus), shapeless.
amphoteric, having both acid and basic characteristics, affecting both blue and red litmus paper.
anaerobe (an-a′er-ōb), any microbe that thrives without oxygen.
anisocytosis, difference in the size of cells, especially red blood cells.
anthrax, an infectious disease of cattle caused by the *Bacillus anthracis.*
antibodies, substances in the body destructive to materials that are harmful to the organism. They may develop naturally or be introduced artificially.
antigen (an′te-jen), a substance which, when introduced into an organism, causes the formation of antibodies.
antioxidant, a substance that delays oxidation.
antitoxin, a substance formed by the body or injected into it to neutralize a poison.
bacillus (*pl.* **bacilli**), a rod-shaped bacterium.
bacteriophage (bak-tēr′e-o-faj), an ultramicroscopic agent which destroys bacteria.
bacterium (*pl.* **bacteria**), a vegetable microorganism. Many bacteria are pathogenic.
basophilic, having an affinity for basic rather than acid dyes.
binary fission, division of cells into two separate parts.
bouillon, a meat broth used as a culture medium.
calibration, the determination of specifications of a given object; correction of graduated apparatus.
carbolfuchsin, a staining fluid.
cast, material that has been molded in a body cavity or the lumen of a tubular structure.
coccus (*pl.* **cocci**), a ball-shaped microorganism.
coefficient, a number or symbol showing the number of times a formula should be multiplied.
conduction, transmission of electrons, heat, or sound waves.
contagion, transmission of disease by direct or indirect contact.
contamination, infection by contact.
cover glass, a thin glass plate used to cover microscopical specimens.
culture, a growth of microorganisms.
  attenuated ~, a culture of microorganisms that have lost their virulence.
cytoplasm (sī′to-plas-m), the protoplasm of a cell other than the nucleus.
Diplococcus (dip-lo-kok′us), a genus of bacteria.

MEDICAL LABORATORY

eosin (e′o-sin), a rose-colored acid stain.
eosinophil, a tissue that is easily stained with eosin.
germicidal (jer-mis-ī′dal), destructive to germs.
glycosuria (glī-ko-su′re-ah), the presence of sugar in the urine.
gonococcus (gon-o-kok′us), the microorganism causing gonorrhea.
Gram, Hans Christian Joachim, Danish bacteriologist who originated a method for staining bacteria.
Gram-negative, not capable of being stained by the Gram method.
Gram-positive, capable of being stained by the Gram method.
Gram's stain, a means of staining bacteria.
hematocrit, (1) a small centrifuge to separate blood cells. (2) a centrifuge tube in which blood cells are separated. (3) the volume and percentage of packed erythrocytes, determined by the reading of a hematocrit tube.
hematology, study of the blood.
hemolysis (hem-ol′is-is), disintegration of red blood corpuscles.
hemolytic, causing disintegration of red blood corpuscles.
hyalin (hī′ă-lin), a glassy material occurring in various body parts.
hyaline (hī′ălin, -lin)′, glassy, translucent.
hypo, common term for sodium hyposulfite, used as photographic fixing solution.
immunity, condition of being protected against a specific disease.
incubation, the growing of a bacterial culture in an incubator. ~ **period,** the time between the infection and the manifestation of a disease.
inoculation, intentional introduction of a disease virus or antitoxin into the body in order to establish immunity to a specific disease.
litmus paper, chemically prepared paper used to test acidity and alkalinity. The blue paper turns red in the presence of acid, and the red paper turns blue in the presence of alkali.
macrocyte, a blood cell that is larger than normal.
medium, (1) the means by which somethings is obtained. (2) (*pl.* **media**) a substance used for the culture of bacteria for study.
meniscus, in laboratory usage, the curved surface of a column of liquid.

methylene (meth′il-ēn), a dye.
Micrococcus (mī-kro-kok′us), a genus of minute bacteria.
microorganism, a minute organism, either plant or animal; especially, a bacterium.
mycology (mī-col′o-je), study of fungi.
neutrophil, a tissue that is easily stained with a neutral dye.
nucleated, having a nucleus.
nucleus, the central protoplasm of a cell.
oxalated, treated with sodium oxalate solution to prevent the coagulation of blood.
oxidant, a substance that supplies oxygen; an oxidizing agent.
oxidation, the process of combining with oxygen.
oxidize, to combine with oxygen.
parasitology (par-ah-sī-tol′ŏ-je), study of parasites.
pasteurization (pas-tūr-īz-a′shun), prevention or delay of fermentation by heating.
pathogenic (path-o-gen′ic), capable of producing a disease.
plasma, liquid part of the blood.
platelet, a small colorless disk in the blood, involved in the coagulation of blood; thrombocyte.
pneumococcus, a microorganism that causes pneumonia and sometimes other diseases.
potential, electric tension or pressure.
protoplasm, the essential substance of the cell body and nucleus of cells.
protozoa, lowest division of the unicellular animal organisms.
reagent, a substance involved in a chemical reaction.
refractivity, the ability to bend or refract light rays.
serum, the clear amber part of the blood that remains after coagulation.
Spirillum, a genus of spiral-shaped bacteria.
Spirochaeta (spī-ro-ke′tah), a genus of spiral microorganisms. ~ **pallida,** the causative agent of syphilis.
Staphylococcus (staf-il-o-kok′us), a genus of bacteria, occurring in clusters, found especially in boils, abscessses, carbuncles, etc.
Streptococcus, a genus of bacteria found in many pathological conditions and occurring in chainlike formation.
symbiosis (sim-be-o′sis), the living together of two dissimilar organisms.

thrombocyte, see *platelet.*
titration, the determination of the strength of a solution by means of standard measurements.
Trichomonas (trick-o-mo'nas), a genus of parasitic organisms causing some intestinal or vaginal infections.

urate, a uric acid salt.
virology, study of viruses.
virus, a microorganism so small that it passes through a porcelain filter; the cause of a variety of diseases.

Neurology and Psychiatry

abasia (ah-ba'zhe-ah), inability to walk because of loss of coördination.
abasic, pertaining to abasia.
affect, a feeling experienced in connection with an emotion.
affect psychosis, affective psychosis, an emotional, mental disorder.
afferent nerves, nerves leading from the periphery to the center.
aggression, a hostile or attacking attitude.
agoraphobia, a dread of open places or of crowds.
agraphia, inability to write, due to a lesion of the brain.
alexia (ah-lek'se-ah), inability to read, due to a lesion of the brain.
alienist, a specialist in treating mental disorders.
amaurotic idiocy (am-aw-rot'ik), a disease of infants and children marked by increasing failure of vision and by paralysis, ending in death.
ambidexterity (am-be-deks-ter'e-te), ability to us either hand effectively.
ambidextrous, being able to use either hand effectively.
ambivalence (am-biv'al-ans), the presence at the same time of opposite or contradictory emotions, such as sympathy and hostility, toward a given person, event, or situation.
amnesia, loss or disturbance of memory.
 anterograde ~, loss of memory for the period since the beginning of the disorder; **retrograde ~,** loss of memory for the period up to the beginning of the disorder.
analgesia (an-al-je'ze-ah), absence of sensitivity to pain.
analytic psychology, the psychotherapeutic method of C. G. Jung.
angioneurosis (an-je-o-nu-ro'sis), angioparalysis, angiospasm, or other neuroses of the blood vessels.

angioparalysis, paralysis of the blood vessels.
angiospasm, spasms of the blood vessels.
anhydrosis, abnormal decrease of sweat.
anorexia, lack or loss of appetite.
antisocial, pertaining to tendencies that are directed against human society.
anxiety neurosis, a form of neurosis characterized by the presence of various fears or a state of general anxiety.
apathy, lack of interest or emotion; indifference.
aphasia (af-a'zhe-ah), impairment or loss of speech or of the ability to write.
apoplexy (ap'o-plex-ē), a stroke.
apperception, the conscious recognition of a sensory impression.
apraxia (ah-prak'se-ah), loss of the power of performing coördinated movements.
aptitude test, a test devised to determine the special skill or ability of a person.
arachnoid (ar-ak'noid), the membrane between the pia mater and the dura mater.
Argyll Robertson pupil, a pupil that does not respond to light but contracts in accommodation.
aspermia, insufficient secretion of semen.
astereognosis (ă-ster-e-og-no'sis), inability to recognize the shape of objects by touch.
asthenia (as-the'ne-ah), feebleness, weakness.
atactic, ataxic, characterized by lack of muscular coördination.
ataxis, one type of lack of muscular coördination.
athetosis (ath-e-to'sis), a disorder characterized by constant twisting movements of the hands and feet.
atonic, without normal tonus.
atonicity, the condition of lacking normal tonus.

atrophy, a wasting or shrinking of a part, due to inadequate nutrition.
autonomic, independent, self-regulating; the autonomic nervous system.
autosuggestion, a mental state in which suggestions that are self-induced are accepted as facts.
Babinski's law, reflex, sign, syndrome, extension of the big toe instead of flexion on stimulating the sole.
basal ganglia, a mass of white or gray matter in each hemisphere of the brain.
behaviorism, a psychological method based on the principle that all behavior is the result of conditioning (learning).
Binet test, a method of testing the mental capacity of children by asking a series of questions graded according to age. The mental capacity of the subjects is judged by the answers given.
Brown-Sequard's disease, a disease of the spinal cord.
catalepsy, a disturbance characterized by rigidity and absence of speech and voluntary motion.
catatonia, a mental disorder marked by severe intellectual and physical deterioration.
catharsis (kath-ar′sis), the part of Freud's psychotherapy in which the patient "purges" himself by telling everything that comes to his mind in association with a given subject.
cerebellum, the small brain, behind the cerebrum.
cerebrospinal, pertaining to the brain and spinal cord.
cerebrum, the large and main part of the brain.
choreo-athetosis (ko-re-o-ath-e-to′sis), a disorder marked by twitching and twisting movements.
chronaxia (kron-ak′se-ah), the time that elapses between a certain stimulus and the nervous response.
claustrophobia (klaw-stro-fo′be-ah), fear of enclosed places.
clonic, pertaining to a clonus.
clonus, spasm with alternating contraction and relaxation of muscles.
column, the gray column of the spinal cord.
compensation, in psychoanalysis the process of emphasizing a favorable character trait in order to hide the existence of a socially disapproved tendency.
complex, in psychoanalysis the term for a group of repressed ideas of emotionally toned content.
conditioned reflex, an automatic response to a certain stimulus that has been developed by training.
continence, sexual abstinence.
conversion, the symbolic expression of an emotional conflict in terms of physical symptoms.
convolution, the rounded eminences on the surface of the brain.
convulsions, clonic, convulsions accompanied by a clonus.
coprophilia (kop-ro-fil′e-ah), a pathologic desire for handling filth and excrement.
cord, the spinal cord.
cortex, cerebellar, the outer layer of the cerebellum.
cortex, cerebral; ∼ **cerebri,** the outer layer of the brain.
cortical, pertaining to the cortex.
cranial, pertaining to the cranium.
cranium, the skull.
d'arsonvalism, d'arsonvalization (dar′-son-val-izm), treatment with high frequency currents.
defense reaction, the Freudian term for a response occasioned by conflicting emotional tendencies and enacted to avoid the conflict.
dejection, same as depression.
delinquency, transgression of the law by a minor.
delirium, transitory disturbance in orientation.
dementia (de-men′she-ah), mental disorder characterized by practically complete loss of the intellectual functions.
dementia praecox (pra′koks), a mental disorder in which the individual withdraws from reality and entertains many morbid concepts or delusions; schizophrenia.
depression, a mental state of sadness and despondency.
deterioration, progressive impairment of mentality.
diplegia (di-ple′je-ah), paralysis of the corresponding parts on each side of the body.

dipsomania (dip-so-ma′ne-ah), uncontrollable desire for alcoholic beverages.

dura mater, the outer of the three membranes of the brain and spinal cord.

dysrhythmia (dis-rith′me-ah), irregularities of the electric brain waves.

EEG, abbreviation for electroencephalogram.

ego, the conscious and responsible element of the mind.

egocentric, self-centered.

electrode, a medium used in the application of electrical currents.

electrodiagnosis, the diagnosis of certain conditions by means of electricity.

electroencephalogram (e-lek-tro-en-sef′a-lo-gram), a tracing that records the changes of electrical potentials occurring in the brain (brain waves).

encephalitis, inflammation of the brain.

encephalitis lethargica, sleeping sickness.

epilepsy, a disease marked by sudden attacks of convulsions and loss of consciousness. ~ **grand mal,** severe case of epilepsy; ~ **petit mal,** mild form of epileptic attacks.

euphoria (u-fo′re-ah) a state of well-being. In psychiatry it indicates an abnormal state of elation.

excitation, an irritation or a stimulation.

exteroceptors, the end organs of the nerves (receptors) in the periphery, which receive stimuli from the outside.

extrovert, a person whose interests are directed toward external matters.

faradic, faradaic, pertaining to faradism.

faradism, (1) an interrupted alternating current. (2) same as faradization.

faradization, the application of a faradic current in the treatment of nerves and muscles.

fasciculus (fas-ik′u-lus), a small bundle of nervous or muscular fibers.

frustration, the thwarting or repression of impulses by forces in the unconscious or the conscious mind.

fugue (fewg), a flight from the patient's usual surroundings of which he later remembers nothing.

galvanic current, unidirectional current for therapeutic purposes.

galvanism, the therapeutic use of a direct current.

galvanometer, an instrument for measuring galvanic current.

ganglion, a small, separate, independent nervous center.

general paralysis (See general paresis.)

general paresis, a degenerative disease of the brain, the result of an earlier syphilitic infection.

Gestalt psychology, a psychological theory according to which the mind experiences objects as wholes (*Gestalten*) not to be broken up into separate parts.

glioma, a tumor of the neuroglia.

globus hystericus, the sensation of having a lump in the throat, a condition frequently seen in hysteria.

group therapy, a method of psychotherapy in which a group of individuals are treated at the same time.

gyrus (ji′rus), a convolution of the brain.

hallucination, the impression of seeing or hearing nonexisting objects or sounds.

hemianesthesia (hem-e-an-es-the′ze-ah), loss of feeling on one side of the body.

hemiplegia (hem-e-ple′je-ah), paralysis of one side of the body.

hemisphere, each half of the brain.

hermaphrodism, hermaphroditism (her-maf′ro-dit-izm), the condition of having both male and female sex organs.

heterosexual, being attracted to the opposite sex.

horn, one of the columns of gray matter in the spinal cord: the anterior horn, containing motor nerve cells; and the posterior horn, containing sensory nerve cells.

hydrocephalus (hi-dro-sef′a-lus), enlargement of the head, due to accumulation of fluid in the brain.

hyperesthesia (hi-per-es-the′ze-ah), abnormally increased sensitivity.

hypnosis, a sleeplike state, induced by another person, in which consciousness is suspended but the subject is receptive to suggestions and commands.

hypochondria (hi-po-kon′dre-ah), a morbid anxiety and preoccupation regarding one's state of health.

hyposensitive, having decreased sensitivity.

hypothalamus (hi-po-thal′am-us), the region in the brain below the thalamus.

hysteria, pathological manifestations and symptoms of mental origin.

id, a psychoanalytic term for that part of the psyche which is regarded as being the source of instinctive energy.

individual psychology, psychotherapeutic method devised by Alfred Adler.

inhibition, the mechanism that restrains or prohibits the enactment of certain instinctual tendencies.

insanity, a collective term given to mental disorders, used mainly in legal parlance.

integration, the combination of separate thoughts or acts for a unified purpose.

intelligence quotient, the intelligence of an individual as measured by a standard intelligence test. I.Q.

introvert, a person whose interests are directed inward.

kleptomania, a compulsion to steal.

Korsakoff's syndrome, a form of psychosis.

leptomeningitis (lep-to-men-in-ji'tis), inflammation of the soft part of the meninges.

lethargy (leth'ar-je), a state of indifference or stupor.

libido, a psychoanalytic term for the energy or urges associated with the erotic instinct.

lobe, a part of the brain.

lobotomy (lo-bot'o-me), separation of the lobes of the brain.

locomotion, movement from one place to another.

locomotor ataxia, a disease of the ganglion cells of the posterior horn, due to syphilis.

malinger (ma-lin'guer), to pretend being ill in order to gain advantages.

mania, a type of emotional disturbance marked by excitement and violent tendencies.

manic depressive psychosis, a mental disorder in which states of elation or mania alternate with those of depression or melancholia.

masochism (maz'o-kizm), a perversion in which sexual pleasure is derived from experiencing pain or abuse.

medulla oblongata, the link between the spinal cord and the brain.

megalomelia (meg-al-o-me'le-ah), abnormally large size of the limbs.

melancholia (mel-an-ko'le-ah), a type of mental disorder in which the patient feels depressed, sad, and hopeless.

meningeal (men-in'je-al), pertaining to the meninges.

meninges, the three membranes that envelop the brain and spinal cord, including the dura, pia, and arachnoid.

meningitis, inflammation of the meninges.

meningomyelitis (men-in-go-mī-e-lī'tis), inflammation of the spinal cord and its membranes.

mental hygiene, systematic endeavors to prevent mental disorders and to maintain mental health.

mesencephalon (mes-en-sef'al-on), the midbrain.

migraine, periodic severe headache.

monomania, a delusion regarding one single subject.

monoplegia (mo-no-ple'je-ah), paralysis of one limb only.

myasthenia gravis (mī-as-the'ne-ah), a condition in which muscular contractions become gradually weaker on repetition.

myelitis (mī-el-ī'tis), inflammation of the bone marrow or the spinal cord.

myelo-encephalitis, inflammation of the brain and spinal cord.

narcissism, liking of one's own body.

narcolepsy, a disorder marked by a desire for and states of frequent sleep.

neuralgia, pain in a nerve or in nerves.

neurasthenia (nu-ras-the'ne-ah), fatigue and weakness without organic cause.

neuritis, inflammation of a nerve.

neuroglia, a special kind of connective tissue supporting the gray matter.

neuron, a nerve cell.

neuropathology, the study of the disorders of the nerves and nerve centers.

neuropsychiatry (nu-ro-sī-kī'a-tre), the study and treatment of disorders of the nervous system that have both neural and mental manifestations.

neurosis, an unbalanced emotional state; a nervous disorder without apparent organic cause.

neurosyphilis, syphilis of the central nervous system.

nostalgia, a longing to return to some former state or abode.

nystagmus, short, rapid, involuntary oscillation of the eyeball.
opisthotonos (o-pis-thot'o-nos), a spasm in which the body is arched backward.
pachymeningitis (pak-e-men-in-jī'tis), inflammation of the dura mater.
palsy, paralysis.
paralysis, loss of motion.
paralytic, (1) pertaining to paralysis. (2) a person affected with paralysis.
paranoia (par-an-oi'ah), a mental disorder marked by systematized delusions, generally of persecution.
paraplegia (par-ah-ple'je-ah), paralysis of the legs and lower part of the body.
parasympathetic, a part of the autonomic nervous system.
paresis (par-e'sis), slight paralysis.
paresthesia, paraesthesia (par-es-the'ze-ah), an abnormal sensation of burning, itching, tingling, etc.
Parkinson's disease, syndrome, a disease of the brain characterized by involuntary motions and muscular rigidity; also called "shaking paralysis."
patellar reflex, the knee reflex.
phobia, fear.
phrenic, (1) pertaining to the brain. (2) pertaining to the diaphragm.
pia mater, the innermost of the three membranes of the brain.
pineal (pī'ne-al), pertaining to the pineal body or gland.
pineal gland, a gland situated at the base of the brain.
plexus, a network of nerves.
poliencephalitis (pol-e-en-sef-al-ī'tis), inflammation of the gray matter of the brain.
polyneuritis, inflammation of many nerves.
polyphagia (pol-ĭ-fa'je-ah), excessive appetite.
pons cerebelli, pons varolii, the organ that connects the cerebrum, cerebellum, and medulla oblongata.
postencephalitis, a disorder following encephalitis.
pseudotabes (su-do-ta'bes), a condition presenting the symptoms of tabes dorsalis but having a favorable course and a different cause.
psyche (sī'ke), the mind.
psychoanalysis, the method of psychotherapy evolved by Sigmund Freud.

psychopathology, the study and treatment of mental disorders.
psychosis, a severe disease or disorder of the mind.
psychosomatic, pertaining to the mind-body relation: to physical symptoms of mental origin, or to mental disorders due to organic causes.
pyknic (pik'nic), a roundish, plump body type.
pyramid, a conical projection on the medulla oblongata.
pyromania (pī-ro-ma'ne-ah), a mania for setting fires.
querulent, a person with an abnormal tendency toward quarreling, a feeling of being misunderstood and of being dissatisfied.
radiculitis, inflammation of the spinal nerve roots.
reflex, the automatic motor response to a sensory stimulus.
relaxation, the decrease of tension; a state of mental and physical rest.
resistance, a psychoanalytic term for the mechanism of repressing unacceptable material and thus preventing it from becoming conscious.
Romberg sign, swaying when standing with eyes closed.
Rorschach test, a psychological test in which ten ink blots are shown to the individual for his interpretation, according to which his emotional make-up is judged.
sadism (sa'dizm), a perversion in which pleasure is derived by inflicting pain and cruelty on another person.
schizoid (skiz'oid), resembling schizophrenia; incipient schizophrenia.
schizophrenia (skiz-o-fre'ne-ah), a mental disorder in which there appears to be a split personality; dementia praecox.
sclerosis (skle-ro'sis), the formation of hard patches of connective tissue in the nervous system. **multiple ~,** sclerosis throughout the central nervous system, particularly the spinal cord.
scotoma, cloudy or blind spots in front of the eyes.
sella turcica (sel'ah tur'se-kah), the depression in the sphenoid bone that contains the hypophysis.
sensory nerves, the nerves that carry impulses from the periphery to the brain.

sexuality, the energies, instincts, and activities that relate to sex.
somatization (so-ma-te-za′shun), the conversion of emotional conflicts into physical symptoms.
somnambulism, sleepwalking.
spasm, a violent, involuntary contraction of a muscle. tonic ~, persistent spasm; clonic ~, spasm alternating with relaxation.
spinal cord, the portion of the central nervous system in the spinal canal.
stroke, a sudden and severe attack, as of apoplexy or paralysis.
subconscious, partially conscious; not perceived by the conscious.
sublimation, the process of substituting purposeful and socially approved activity for instinctual desires.
sympathetic nervous system, a part of the vegetative nervous system.
sympathicus, the sympathetic nervous system.
synapse, synapsis, the connection between the fibers of nerves.
syringomyelia (si-rin-go-mī-e′le-ah), a disorder marked by the formation of abnormal cavities filled with liquid in the spinal cord.
syringomyelitis, syringomyelia complicated by inflammation of the spinal cord.
tabes (ta′bez), a progressive wasting of the body.
tabes dorsalis, same as locomotor ataxia.
tetany, a disease marked by spasms of the muscles, particularly of the hands, due to a disease of the parathyroid gland.
thalamic, pertaining to the thalamus.
thalamus, a part of the midbrain.
tic, involuntary contraction or twitching of certain muscles; automatically repeated motions.
tonic, (1) characterized by continuous tension. (2) pertaining to or producing normal tone.
tonicity, the healthy state of the body in regard to tension.
transference, in psychoanalysis, the mechanisms of transferring to the psychiatrist the feelings which the patient had as a child toward his parents.
transvestism, the urge to wear clothing of the opposite sex.
trigeminus (trī-jem′in-us), the trifacial nerve, the fifth cranial nerve.
vegetative nervous system, the sympathetic and parasympathetic nervous system.
vertigo, dizziness.

Ophthalmology

ablatio retinae (ab-la′she-o ret′in-a), detachment of the retina.
accommodation, adjustment of the eye for vision at various distances.
achromate (ah-kro′māt), a colorblind person.
adaptation, accommodation of the eyes to light.
amaurosis (am-aw-ro′sis), blindness.
amblyopia (am-ble-o′pe-ah), the dim vision in a squinting eye.
ametropia (am-e-tro′pe-ah), the condition in which the eye is unable to focus on the retina the image of distant objects.
aniseikonia (an-e-sĭ-ko′ne-ah), the condition in which retinal images are unequal in size or shape in the two eyes.
anisocoria (an-ī-so-ko′re-ah), inequality of the size of the pupils.
anisometropia (an-is-o-met-ro′pe-ah), marked inequality in the state of refraction of the two eyes.
anophthalmos (an-of-thal′mos), one who is born without eyes.
anopsia, defect of vision.
aqueous humor (ak′wee-us), the fluid between the cornea and the lens.
asthenopia, weak eyes.
astigmatism, a defect in the refractory mechanism of the eye, generally due to an abnormal curvature of the cornea.
atropine, a drug used for the dilatation of the pupils.
axis, the line of vision.
bifocal lens, a lens the upper part of which has one focus and the lower part another.
binocular, pertaining to both eyes.
binocular vision, the fusion of vision of both eyes.

blepharitis (blef-ar-i'tis), inflammation of the eyelids.
blepharoplasty (blef'a-ro-plas-te), surgery of the eyelid.
canthus (kan'thus), the slit between the eyelids at the inner and outer end.
cataract, opacity of the lens of the eye.
choked disk (See papilledema.)
choroid (ko'roid), the vascular structure of the eye between the sclera and the retina.
choroiditis, inflammation of the choroid.
choroidocyclitis (ko-roi-do-sik-li'tis), inflammation of the choroid and ciliary processes.
choroidoretinitis (ko-roi-do-ret-in-i'tis), inflammation of the choroid and retina.
cilia, (1) the eyelashes. (2) the eyelids.
ciliary, pertaining to the eyelids or the eyelashes.
ciliary body, a mass of tissue between iris, sclera, and cornea.
cilium, (1) an eyelash. (2) the eyelid.
conjunctiva, the membrane covering the eyeball and lining the eyelid.
conjunctivitis, inflammation of the conjunctiva.
convergence, the ability to direct the visual lines of the two eyes to a near point.
convex, curved outward.
cornea, the glasslike part of the eyeball.
cyclitis (sik-li'tis), inflammation of the ciliary body.
cycloplegia (ci-klo-ple'je-ah), paralysis of the ciliary muscle.
dacrocystitis, dacryocystitis (dak-re-o-sis-ti'tis), inflammation of the tear sac.
diopter, dioptre, dioptric, dioptry, the unit of refractive power of a lens used in the prescription of eyeglasses.
diplopia (dip-lo'pe-ah), double vision.
disk, the area of the retina where the optic nerve enters it.
divergence, a pathological deviation of the visual lines.
emmetropia (em-et-ro'pe-ah), the exact focusing of parallel lines on the retina, which represents the normal condition of the eye.
enophthalmos (en-of-thal'mos), recession of the eyeball into the orbit.
enucleation (e-nu-kle-a'shun), removal of the eyeball.
epicanthus (ep-e-kan'thus), a condition in which a piece of skin extends over the inner slit between the eyelids.
epiphora (e-pif'o-rah), an overflow of tears due to a pathological narrowing of the tear duct and insufficient drainage.
esophoria (es-o-fo're-ah), an inward squint.
exophoria (eks-o-fo're-ah), an outward squint.
exophthalmos, protrusion of the eyeball.
fovea, the central depression of the retina.
fundus oculi, the rear of the eye opposite the cornea.
glaucoma, a disease characterized by abnormally high pressure within the eye, resulting in blindness.
glioma (of the retina) (gli-o'mah), a malignant growth of the retina.
hemeralopia (hem-er-al-o'pe-ah), day blindness; incorrectly, night blindness.
hemianopia (hem-e-an-o'pe-ah), blindness confined to one-half of each eye.
heterophoria (het-er-o-fo're-ah), deviation of the movements of the two eyes.
hordeolum (hor-de'o-lum), a sty.
humor, the fluids of the eyes.
hyalitis (hi-a-li'tis), inflammation of the vitreous body.
hypermetropia (hi-per-me-tro'pe-ah), farsightedness; hyperopia.
hyperopia, farsightedness.
iridectomy, excision of a part of the iris.
iridocyclitis (ir-id-o-sik-li'tis), inflammation of the iris and of the ciliary structures.
iris, the contractile circle around the pupil, which determines the color of the eyes.
iritis, inflammation of the iris.
keratectomy (ker-at-ek'to-me), removal of part of the cornea.
keratitis, inflammation of the cornea.
keratocentesis (ker-at-o-sen-te'sis), puncture of the cornea.
lacrimal, pertaining to tears.
lacrimal glands, the glands that secrete tears.
lacrimation, the secretion of tears.
lacrimotomy (lak-rim-ot'o-me), incision of the lacrimal sac or duct.
macula corneae (mak'u-lah kor'ne-a), a corneal opacity.
microphthalmos (mi-krof-thal'mus), abnormal smallness of the eye.

miosis (mī-o'sis), extreme contraction of the pupil.
miotic, an agent that causes the contraction of the pupil.
mydriasis (mid-rī'as-is), extreme dilation of the pupil.
mydriatic, an agent that causes the dilation of the pupil.
myopia (mī-o'pe-ah), nearsightedness.
nebula, in ophthalmology, an opacity of the cornea.
nystagmus (nis-tag'mus), involuntary oscillations of the eyeballs.
ocular, pertaining to the eye.
ophthalmia (of-thal'me-ah), infectious inflammation of the eye or of the conjunctiva; conjunctivitis.
ophthalmic, pertaining to the eye.
ophthalmitis, inflammation of an eye.
ophthalmometer, an instrument for measuring and examining the eye.
ophthalmopathy (of-thal-mop'ath-e), any disease of the eye.
ophthalmoplegia, paralysis of the ocular muscles.
ophthalmoscope, an instrument for examining the interior of the eye.
orbit, the eye socket.
pannus, the spread of granulation tissue over the cornea.
papilla (nervi optici), the optic disk.
papilledema, a swelling of the optic disk.
perimeter (per-im'e-ter), an instrument for measuring the extent of the visual field.
photophobia, fear of light or pain caused by bright light.
presbyopia (pres-be-o'pe-ah), increasingly defective vision characteristic of advanced age.
proptosis (See exophthalmos.)
pterygium (ter-ij'e-um), a thickening of the conjunctiva.
ptosis (to'sis), a pathological drooping of the eyelid.
pupil, the round opening in the iris.
refraction, (1) the deflection of light rays by the transparent eye structures. (2) correction of refractional error.
retina, the inner structure of the eye, which receives the optical images and which is connected with the brain by the optical nerve.
retinitis, inflammation of the retina.
retinoblastoma (ret-ī-no-blas-to'mah), a malignant tumor of the retina.
retinopathy (ret-i-nop'a-the), any diseased condition of the retina.
retinoscopy, inspection of the retina.
retrobulbar, behind the eyeball.
sclera, the hard, white part of the eye.
sclerectomy, the cutting out of a part of the sclera.
scotoma (sko-to'mah), cloudy or blind spots in front of the eyes.
staphyloma (staf-il-o'mah), protrusion of the cornea or sclera.
strabismus, a squint.
sty, a furuncle or inflammation on the eyelid.
tenotomy (ten-ot'o-me), the cutting of an eye muscle to correct a squint.
trachoma (tra-ko'mah), a contagious disease of the conjunctiva.
vitreous, the transparent gelatinous substance between the retina and the lens.

Orthopedics (including Physical Medicine)

abduction, drawing away from the middle line or center.
ankylosis (ang-kil-o'sis), pathological immobility of a joint.
antagonist, a muscle that balances the effects of another muscle.
arthrosis, a disease of a joint.
articulate, to unite by joints.
articulation, union by joints.
astragalectomy (as-trag-al-ek'to-me), surgical removal of the astragalus.
astragalus, one of the bones forming the ankle joint.
atrophia, atrophy.
atrophic, pertaining to atrophy.
atrophy of disuse, a wasting caused by lack of exercise.
bursitis, inflammation of a bursa.
calcification, hardening of the tissues by deposits of calcium salts.
calisthenics, a system of gymnastics.
capsule, any capsular ligament.

cartilage, an elastic substance covering the end of bones and forming joints or a connection between bones.
circumduction, the circular movement of a limb.
coccygodynia (kok-sig-o-din'e-ah), pain in and around the coccyx.
Colles fracture, break above the wrist joint.
collum, the neck; any necklike part.
compound fracture, a fracture in which the bones penetrate the skin.
condyle (kon'dīl), a rounded eminence at the end of some bones, e.g., in the knee joint.
contraction, (1) the normal shortening of a muscle in motion. (2) a pathological shortening due to injury or disease.
coraco-acromial (kor-ak-o-ak-ro'me-al), relating to the coracoid and acromion processes. (Both are bony processes of the scapula.)
coxa (kok'sah), the hip or hip joint.
coxa valga, deformity of the hip joint.
coxalgia, coxalgy, pain in or disease of the hip joint.
cubitus (ku'bit-us), the forearm.
cubitus valgus, inward deviation of the forearm.
cubitus varus, outward deviation of the forearm.
cuneiform (ku-ne'if-orm), wedge shaped; a wedge-shaped bone. (Applied to three bones in the foot and one in the wrist.)
curvature, Pott's, abnormal bending of the spine, due to a disease of the vertebrae.
decalcification, loss of calcium from the bones.
deformation, deformity, disfigurement or malformation of the body.
diaphysis (dī-af'is-is), the shaft of a long bone.
dislocation, displacement, especially of a broken bone.
disseminated, widely spread (said of a disease).
disuse atrophy, a wasting due to lack of function.
dorsal, pertaining to the back.
dorsum, the back; the back of any part or organ.
dystonia (dis-to'ne-ah), abnormality in muscle tone.

dystrophy (dis'tro-fe), a special disease of the muscles.
epicondyle (ep-e-kon'dīl), bony processes at the elbow.
extension, stretching of a limb.
extensor, a muscle that effects an extension.
fascia (fash'e-ah), a sheet or strip of fibrous tissue that covers the muscles.
fibrosis, the formation of fibrous tissue
flexor, a muscle that bends a joint.
fracture, a break.
genu, (jen'u), the knee.
gonitis (go-nī'tis), inflammation of the knee.
greenstick fracture, an incomplete break of one side of a bone.
insertion, the place where a muscle is attached to the part that it moves.
kyphosis (kī-fo'sis), humpback.
lordosis, curvature of the spinal column toward the front.
lumbago, lower back pain.
lumbosacral, pertaining to the loins and sacrum.
luxation, dislocation.
malleolus, the rounded processes of the tibia and fibula.
microtherm, an apparatus for the production of heat rays by means of electric waves.
mobilization, the process of moving a stiff joint.
muscularis, the muscular coat of an organ.
myopathy (mī-op'a-the), any disease of the muscles.
myositis (mī-o-sī'tis), inflammation of a muscle, generally a voluntary muscle.
olecranon (o-lek'ran-on), a part of the ulna forming the elbow.
os (pl. ossa), bone, bones.
osseous (os'e-us), bony.
ossification, the formation of bony tissue.
osteochondritis (os-te-o-kon-drī'tis), inflammation of bone and cartilage.
osteoporosis, the condition in which a bone becomes abnormally porous.
periarthric (per-e-ar'thrik), around a joint.
perichondrium (per-e-kon'dre-um), the membrane that envelops cartilage.
periosteum (per-e-os'te-um), the fibrous membrane covering a bone.
poliomyelitis (pōl-e-o-mī-el-ī'tis), inflammation of the gray substance of

the spine, especially of the anterior horns; infantile paralysis.
polyarthritis, inflammation of several joints.
Potts fracture, break above the ankle joint.
pyarthrosis (pī-ar-thro'sis), pus in a joint.
recalcification, the process of restoring calcium to the bones.
reduction, the process of setting a fracture or a dislocation.
rehabilitation, the process of restoring a physically handicapped patient to a useful life and possibly a gainful occupation.
resection, the cutting out of part of a bone (or a nerve).
rickets, a softening of the bones, due to lack of calcium caused by vitamin D deficiency.
sacroiliac, pertaining to the sacrum and ilium.
slipped disk, a displacement of the disk between two vertebrae.
spina, the spine.

splint, an appliance for the support or immobilization of injured parts.
spondylitis (spon-dil-ī'tis), inflammation of a vertebra.
stellar fracture, a star-shaped break.
styloid, a pencil-shaped prominence on a bone.
supination, rotating the hands outward.
synchondrosis (sin-kon-dro'sis), the connection of bones by cartilage.
synovia (sin-o've-ah), the fluid in a joint cavity, which serves as a lubricant.
synovial, pertaining to synovia.
synovitis, inflammation of a synovial membrane.
talipes (tal'ip-ez), clubfoot.
tendon, the fibrous end of a muscle attached to a movable part.
tendovaginal, pertaining to a tendon sheath.
tendovaginitis, inflammation of a tendon sheath.
traction, a drawing or pulling, as of a leg to keep it from shortening.
ultrasonic, pertaining to air waves with a higher frequency than sound waves.

Otology, Rhinology, and Laryngology

acusticus (a-kus'tik-us), the auditory nerve.
adenoids (ad'en-oids), enlargement of the adenoid tissue in the nasal pharynx of children.
alveolus (*pl.* alveoli) (al-ve'o-lus), (1) the small air cells of the lung. (2) the socket of a tooth.
anosmia (an-os'me-ah), lack or loss of the sense of smell.
antrum (*pl.* antra), a cavity in a bone, especially in the upper jawbone.
aphonia, loss of voice.
audiogram, the record or chart of the information obtained by means of the audiometer.
audiometer, an instrument for testing hearing capacity and determining hearing defects.
auditory, pertaining to the sense of hearing.
auricle, the external ear.
bronchi (bron'ki), the two main branches of the trachea.

bronchia, the bronchial tubes smaller than the bronchi.
bronchioles, very small bronchial tubes.
bronchiolitis, inflammation of the bronchioles.
bronchitis, inflammation of the bronchi.
cannula, a small tube.
cerumen (se-ru'men), earwax.
cochlea (kok'le-ah), a spiral-formed tube in the inner ear.
concha (a shell), (1) the hollow part of the external ear; (2) one of the turbinated bones.
coryza (ko-rī'zah), the common cold.
decibel, a unit used for the measurement of hearing. It is the smallest increase in sound intensity perceived by the human ear.
diplacusis (dip-la-ku'sis), hearing a sound differently in each ear.
epiglottis, the fold of tissue at the entrance of the larynx.
epiglottitis, inflammation of the epiglottis.

epistaxis (ep-is-tak'sis), nosebleed.
ethmoid bone, the spongelike bone separating the nasal cavities from the brain cavity.
ethmoid sinus, the sinuses in the ethmoid bone.
ethmoiditis (eth-moi-di'tis), inflammation of the ethmoid bone.
eustachian tube (u-sta'ke-an), the tube connecting the pharynx with the middle ear.
fenestration, the making of an opening (window) in the bone forming one of the semicircular canals in the ear.
frontal sinus, the sinuses located in the forehead.
glottis, the opening of the larynx.
labyrinth (lab'ir-inth), a part of the internal ear.
laryngitis, inflammation of the larynx.
laryngoscopy (lar-in-gos'ko-pe), inspection of the interior of the larynx by means of the laryngoscope.
larynx, the organ containing the vocal cords.
mastoid, the part of the temporal bone behind the external ear.
mastoidectomy (mas toi dek'to-me), excision of part or all of the mastoid process.
mastoiditis (mas-toi-di'tis), inflammation within the mastoid process.
maxillary sinuses, the sinuses in the upper jaw connecting with the nose, also called antrum or antra.
meatus acusticus (me-a'tus a-kus'tik-us), the opening of the outer ear.
myringitis (mir-in-ji'tis), inflammation of the eardrum.
myringotomy (mir-in-got'o-me), incision of the eardrum.
naris (*pl.* **nares**), a nostril.
nasofrontal, pertaining to the nasal and frontal bones.
olfaction, the sense of smell.
otalgia, pain in the ear.
otic, pertaining to the ear.
otitis, inflammation of the ear.
otorrhea (o-to-re'ah), a discharge from the ear.
otoscope, an instrument for inspecting the ear.
ozena, a disease of the nose with an ill-smelling discharge.
pansinusitis, inflammation of all the sinuses.

paracentesis (par-ah-sen-te'sis), surgical puncture of the eardrum.
parotid, situated near the ear.
parotis, the salivary gland below the ear.
peritonsillar (per-it-on'sil-ar), around the tonsils.
petrosa, a part of the temporal bone.
petrositis, inflammation of cells within the petrosa.
pharyngitis (far-in-ji'tis), inflammation of the pharynx.
pharynx, the sac between the mouth, nose, and esophagus.
polypus, a tumor which grows on mucous membranes.
pretracheal (pre-tra'ke-al), in front of the trachea.
retropharyngeal (re-tro-far-in'je-al), behind the pharynx.
rheum, rheuma, any watery or catarrhal discharge.
rhinitis (ri-ni'tis), inflammation of the nasal mucous membrane.
rhinoscopy (ri-nos'ko-pe), the inspection of the nasal passages by means of a rhinoscope.
salpingitis (sal-pin-ji'tis), inflammation of the eustachian tube.
septum, the partition that separates the two nasal cavities.
septum alveoli, the thin bony plate between the tooth sockets (alveoli).
sinus, a cavity in one of the cranial bones communicating with the nose. These are the ethmoid, frontal, maxillary, and sphenoid sinuses.
sinusitis, inflammation of a sinus.
sphenoid bone (sfe'noid), a bone at the base of the skull over the nasal cavities behind the ethmoid bone.
sphenoid sinus, the sinuses within the sphenoid bone.
sphenoiditis (sfe-noi-di'tis), inflammation of the sphenoid sinus.
tinnitus (tin-it'us), a ringing sound in the ears.
tonsil, a small lobe-shaped organ on each side within the throat.
tonsillectomy, removal of tonsils.
tonsillitis, inflammation of a tonsil.
trachea (tra'ke-ah), the windpipe.
tracheitis (tra-ke-i'tis), inflammation of the trachea.
turbinated bone, turbinal, one of three shell-like bones of the nasal structure originating from the upper jawbone.

tympanic, pertaining to the tympanum.
tympanum, the middle ear; also the eardrum.
uvula, the small cone-shaped body hanging from the palate.

vestibule, the oval cavity at the entrance of the internal ear.
Vincent's angina, an infectious disease affecting the throat, mouth, and gums. Same as trench mouth.

Pediatrics

angina (an-jī'na), a severe sore throat with symptoms of strangling.
Binet-Simon test (be-na'se-mon'), a test to determine the intelligence of children in relation to their age level.
chickenpox, an infectious disease with blister formation.
chorea (ko-re'ah), a disease marked by involuntary and irregular movements; St. Vitus's dance.
choreiform (ko-re'if-orm), resembling chorea.
convulsions, violent involuntary muscular contractions.
croup (kroop), an inflammation of the throat marked by difficulty of breathing and spasms of coughing.
dextrinized food, food that has been prepared so that the starchy base has been converted into soluble carbohydrates.
Dick test, a test for determining the degree of susceptibility or immunity to scarlet fever.
diphtheria (dif-the're-ah), an infectious disease due to the diphtheria (Loeffler) bacillus.
encephalitis (en-sef-al-ī'tis), inflammation of the brain due to a virus.
enuresis (en-u-re'sis), lack of control regarding the voiding of urine.
erythroblastosis foetalis (e-rith-ro-blas-tō'sis fe-tal'is), a pathological blood condition in the newborn due to negative Rh in the mother and positive Rh in the father and child.
gamma globulin (glob'u-lin), a protein used at present as prophylaxis in poliomyelitis.
German measles, a disease resembling measles, with light pink eruptions and a short course.
hydrocephalus (hī-dro-sef'a-lus), an abnormally enlarged head, due to an excessive amount of fluid in the brain.
intussusception (in-tus-sus-sĕp'shun), the slipping of one part of the intestine into another.
idioglossia (id-e-o-glos'e-ah), a condition in which speech is infantile and unintelligible.
lalling, the persistence of infantile speech.
measles (me'zelz), a contagious fever due to a virus.
mongolism, a form of idiocy in children.
nanism (na'nizm), stunted growth; dwarfism.
parotitis (par-ot-ī'tis), inflammation of the parotid gland; mumps.
pertussis (per-tus'is), whooping cough.
poliomyelitis (pol-e-ō-mī-el-ī'tis), inflammation of the gray matter of the spinal cord, especially of the anterior horns; infantile paralysis.
puberty, the age at which reproduction becomes possible.
pyknolepsy (pik'no-lep-se), frequent brief attacks of loss of consciousness occurring in children, resembling very mild epilepsy.
rachitis (ra-kī'tis), same as rickets.
Rh factor. If the father and the child are Rh positive and the mother Rh negative, mother and child are antagonistic. As a result destruction of red blood cells takes place in the child, called erythroblastosis (formerly "blue baby").
(See also General Medicine, page 378.)
rickets, a condition in which the bones do not harden normally owing to insufficient deposition of calcium salts in the bones.
roseola infantum (ro-ze'o-lah in-fan'-tum), a fever with a rose-colored rash.
rubella, German measles.
rubeola (ru-be'o-lah), (1) measles. (2) rubella.
St. Vitus's dance, same as chorea.
scarlatina, a contagious, infectious fever with a scarlet rash; scarlet fever.

scarlet fever (See scarlatina.)
Schick test, a test for the determination of susceptibility to diphtheria.
scorbutus (skor-bu′tus), same as scurvy.
scurvy, a disease due to a deficient diet.
tapeworm, a parasitic worm in the intestines.

toxin-antitoxin, a mixture used for vaccination against diphtheria.
varicella (var-is-el′ah), chickenpox.
variola (var-i′o-lah), smallpox.
whooping cough (hoop′ing), an infection of the respiratory tract with spasms of coughing; pertussis.

Proctology

anal (a′nal), pertaining to the anus.
anoscope, an instrument for inspecting the lower part of the rectum.
anus, the opening of the rectum.
Ascaris, an intestinal parasite.
ataxic sphincter, slow or incomplete contraction of the anus.
cecostomy (se-kos′to-me), making an artificial opening into the cecum.
colitis, inflammation of the colon.
colopexy (kol′o-pek-se), the attaching of the lower part of the colon to the abdominal wall by surgical means.
condyloma (kon-dil-o′mah), a wartlike growth in or around the anus or vulva.
dermoid, rectal, a cyst in the rectum.
fissure, anal, a painful ulcer at the margin of the anus.
fistula, anal, a deep ulcer near the anus, sometimes extending to the rectum.
giardiasis (ge-ar-di′as-is), infestation of the intestines with the Giardia microorganism.
hemorrhoid, a tumor consisting of varicose veins at the anus; a pile. **external** ∼, hemorrhoids situated outside the anus; **internal** ∼, hemorrhoids situated above the anus.
hemorrhoidectomy, the cutting out of hemorrhoids.
levator ani, the muscle that lifts the rectum.
pararectal, next to the rectum.
pectenosis, an abnormal narrowing of the anal canal caused by contracting scar tissue.
perianal, situated around the anus.
perineum, the space between the anus and the genital organs.
piles, see hemorrhoid.
procidentia (pro-sid-en′she-ah), a complete prolapse of an organ.
proctectasia (prok-tek-ta′ze-ah), dilatation of the rectum.

proctectomy, excision of the rectum.
proctitis, inflammation of the rectum.
proctodynia (prok-to-din′e-ah), pain in or around the anus or the rectum.
proctoparalysis, paralysis of the rectal and anal muscles.
proctoptosis (prok-top-to′sis), prolapse of the rectum.
proctoscope, an instrument for inspecting the rectum.
proctosigmoiditis (prok-to-sig-moi-di′tis), inflammation of both the rectum and the sigmoid.
proctotomy (prok-tot′o-me), the surgical incision through an anal or a rectal stricture.
prolapse, the protrusion of an organ (anus, rectum, or colon).
pruritus ani, itching at the anus.
raphe, anal (ra′fe), the ridge of skin extending from the anus to the coccyx.
raphe, perineal, the ridge of skin extending from the anus across the perineum.
rectitis, inflammation of the rectum.
rectum, the lowest part of the large intestine.
sigmoid, (1) the lower end of the colon, ending in the rectum. (2) shaped like the letter s.
sigmoiditis, inflammation of the lower end of the colon.
sigmoidoscope, an instrument for examining the interior of the sigmoid.
sigmoidoscopy, examination of the sigmoid by means of the sigmoidoscope.
sphincter ani, the ringlike muscle which closes the anus.
suppository, a cone-shaped, medicated preparation for insertion into the rectum or the urethra.
tenesmus (te-nez′mus), straining while trying to urinate or to empty the bowels.

Radiology

actinic rays, the rays of radiant energy capable of producing chemical and thermal changes.
alpha particles, positively charged particles given off from radioactive substances.
alpha rays, streams of matter made up of alpha particles.
ammeter, same as amperemeter.
ampere, the unit used in the measurement of the amount of electricity.
amperemeter, an instrument for measuring amperage.
angiocardiography (an-je-o-car-de-og'ra-fe), radiographic visualization of the heart and vessels.
angstrom unit, a unit of wave length.
anode, the positive electrode.
anteroposterior, pertaining to x-rays that penetrate the body from the front toward the back.
applicators, instruments for the use of radium and other radioactive substances in local application. They may be tubes, needles, or glazed-surface plaques.
arteriography (ar-te-re-og'ra-fe), radiographic visualization of the arteries.
atom, the smallest particle into which an element can be broken up.
atomic energy, the energy released by disintegrating atoms.
atomic fission, a process during which the nucleus of an atom is split.
atomic number, a number assigned to all the elements, based upon atomic structure.
atomic weight, a number which represents the actual weight of the nucleus.
barium sulphate, a compound used in roentgenology because of its opacity to roentgen rays.
beta rays, electrons thrown out at high speed from radioactive atoms.
bronchography (bron-kog'ra-fe), radiographic examination of the bronchial tree.
Bucky diaphragm, Bucky-Potter diaphragm, a grid used in roentgenology to filter out secondary rays.
cassette, the container in which the film is placed when taking an x-ray picture.
cathode, the negative electrode.
choke coil, an instrument to control the strength of alternating current.
cholecystography (ko-le-sis-tog'raf-e), examination of the gall bladder with roentgen rays by means of injecting or swallowing x-ray opaque substances that are excreted into the bile and that thus make the gall bladder visible on x-ray films.
circuit, the round or course traveled by an electrical current.
coil, windings of insulated wire.
condenser, an apparatus by which charges of electricity can be accumulated.
conduction, the transfer of electricity.
conductivity, the capacity of a body to conduct an electrical current.
Coolidge tube, a vacuum tube for the generation of x-rays.
curie (ku're), the quantity of radium emanation in equilibrium with 1 gram of radium element. Used as a unit of measurement (named after the discoverers of radium).
current, the stream of electricity that moves along a conductor. **alternating ~,** a current that periodically flows in opposite directions. **direct ~,** a current flowing in one direction.
cycle, the unit of frequency of alternating current.
damping, decreasing the amplitude of the oscillations of an electric current.
density, (1) the number or quantity of rays per square unit. (2) the degree of blackening of the x-ray film.
diaphragm, Bucky (See Bucky diaphragm.)
dielectric (di-e-lek'trik), an insulating substance.
dosimetry, a method for determining the amount of energy.
electron, a particle of matter carrying a negative charge.
electron microscope, a microscope which uses streams of electrons instead of light to dissolve details, thereby making visible submicroscopic structures.
emanation, a gaseous substance given off from radioactive matter.

encephalography (en-cef-a-log′ra-fe), radiographic examination of the brain.

erythema (er-ith-e′mah), a redness of the skin, such as develops in sunburn or after intense x-ray treatments.

erythema dose, the minimum amount of application of rays that produces erythema.

filament, the thread of wire in the tube which, when heated up, is the origin of the high-speed free electrons that bombard the target and produce the x-rays.

filter, a metal screen used to filter out certain rays that may produce harmful effects.

fluorescence (flu-or-es′ens), the ability of a substance to emit a bluish light after being exposed to certain rays.

fluoroscope, an apparatus for examining internal structures and organs by means of the roentgen rays.

gamma rays, very short and therefore highly penetrating rays given off by radioactive substances.

Geiger counter, an instrument for the detection and measurement of radiation (alpha, beta, and gamma rays).

grenz rays, rays whose wave length lies somewhere between the x-rays and ultraviolet rays.

high frequency, a term applied to an alternating current having a rate of alternation or oscillation exceeding the rate at which muscular contraction ceases; that is, more than 40,000 per second.

impedance (im-pe′dans), the opposition offered in a coil to the flow of an alternating current.

implantation, the introduction of applicators containing radioactive substances into the tissues.

inductance, the generation of an electrical current in a coil by a magnetic field.

insulator, any substance or appliance made of some nonconducting material used in preventing the passage of electricity.

ion, an atom or group of atoms being positively or negatively electrified.

irradiation, treatment by roentgen rays or other forms of radioactivity.

isotope (ī′so-tōp), an atom of the same atomic number and chemical properties but different atomic weight. **radioactive** ∼, an element or a substance which has been made radioactive.

kilovolt, a unit of 1,000 volts.

meson, a particle of the atom, about 300 times the mass of an electron, with either a negative or a positive electric charge.

microcurie (mī-kro-ku′re), one-millionth of a curie.

microgram, one-millionth of a gram.

milliampere, one-thousandth part of an ampere.

milliamperemeter, an instrument to measure amperage in units of milliamperes.

millicurie, one-thousandth of a curie.

milligram, one-thousandth of a gram.

molecule, an aggregation of atoms.

myelography (mī-e-log′ra-fe), a method of taking x-rays of the spinal subarachnoid space.

neutron, a particle of matter which carries no electric charge.

nuclear energy, the energy stored by the nucleus in the atom and which is released when the nucleus disintegrates, or is split.

nucleus (new′kle-us), the core of the atom, which is said to contain the protons and neutrons.

ohm, the unit of electric resistance.

orthodiagraph (or-tho-dī′a-graf), an apparatus for determining the size of an organ in fluoroscopy.

pneumography (nu-mog′ra-fe), a method of taking x-rays of the lungs.

polarity, the positive or negative state with reference to the two poles of electricity.

positioning, the placing of the part to be x-rayed in that position which is known to give the best photographic results.

positron, a particle of matter which is said to have the same mass and an equal amount of electrical charge as an electron but which is charged positively.

posterior-anterior, pertaining to x-rays penetrating the body from the back toward the front.

potential, the degree of electrification in reference to some standard (as of the earth).

proton, a part of the nucleus of an atom bearing a positive charge of electricity.
pyelography (pī-e-log'ra-fe), a method of taking x-rays of the kidneys.
quantum, the basic unit of radiant energy.
radiant, emitting rays.
radiation, the transfer through space of any form of energy, such as light, heat, or x-rays.
radioactive, pertaining to radioactivity.
radioactivity, the process of emitting energy, such as alpha, beta, and gamma rays.
radiogram, same as radiograph.
radiograph, a photograph made by x-rays; an x-ray picture.
radiosensitivity, the standard by which the reaction of a cell to irradiation is judged.
radiothermy, therapeutical use of radiant energy.
radium, a radioactive element.
radiumologist, a specialist in treatment with radium.
rectifier, an apparatus for changing an alternating current into direct current.
resistance, the opposition of a substance to the passage of an electric current.
Roentgen, W. K., German physicist and discoverer of x-rays.
roentgen, a unit used as x-ray dosage.
roentgen rays, electromagnetic waves of very short wave length, which penetrate many substances, affect a photographic film, cause chemical reactions, and produce changes in living matter; x-rays.
roentgenization (runt-gen-iz-a'shun), exposure to roentgen rays.

roentgenograph (runt-gen'o-graf), same as radiograph, radiogram, or roentgenogram.
roentgenology (runt-gen-ol'o-je), the diagnostic and therapeutical application of roentgen rays.
roentgenotherapy, the use of roentgen rays in the treatment of disease.
shadow box, an apparatus with an illuminator for viewing x-ray films.
spectrum, a chart of electromagnetic waves arranged in the order of wave length.
stereoscope (ster'e-o-skōp), an apparatus that combines two radiographs in such a way that the eyes see the picture in three dimensions.
tracer substance, a substance which is radioactive and which therefore can be traced by means of a Geiger counter in its course through the organism.
transformer, an apparatus for changing electrical energy at one voltage to electrical energy at another voltage. A transformer is needed for obtaining the high voltage necessary for the generation of x-rays.
tube, a sealed glass bulb that emits the x-rays.
urography (u-rog'ra-fe), a method of taking x-rays of the urinary tract.
ventriculography (ven-trik-u-log'ra-fe), radiographic examination of the ventricles of the brain.
volt, a unit of electrical tension.
voltmeter, an instrument to measure voltage.
watt, a unit of electrical energy.
x-rays, see **roentgen rays.**

Urology

anuresis (an-u-re'sis), complete suppression of the voiding of urine.
anuria, same as **anuresis.**
aspermia, lack or insufficient secretion of semen.
balanitis, inflammation of the glans penis.
bladder, the sac that holds the urine.
bougie, a narrow, rigid cylinder for introduction into the urethra, cervix, or any other orifice.

Bright's disease, nephritis.
calculus, an abnormal solid mass in the bladder, gall bladder, biliary passages, or the kidneys, commonly called a stone.
catheter, a narrow tube of rubber, metal, or glass for emptying the bladder or the kidney.
catheterization (kath-e-ter-iz-a'shun), emptying the bladder by means of a catheter.

chancre, the primary syphilitic sore.
circumcision, removal of the foreskin.
cystitis (sis-tī'tis), inflammation of the bladder.
cystopyelonephritis (sis-to-pī-e-lo-nef-rī'tis), inflammation of both the bladder and the pelvis of the kidney.
cystoscope (sis'to-skōp), an instrument for inspection of the interior of the bladder.
cystospasm, spasm of the bladder.
cystotomy (sis-tot'o-me), making an incision into the bladder.
diuretic (dī-u-ret'ik), that which increases the secretion of urine.
dysuria (dis-u're-ah), difficult or painful urination.
enuresis (en-u-rē'sis), involuntary voiding of urine.
epididymis (ep-id-id'im-is), an oval body on the upper part of each testicle.
epididymitis, inflammation of the epididymis.
fibrolipoma, a tumor composed of fibrous tissue and fat.
glans penis, the end of the penis.
gonorrhea, a venereal disease due to the gonococcus.
gravel, sandlike concrete matter in the kidney or bladder.
gumma, a soft, gummy tumor, the tertiary form of syphilis.
hydrocele (hī'dro-sēl), an abnormal collection of fluid within the capsule of a testis.
hydronephrosis (hī-dro-nef-ro'sis), an abnormal accumulation of urine in the kidney, which causes the formation of a cyst.
kidneys, the two organs that secrete the urine.
micturition (mik-tu-re'shun), the voiding of urine.
Neisseria, the gonococcus.
nephralgia, pain in a kidney.
nephritis, inflammation of the kidneys.
nephrolithiasis (nef-ro-lī-thī'a-sis), the formation of kidney stones.
nephrolithotomy (nef-ro-lith-ot'o-me), the surgical removal of a stone from the kidney.
nephroptosis (nef-rop-to'sis), "floating kidney."
nephrosis, any degenerative disease of the kidney.
orchidectomy, orchiectomy (or-kid-ek'to-me, or-ke-ek'to-me), removal of a testis.
orchiditis, same as **orchitis.**
orchidoncus (or-kid-ong'kus), a tumor of a testicle.
orchidopathy (or-kid-op'ath-e), any disease of a testis.
orchiodynia (or-ke-o-din'e-ah), pain in a testicle.
orchitis (or-kī'tis), inflammation of a testis.
penis, the male organ.
perinephritis (per-e-nef-rī'tis), inflammation of the perinephrium.
perinephrium, the tissues around the kidneys.
periureteric (per-e-u-re-ter'ik), around the ureter.
periurethral (per-e-u-reth'ral), around the urethra.
phimosis (fi-mo'sis), an abnormally narrow opening of the foreskin.
posthitis (pos-thī'tis), inflammation of the foreskin.
prepuce, the circular fold of skin surrounding the glans penis; the foreskin.
prostate, a gland in the male located around the neck of the bladder and the urethra.
prostatectomy (pros-tat-ek'to-me), excision of a part of the prostate.
prostatic, pertaining to the prostate gland.
prostatitis, inflammation of the prostate gland.
pyelitis (pī-el-ī'tis), inflammation of the pelvis of the kidney.
pyelograph, a roentgenogram (x-ray picture) of the kidney and ureter.
pyelolithotomy (pī-el-o-lith-ot'o-me), the surgical removal of a stone from the pelvis of the kidney.
pyelonephritis, inflammation of the kidney and its pelvis.
pyelonephrosis (pī-el-o-nef-ro'sis), a disease of the kidney and its pelvis.
pyonephritis (pī-o-nef-rī'tis), inflammation of the kidney with pus formation.
pyonephrosis, pus formation in the pelvis of the kidney.
pyuria (pī-u're-ah) pus in the urine.
renal, pertaining to the kidney.
scrotal, pertaining to the scrotum.
scrotum, the pouch containing the testicles.

semen, the fluid produced by the testes containing the spermatozoa.

spermatozoa (*sing.* **spermatozoon**) (sper-mah-to-zo′ah), the motile constituents of the semen that fertilize the ovum.

stricture, the pathologic narrowing or closure of any passage.

testicles, the testes.

testis, the male reproductive gland.

ureter (u-re′ter), the tube connecting the kidney with the bladder.

ureteral, pertaining to the ureter.

ureteritis, inflammation of the ureter.

urethra, the canal through which the urine is voided.

urethrophraxis (u-re-thro-frak′sis), obstruction of the urethra.

urethroscope (u-re′thro-skōp), an instrument for inspecting the interior of the urethra.

urinalysis, the chemical analysis of the urine.

urolithiasis (u-ro-lith-ī′as-is), a pathologic condition marked by the formation of stones in the urinary tract.

vas deferens, a tube connecting the testicles with the urethra.

Check Lists

(This space may be used by the assistant for her own check lists, as has been suggested throughout the book.)

TABLE 1. *Centigrade and Fahrenheit Equivalents*

Centigrade, degrees	Fahrenheit, degrees	Centigrade, degrees	Fahrenheit, degrees
50	122	37.5	99.5
45	113	37	98.6
44	111.2	36.5	97.7
43	109.4	36	96.8
42	107.6	35.5	95.9
41	105.8	35	95
40.5	104.9	34	93.2
40	104	33	91.4
39.5	103.1	32	89.6
39	102.2	31	87.8
38.5	101.3	30	86
38	100.4		

To change degrees Fahrenheit to degrees centigrade, subtract 32 from the Fahrenheit reading and multiply the result by 0.555.

To change centigrade degrees to Fahrenheit degrees, multiply the centigrade reading by 1.8 and add 32 to the result.

TABLE 2. *Equivalent Values of Avoirdupois and Metric Weights*

Av. Ounces	Grams	Av. Pounds	Grams
1/16	1.772	1	453.59
1/8	3.544	2	907.18
1/4	7.088	2.2	1000.00
1/2	14.175	3	1360.78
1	28.350	4	1814.37
2	56.699	5	2267.96
3	85.049	6	2721.55
4	113.398	7	3175.15
5	141.748	8	3628.74
6	170.097	9	4082.33
7	198.447	10	4535.92
8	226.796		
9	255.146		
10	283.495		
11	311.845		
12	340.194		
13	368.544		
14	396.893		
15	425.243		

TABLE 3. *Metric Equivalents for Apothecaries' Measures (Volume, usually fluid)*

Minims	Cubic Centimeters	Fluidrachms	Cubic Centimeters	Fluidounces	Cubic Centimeters
1	0.06	1	3.70	1	29.57
2	0.12	2	7.39	2	59.15
3	0.19	3	11.09	3	88.72
4	0.25	4	14.79	4	118.29
5	0.31	5	18.48	5	147.87
6	0.37	6	22.18	6	177.44
7	0.43	7	25.88	7	207.01
8	0.49			8	236.58
9	0.55			9	266.16
10	0.62			10	295.73
11	0.68			11	325.30
12	0.74			12	354.88
13	0.80			13	384.45
14	0.86			14	414.02
15	0.92			15	443.59
16	0.99			16	473.17
17	1.05			17	502.74
18	1.11			18	532.31
19	1.17			19	561.89
20	1.23			20	591.46
25	1.54			21	621.03
30	1.85			22	650.60
35	2.16			23	680.18
40	2.46			24	709.75
45	2.77			25	739.32
50	3.08			26	768.90
55	3.39			27	798.47
				28	828.04
				29	857.61
				30	887.19
				31	916.76
				32	946.33
				48	1419.49
				56	1656.08
				64	1892.66
				72	2129.25
				80	2365.83
				96	2839.00
				112	3312.16
				128	3785.32

TABLE 4. *Apothecaries' Equivalents for Metric Measures (Volume, usually fluid)*

Cubic Centimeters	Fluidounces	Cubic Centimeters	Fluidrachms	Cubic Centimeters	Minims
30	1.01	5	1.35	0.05	0.81
50	1.69	6	1.62	0.07	1.14
75	2.54	7	1.89	0.09	1.46
100	3.38	8	2.17	1	16.23
200	6.76	9	2.43	2	32.5
300	10.15	10	2.71	3	48.7
400	13.53	25	6.76	4	64.9
473	16.00				
500	16.91				
600	20.29				
700	23.67				
800	27.05				
900	30.43				
1000	33.82				

TABLE 5. *Apothecaries' Equivalents for Metric Weights*

Grams	Exact Equivalents in Grains	Grams	Exact Equivalents in Grains
0.01	0.1543	12.0	185.189
0.02	0.3086	13.0	200.621
0.03	0.4630	14.0	216.054
0.04	0.6173	15.0	231.486
0.05	0.7716	16.0	246.918
0.06	0.9259	17.0	262.351
0.07	1.0803	18.0	277.783
0.08	1.2346	19.0	293.216
0.09	1.3889	20.0	308.648
0.1	1.543	21.0	324.080
0.2	3.086	22.0	339.513
0.3	4.630	23.0	354.945
0.4	6.173	24.0	370.378
0.5	7.716	25.0	385.810
0.6	9.259	26.0	401.242
0.7	10.803	27.0	416.674
0.8	12.346	28.0	432.107
0.9	13.889	29.0	447.538
1.0	15.432	30.0	462.971
2.0	30.865	31.0	478.403
3.0	46.297	32.0	493.835
4.0	61.730	40.0	617.294
5.0	77.162	45.0	694.456
6.0	92.594	50.0	771.618
7.0	108.027	60.0	925.942
8.0	123.459	70.0	1080.265
9.0	138.892	80.0	1234.589
10.0	154.324	90.0	1388.912
11.0	169.756	100.0	1543.236

TABLE 6. *Metric Equivalents for Apothecaries' Weights*

Grains	Grams	Grains	Grams
1/50	0.00130	50	3.240
1/32	0.00202	51	3.305
1/20	0.00324	52	3.370
1/18	0.00360	53	3.434
1/16	0.00405	54	3.499
1/15	0.00432	55	3.564
1/12	0.00540	56	3.629
1/10	0.00648	57	3.694
1/8	0.00810	58	3.758
1/6	0.01080	59	3.823
1/5	0.01296	60	3.888
1/4	0.01620	61	3.953
1/3	0.02160	62	4.018
1/2	0.03240	63	4.082
3/4	0.04860	64	4.147
1	0.0648	65	4.212
2	0.1296	66	4.277
3	0.1944	67	4.342
4	0.2592	68	4.406
5	0.3240	69	4.471
6	0.3888	70	4.536
7	0.4536	71	4.601
8	0.5184	72	4.666
9	0.5832	73	4.730
10	0.6480	74	4.795
11	0.7128	75	4.860
12	0.7776	76	4.925
13	0.8424	77	4.990
14	0.9072	78	5.054
15	0.9720	79	5.119
16	1.037	80	5.184
17	1.102	81	5.249
18	1.166	82	5.314
19	1.231	83	5.378
20	1.296	84	5.443
21	1.361	85	5.508
22	1.426	86	5.573
23	1.490	87	5.638
24	1.555	88	5.702
25	1.620	89	5.767
26	1.685	90	5.832
27	1.749	91	5.897
28	1.814	92	5.962
29	1.879	93	6.026
30	1.944	94	6.091
31	2.009	95	6.156
32	2.074	96	6.221
33	2.138	97	6.286
34	2.203	98	6.350
35	2.268	99	6.415
36	2.333	100	6.480
37	2.398	120	7.776
38	2.462	150	9.720
39	2.527	180	11.664
40	2.592	200	12.958
41	2.657	480	31.103
42	2.722	500	32.396
43	2.786	600	38.875
44	2.851	700	45.354
45	2.916	800	51.833
46	2.981	900	58.313
47	3.046	960	62.207
48	3.110	1000	64.799
49	3.175		

TABLE 7. *Equivalent Values of Metric and Linear Measures*

Inches	Centimeters	Inches	Millimeters
1	2.54	1/25	1.00
2	5.08	1/12	2.12
3	7.62	1/8	3.18
4	10.16	1/4	6.35
5	12.70	1/3	8.47
6	15.24	1/2	12.70
7	17.78	5/8	15.88
8	20.32	2/3	16.93
9	22.86	3/4	19.05
10	25.40	5/6	21.16
11	27.94	7/8	22.22
12	30.48	11/12	23.28

TABLE 8. *Equivalents of Common Household Measures*

1 drop	= 1 minim
1 teaspoonful	= 1 dram or 4 cc.
1 tablespoonful	= 4 dram or 16 cc.
1 wineglassful	= 2 fluidounces or 60 cc.
1 teacupful	= 4 fluidounces or 120 cc.
1 tumblerful	= 8 fluidounces or 240 cc.
12 tablespoonfuls	= 1 cup (powder)
16 tablespoonfuls	= 1 cup (liquid)

TABLE 9. *Preparation of Solutions*

Prescribed Strength	Amount of Full-strength Drug	Fluid to Be Added
1:1000	1 teaspoonful	1 gallon
1:1000	15 drops	1 quart
1/10 of 1%	15 drops	1 quart
1:500	2 teaspoonfuls	1 gallon
1:500	30 drops	1 quart
1/5 of 1%	30 drops	1 quart
1:200	5 teaspoonfuls	1 gallon
1:200	1¼ teaspoonfuls	1 quart
1/2 of 1%	1¼ teaspoonfuls	1 quart
1:100 (1%)	2½ teaspoonfuls	1 quart
1:50 (2%)	5 teaspoonfuls	1 quart
1:25 (4%)	2½ tablespoonfuls	1 quart
1:20 (5%)	3 tablespoonfuls	1 quart

Index

Abbreviations, medical, 367
Abdominal pain, first aid in, 207
  in pregnancy, 174
Accounts, doctors' (*see* Bookkeeping)
  patients' (*see* Bills; Ledger cards)
Acetest, 297
Acetone determination in urine, 297
Albumin determination in urine, 297–298
Albutest, 298
Allergy, definition of, 162–163
  diagnosis of, 163–164
  intradermal skin test in, 167
  patch test in, 165–167
  scratch test in, 164–165
Amorphous material in urine, *illus.*, 297
Anesthesia, general, 109–110
  inhaler for, *illus.*, 111
  local, 110–112
  in office, 109–112
Animal bites, first aid in, 207
Antigen-antibody reaction, 163
  (*see also* Allergy)
Antiseptics, 90
Apoplexy, first aid in, 208
Apothecaries' measures, metric equivalents of, 416–417
Apothecaries' weights, metric equivalents of, 417
Appearance of medical asistant, 11
Appointment book, page in, *illus.*, 225
Appointment cards, 226
Appointment system, 221–226

Appointments, canceled, by doctor, 228
  by patient, 227
  doctor's lateness for, 227–228
  making of, 221–227
  for out-of-office visits, 229–230
  scheduling of, 17, 19
Arch supports, making of model for, 195–196
Assistant, medical (*see* Medical assistant)
Attitude toward patients, 20–22
Audiogram, 203; *illus.*, 204
Audiometer, 201–204
Autoclave, *illus.*, 38, 43
Autoclaving, 38–44
  material prepared for, *illus.*, 41, 42
  (*See also* Sterilization)
Avoirdupois, metric equivalents of, 415

Bacteria, kinds of, 25–27
Bacteriologic smears (*see* Smears, bacteriologic)
Bacteriology, 23–27
Bag, doctor's, care of, 289
Bandages, reason for, 119
  types of, 119–123
    cravat, 123; *illus.*, 122
    plaster-impregnated, 194
    roller, 119–121; *illus.*, 120
    triangular, 121–122; *illus.*, 122
Basal metabolism rate, 325–326
Basal metabolism test, 325–341
  general instructions, 326–327

Basal metabolism test, Jones Air-Basal metabolism unit, 340; *illus.*, 341
  Jones Motor-Basal, 327–333; *illus.*, 328
    computation of results, 329–332
    connecting the patient, 327; *illus.*, 328
    making the test, 328–329
    preparation of apparatus, 327
    specimen tracings, 331–333; *illus.*, 331
  Sanborn Metabulator, 333–340; *illus.*, 333
    computation of results, 337–339
    connecting the patient, 335–336; *illus.*, 335
    making the test, 336–337
    operation of, 333
    preparing the apparatus, 334–335
    scale for computing results, *illus.*, 340
Bills, 254–256; *illus.*, 256
  collection of, 255–258
  in health insurance, 272–274
  itemized, 254–255
  in Workmen's Compensation, 276
Biopsy, gynecological, 170
Bleeding, first aid in, 208
Blood, composition of, 53–54
  occult, in urine, 298
Blood counts (*see* Hematology)
Blood diseases, 70–71
Blood pressure, average, 54–55
  meaning of, 54–56
  taking of, 53–58
    apparatus for, *illus.*, 57
    technique, 56–58; *illus.*, 58
Blue Cross insurance, 271, 277
Blue Shield insurance, 271–274, 277
Bookkeeping, 258–268
  cash and checks, handling of, 265–266
  payroll records, 264, 266–267
  petty cash, 267–268
Bookkeeping systems for doctors, 260
  Fagell system, 260–265
    analysis of office expenses, 262

Bookkeeping systems for doctors, Fagell system, annual summary of accounts, 262–263; *illus.*, 263–265
  daily record of disbursements, 261–262; *illus.*, 262–263
  daily record of receipts and charges, 260–261; *illus.*, 261
  employees' earning record, *illus.*, 267
  schedule of depreciation, 262–263
Braces, prescription of, 196
Bumintest, 297
Burns, first aid in, 210–211

Calorie, definition of, 153–154
  (*See also* Diet)
Canceling appointments, 227–228
Cardiology, terms pertaining to, 383–385
  (*See also* Electrocardiography)
Case history (*see* Medical history)
Centigrade, conversion of, to Fahrenheit, 415
  equivalents of, 415
Cervical coagulation, 172
Cholecystography, preparation of patient for, 146
Clinitest, 299–300
Collections (*see* Bills)
Convulsions, first aid in, 211
Convulsive treatment (*see* Shock therapy)
Cravat bandage, 123; *illus.*, 122
Crutches, teaching use of, 196–197

Decibel, definition of, 210
Deficiency diseases, 71
Degenerative diseases, 71–72
Dermatology, terms pertaining to, 385–387
  (*See also* Allergy)
Diabetes, test for determination of, 299–300
Diathermy, reason for use of, 130
  technique of application of, 131–134; *illus.*, 131–133
Diet, discussion of, 156–157
  prescription of, 156

INDEX

Diet, superstitions relating to, 149
  treatment by, 149–159
  types of, 155
Diet lists, 156–157
Dietary requirements, 153; *chart*, 154
Diopter, definition of, 188–189
Diplomates, 160–161
Disease, contagious, 5–6
  infectious, 5–6
  nature of, 68–72
  protection against, 5
  transmission of, 4–6
Disease groups, 68
Doctor and medical assistant, 9–10
Doctor's bag, care of, 289
  contents of, 289
Dosage (*see* Medications)
Dressings, application of, 118
  removal of, 119
  types of, 117–118
  (*See also* Bandages)
Drugs, for emergencies, 89
  types of, 77–79
  (*See also* Medications)
Dry heat, sterilization by, 44

Ear, *illus.*, 199
Ear specialist (*see* Otology)
Electrocardiogram, definition of, 340–343
Electrocardiography, 341–366
  apparatus for, 348–366
    Beck-Lee Cardi-all, 357–360
      completed record, 359–360; *illus.*, 359
      connecting the patient, 358
      making the test, 358–359
      paper, changing of, 360; *illus.*, 360
      preparing the apparatus, 358
    Beck-Lee string galvanometer, 348–356
      calibration of, 349–351
      camera, loading of, 356–357; *illus.*, 356, 357
      description of, 348–349
      developing of electrocardiogram, 355–356
      leads, identification of, 352–355

Electrocardiography, apparatus for, Sanborn Viso-Cardiette, 360–366; *illus.*, 361
    connecting the patient, 361–362
    leads, marking of, 363–364
    making the test, 362–363
    paper, changing of, 364–366; *illus.*, 364, 365
    preparing the apparatus, 361
    sample tracing, 363
  cardiac cycle, correlation of, with electrocardiogram, *illus.*, 345
  currents, direction of, 343–344; *illus.*, 344
  electrodes, application of, 346
  heart, *illus.*, 342, 343
  leads, position of, 346–348; *illus.*, 347
Electrosurgery, 139
  cervical coagulation by, 172
Electrotherapy (*see* Physical therapy)
Emergencies, first aid in (*see* First aid)
  during pregnancy, 174
Emergency drugs, 89
Emergency telephone calls, 234–235
Employees' earning records, 266–267
Enamelware, sterilization of, 34–35
Endocrinology, terms pertaining to, 387–389
Epileptic fits, first aid in, 211
Equipment, medical, care of, 281–282
Erythrocyte count, technique of, 305–308
Erythrocyte sedimentation rate, 316–317
Examination, of blood (*see* Hematology)
  of ear (*see* Otology)
  of eye (*see* Ophthalmology)
  gynecological, 169
  neurological, 176–177
  routine general, 48
    setup for, 47–48
  of urine (*see* Urine)

Examinations, helping with, 45–66
  methods of, 45–47
  preparing patient for, 49–50
    draping, *illus.*, 52
  (*See also* Specialist, assistant to)
Exercises, 137–138
  in orthopedics, 192–193
Eye, *illus.*, 184
Eye diseases, 191–192
Eye drops, instillation of, *illus.*, 187
Eye specialist (*see* Ophthalmology)
Eyeglasses, prescription of, 185–190

Fahrenheit, conversion of, to centigrade, 415
  equivalents of, 415
Fagell bookkeeping system (*see* Bookkeeping systems for doctors)
Fainting, first aid in, 211–212
Faradic current, 128
Fees, collection of (*see* Bills)
  discussion of, 252–253
  payment of, in cash, 253–254
Fever, meaning of, 61–62
  (*See also* Temperature)
Fever chart, *illus.*, 65
Fever thermometer (*see* Thermometer)
Filing practices, 247–248
  cross references in, 247
  for medical history, 245–247
  for out card, 247
  by subject, 247–248
First aid, 206–218
  do's and don'ts in, 217–218
  emergencies requiring, 206–217
    abdominal pain, 207
    animal bites, 207
    apoplexy, 208
    bleeding, 208
    burns, 210–211
    convulsions, 211
    epileptic fits, 211
    fainting, 211–212
    foreign bodies, 212–213
    heart attack, 213–214
    insect bites, 214–215
    poison ivy, 216
    poisoning, 215–216

First aid, emergencies requiring,
    shock, 216
    wounds, 216–217
  pressure points, *illus.*, 209
  supplies in, 218
Food, constituents of, 151
  (*See also* Diet)
Foods, basic, chart of, 154
Foreign bodies, in ear, 212
  in eye, 212–213
  swallowed, 213
Fungi, 27

Galvanic current, 128
  hand interrupter for, *illus.*, 129
Gastroenterology, terms pertaining to, 389–391
Gastrointestinal series, preparation of patient for, 145–146
General medicine, terms pertaining to, 370–381
Glandular disturbances, 71
Glasses, prescription of, 185–190
Glassware, sterilization of, 34
Gloves (*see* Rubber gloves)
Glycosuria, determination of, 299–300
Gram's-stain reaction, 323
Gram's-stain technique, 321–322
Grooming, 10–12
Gynecology, 167–172
  biopsy in, 170
  cervical coagulation, 172
  examination in, 169
  female reproductive organs, *illus.*, 168
  hysterosalpingography, 172
  infertility, examination for, 171
  smears in, taking of, 170
  (*See also* Obstetrics)

Health insurance, 269–271
  Blue Cross, 271, 277
  Blue Shield, 271–274, 277
  claim forms, 272–274
  contracts, types of, 272
  fees paid, 272–274
Hearing tests (*see* Otology)
Heart, *illus.*, 342, 343
  (*See also* Electrocardiography)

INDEX

Heart attack, first aid in, 213-214
Heat, application of, 127-128
Height, taking of, 58-59
Hematest, 298
Hematology, 300-317
  blood counts, 304-316
    counting chamber, 304-305; *illus.*, 304
    differential count smears, 311-316
      equipment for, 311
      examining the smear, 314-316
      procedure, 311-313
      sample report, 316
      staining rack, *illus.*, 314
      staining the smear, 313-314
    method of counting cells, 304-305; *illus.*, 305
    red blood cell (erythrocyte) count, 305-308
    white blood cell (leukocyte) count, 308-309
  erythrocyte sedimentation rate, 316-317
    equipment for, 317
    procedure, 317
  hemoglobin estimation, 309-311
    equipment for, 309
    hemometer tube, *illus.*, 309
    procedure, 310
    reporting results, 310-311
  obtaining blood, 300-304
    equipment for, 300-302
    instruments for skin puncture, 300-301
    procedure, 302-304
    sites for skin puncture, 300
    technique for using lancet, *illus.*, 302
Holmes, Oliver Wendell, 24
Hospitalization insurance, 271
  (*See also* Health insurance)
House calls, appointments for, 229-230
  record of, 229-230
Household measures, equivalents of, 419
Housekeeping hints, 279-289
Hydrotherapy, 138

Hypodermic needles, care of, 104-107
  construction of, *illus.*, 33
  sharpening of, *illus.*, 105
  sterilization of, 33
  stuck, removal of, *illus.*, 106
Hysterosalpingography, 172

Infections, 68
  (*See also* Bacteriology)
Infectious diseases, 5-6
Infertility, examination for, 171
Inflammation, 68-69
Inhalation therapy, 197-198
Injections, materials for, 98
  reasons for, 94-95
  technique for, 96, 99-102; *illus.*, 96
  types of, 95-97
    into a fracture, 97
    intra-articular, 97, 101-102
    intradermal, 97
    intramuscular, 96
    intravenous, 97, 101
    subcutaneous, 95
Insect bites, first aid in, 214-215
Instruments, care of, after surgery, 115-117
  for doctor's bag, 289-290
  sterilization of, 31-34, 40-43
  used in surgery, 113-114
Insurance in medical practice, 269-278
  health, 271-274
  hospitalization, 271
  malpractice, 277-278
  Workmen's Compensation, 274-276
Intradermal skin test, 167
Irrigation, of ear, 200
  of nose, 198-199
  syringe for, *illus.*, 200
  (*See also* Solutions)

Koch, Robert, 24

Labeling of medications, 92
Laboratory (*see* Medical laboratory techniques)

Laryngology, 197–199
  inhalation therapy in, 197–198
  irrigations in, setup for, 198–199
    technique of giving, 198–199
  terms pertaining to, 404–406
Laundry, handling of, 285–286
  type of, 284
Ledger card, patients', entries made on, 249–250
  filing of, 250–251
  (See also Bills)
Leeuwenhoek, Antonj van, 23
Lenses (see Ophthalmology)
Lensometer, illus., 191
Leukocyte count, technique of, 308–309
Linear measures, metric equivalents of, 419
Lister, Joseph, 24

Malpractice insurance, 277–278
Massage, contraindications for, 137
  position of hands for, illus., 136
  types of, 135
Medical assistant, appearance of, 11
  duties of, 4, 7–9
  position of, 3
  privileges of, 6
  relations of, to coworkers, 14
    to doctor, 9–10
    to patients, 17–20
  role of, in office surgery, 116–117
  (See also Specialist, assistant to)
Medical assistant societies, 2
Medical history, contents of, 238
  filing of, 245–247
  forms for, 238–243; illus., 240–243
  taking of, by assistant, 239–245
Medical laboratory techniques, 291–366
  bacteriologic smears, 317–324
  basal metabolism test, 325–340
  electrocardiography, 340–366
  hematology, 300–317
  terms pertaining to, 394–396
  urinalysis, 292–300
Medical terminology, 367–413
  abbreviations in, 367
  classified list of terms, 370–413

Medical terminology, prefixes in, 367–369
  suffixes in, 367–369
  word elements in, 367–369
Medicare, 276–277
Medications, for doctor's bag, 289
  dosage of, 85–86
  equivalent metric values, 415–419
  labeling of, 92
  methods of administration of, 84–85
  prescription for, 86–88
  principles of, 75–92
  standards for, 75–76
  storage of, 91–92
  types of, 77–79
Metric equivalents, of apothecaries' measures, 416–417
  of apothecaries' weights, 418
  of avoirdupois, 415
  of linear measures, 419
Minor surgery (see Surgery)

Narcotics, handling of, 79–83
  law governing, 80–81
  license for prescribing, 80
  records of, 82
Needles (see Hypodermic needles)
Neurological examination, 176–177
Neurology, 175–183
  terms pertaining to, 396–400
Neuroses, 72, 175–176
Nosebleed, first aid in, 214–215

Obstetrics, assisting in, 167–175
  emergencies in, 174
  prenatal care in, 172–175
  terms pertaining to, 391–394
Office, doctor's, care of, 279–281
Office hours, 226–227
Operating room in doctor's office, 113
Ophthalmology, 184–192
  eye, illus., 184
  eye diseases, 190–191
  eye drops, application of, 186–187; illus., 187
  eyeglasses, checking of, 190–191
    prescribing of, 185–190

INDEX

Ophthalmology, eyeglasses, prescription for, explanation of, 189–190; *illus.*, 189
  instruments used in examinations, 185
  lenses, 188–190
    diopter, definition of, 188–190
    lensometer, *illus.*, 191
    types of, 188
  refraction, 185–186
  terms pertaining to, 400–402
  vision, definition of, 187
    testing and correction of, 185–190
Ophthalmoscope, *illus.*, 185
Orthopedics, assisting in, 192–197
  arch supports, making model for, 195–196
  braces, prescription of, 196
  crutches, teaching use of, 196–197
  exercises in, 192–193
  plaster casts, making of, 193–195
  splints, types of, 196
  terms pertaining to, 402–404
Otolaryngology, assisting in, 197–205
  terms pertaining to, 404–406
  (*See also* Laryngology; Otology)
Otology, assisting in, 199–205
  audiogram, *illus.*, 204
    recording results on, 203
  audiometer, 201–204
  decibel, definition of, 201
  ear, *illus.*, 199
  hearing tests, 200–205
    administration of, *illus.*, 202
  irrigation of ear, 200
  otoscope, *illus.*, 200
  Rinne test, 205

Papanicolaou test, kit for, *illus.*, 171
Pasteur, Louis, 23–24
Patch test, 165–167; *illus.*, 166–167
Patient, attitude toward, 20–22
    while taking x-rays, 141–142
  draping of, *illus.*, 52
  first visit of, 219, 222
  preparation of, for cholecystography, 146
    for gastrointestinal series, 145–146

Patient, preparation of, for general examination, 49–50
  for minor surgery, 108–109
  for x-rays, 142–146
  psychology of, 17–20
  reception of, 219–221
Patients' records, 237–251
  personal-health record, 245
  (*See also* Medical history)
Payroll records, 266–267
Pediatrics, terms pertaining to, 406–408
Personality of medical assistant, 13
Petty cash, 267–268
Physical therapy, application of, diathermy, 129–134
  electrosurgery, 139
  exercises, 137–138
  faradic current, 128
  galvanic current, 128
  heat, 127–128
  hydrotherapy, 138
  massage, 134–138
  sinusoidal current, 128
  utrasonic therapy, 134
  ultraviolet light, 125–127
  terms pertaining to, 402–404
  (*See also* Orthopedics)
Plaster casts, making of, 193–195
Poison ivy, first aid in, 216
Poisoning, first aid in, 215–216
Poultices, application of, 128
Prefixes and suffixes, 367–369
Pregnancy, care during (*see* Obstetrics)
Prenatal care (*see* Obstetrics)
Preparation of patient (*see* Patient, preparation of)
Prescription, of diet, 156
  of eyeglasses, 185–190
  of medications, 86–88
Prescription blanks, 81; *illus.*, 87
Pressure points, *illus.*, 209
Proctology, terms pertaining to, 408–409
Psychiatric disorders, 175–176
Psychiatry, 175–183
  terms pertaining to, 396–400
Psychology, of patient, 17–20
  personal, 14–17

Psychosis, 176
Public relations, 20-22, 280-281
Pulse, taking of, 59
Pulse rate, 59

Radiology, terms pertaining to, 409-411
  (*See also* X-rays)
Records, financial, 258-268
  patients', 237-251
Refraction, 185-186
Removal of stains, 286-288
Reproductive organs, female, *illus.*, 168
Respiration, method of taking, 60-61
  rate of, 60
Rhinology, terms pertaining to, 404-406
  (*See also* Otolaryngology)
Roentgenology (*see* X-rays)
Roller bandages, 119-121; *illus.*, 120
Rubber gloves, care of, 35-36
  sterilization of, by autoclaving, 40
    by boiling, 35-36
Rubber goods, sterilization of, 35-36, 40

Scratch test, 164-165; *illus.*, 165
Secretarial duties, medical, 219-236
Sedimentation rate, erythrocyte, determination of, 316-317
Sediments in urine, obtaining of, 295-296; *illus.*, 296
Semmelweis, Ignaz, 24
Shock, first aid in, 216
Shock therapy, aftercare in, 182-183
  assistant's role during, 181-183
  preparation of patient for, 178-179
  release for, 180
  setup for, 179
  technique of, 178-183
Sinusoidal current, 128
Skin test, intradermal, 167
Smears, bacteriologic, equipment for making, 317-318
  examination of, 321-323

Smears, bacteriologic, Gram's-stain reaction, 323
  Gram's-stain technique, 321-322
  procedure for, 318-321; *illus.*, 318-320
  staining of, 321
differential blood count, criteria for, 313
  equipment for making, 311
  examination of, 314-316
  procedure for, 311-314
  staining of, 313-314
gynecological, 170
Solids in urine, determination of, 293-294
Solutions, percentages for, 419
  preparation of, 90-91
Specialist, assistant to, in allergy tests, 164-167
  in gynecology, 167-174
  in neurology and psychiatry, 175-183
  in ophthalmology, 184-186, 190-192
  in orthopedics, 192-197
  in otolaryngology, 198-205
Specific gravity of urine, determination of, 293-294
Splints, 196
Stainless-steel ware, sterilization of, 34-35
Stains, removal of, 286-288
Stefansson, Vilhjalmur, 159
Sterilization, of enamelware, 34-35
  of glassware, 34
  of hypodermic needles, 33
  of instruments, 33-34
  methods of, 31-44
    by boiling, 31
    by chemical means, 36-38
    by dry heat, 44
    by steam (autoclave), 38-44
  need for, 27-28
  purpose of, 30
  of rubber goods, 35-36, 40
  of stainless-steel ware, 34-35
  of syringes, 32-33
  terms used in, 29

INDEX

Sterilizers, autoclave, *illus.*, 38, 43
  for boiling, *illus.*, 31
  care of, 31–32
  for cold sterilization, *illus.*, 37
Storage of medications, 91–92
Suffixes and prefixes, 367–369
Supplies, administrative, 283–284
  for doctor's bag, 289
  for first aid, 218
  medical, 282–283
Surgery, 108–123
  anesthesia in, 109–112
  assistant's role in, 116–117
  bandages in, 119–123
  dressings in, 117–119
  instruments used in, 113–114
  setup for, 113
  terms pertaining to, 381–383
  (*See also* Electrosurgery)
Syringes, care of, 102–103
  construction of, 32; *illus.*, 32
  opener for, *illus.*, 104
  sterilization of, 32–33

Taub, Samuel J., 163
Telephone, consultation by, 228–229
Telephone calls, emergency, 234–235
  handling of, 230–236
    summary of technique of, 235–236
  memorandum of, 234
  outgoing, 236
  from patients, 230–233
  from strangers, 233–234
Telephone hour for patients, 228–229
Temperature, conversion of Fahrenheit to centigrade, 415
  normal, 61
  taking, methods of, 62–63
    technique of, 62–64
  (*See also* Thermometer)
Tests, routine, 53–66
  special, basal metabolism, 325–341
    electrocardiogram, 341–366
    hearing, 200–205
    laboratory, 291–340
    skin, 164–167

Therapy (*see* Treatment)
Thermometer, care of, 64; *illus.*, 62
  reading of, 64
  types of, 64
Treatment, by allergist, 162–167
  by diet, 149–159
  by gynecologist, 167–172
  by injections, 94–107
  by irrigations, 198–199, 200
  by laryngologist, 197–199
  by neurologist, 175–183
  by obstetrician, 172–175
  by ophthalmologist, 184–192
  by orthopedist, 192–197
  by otologist, 199–205
  by physical therapy, 124–139
  by shock therapy, 177–183
  by surgery, 108–123
  types of, 72–74
Triangular bandages, 121–122; *illus.*, 122
Tumors, 68–70

Ultrasonic therapy, 134
  application of, *illus.*, 135
Ultraviolet light, application of, 125–127
Uniforms, 11–12
Urinalysis, 291–300
Urine, amorphous material in, *illus.*, 297
  appearance of, 292
  chemical examination of, 296–300
    for acetone, 297
    for albumin, 297–298
    for blood, occult, 298–299
    for sugar (glycosuria), 299–300
  collection of specimen of, 292
  color of, 292
  miscroscopic examination of, 295–297
    sediment in, obtaining of, 295–296; *illus.*, 296
  odor of, 292
  physical examination of, 292–294
  quantity of, 292
  reaction of, 292–293
  solids in, determination of, 293–294

Urine, specific gravity of, determination of, 293-294
Urology, terms pertaining to, 411-413

Viruses, 27
Vision, testing and correction of, 185-190
(*See also* Ophthalmology)
Vitamins, types of, 152-153
(*See also* Diet)

Weight, taking of, 58-59
Wet dressings, application of, 138
Wolf, H. F., 68, 126, 130
Word elements of medical terms, 367-369
Workmen's Compensation insurance, bills in, 276
  claim forms, 275-276
Workmen's Compensation insurance, law regarding, 274
  medical history in, 275
Wounds, first aid in, 216-217

X-ray department, administrative routine of, 147
X-ray films, developing solution for, 148
  fixer for, 148
  supply of, 147
X-rays, attitude toward patient while taking, 141-142
  danger of, 141
  preparations for, 140-148
  special examinations by, 144-148
    cholecystography, 146
    gastrointestinal series, 145-146
    hysterosalpingography, 172
    pyelography, 146
  terms pertaining to, 409-411